ADOLESCENT MEDICINE: STATE OF THE ART REVIEWS

Acute Emergencies in Adolescents

GUEST EDITORS

Monika K. Goyal, MD, MSCE

John D. Rowlett, MD

Donald E. Greydanus, MD, Dr HC (ATHENS)

December 2015 • Volume 26 • Number 3

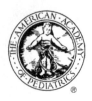

ADOLESCENT MEDICINE:
STATE OF THE ART REVIEWS
December 2015
Editor: Carrie Peters
Marketing Manager: Linda Smessaert
Production Manager: Shannan Martin
eBook Developer: Houston Adams

Volume 26, Number 3
ISBN 978-1-58110-888-0
ISSN 1934-4287
MA0731
SUB1006

The recommendations in this publication do not indicate an exclusive course of treatment or serve as a standard of medical care. Variations, taking into account individual circumstances, may be appropriate.

Statements and opinions expressed are those of the author and not necessarily those of the American Academy of Pediatrics.

Products and Web sites are mentioned for informational purposes only. Inclusion in this publication does not imply endorsement by the American Academy of Pediatrics. The American Academy of Pediatrics is not responsible for the content of the resources mentioned in this publication. Web site addresses are as current as possible but may change at any time.

Every effort has been made to ensure that the drug selection and dosage set forth in this text are in accordance with the current recommendations and practice at the time of publication. It is the responsibility of the health care provider to check the package insert of each drug for any change in indications and dosage and for added warnings and precautions.

Adolescent Medicine: State of the Art Reviews is published three times per year by the American Academy of Pediatrics, 141 Northwest Point Blvd, Elk Grove Village, IL 60007-1019. Periodicals postage paid at Arlington Heights, IL.

POSTMASTER: Send address changes to American Academy of Pediatrics, Department of Marketing and Publications, Attn: AM:STARs, 141 Northwest Point Blvd, Elk Grove Village, IL 60007-1019.

Subscriptions: Subscriptions to *Adolescent Medicine: State of the Art Reviews* (AM:STARs) are provided to members of the American Academy of Pediatrics' Section on Adolescent Health as part of annual section membership dues. All others, please contact the AAP Customer Service Center at 866/843-2271 (7:00 am–5:30 pm Central Time, Monday–Friday) for pricing and information.

Adolescent Medicine: State of the Art Reviews

Official Journal of the American Academy of Pediatrics
Section on Adolescent Health

EDITORS-IN-CHIEF

VICTOR C. STRASBURGER, MD, Distinguished Professor Emeritus of Pediatrics, Founding Chief, Division of Adolescent Medicine, University of New Mexico, School of Medicine, Albuquerque, New Mexico

DONALD E. GREYDANUS, MD, Dr HC (ATHENS), Professor & Founding Chair, Department of Pediatric & Adolescent Medicine, Western Michigan University Homer Stryker M.D. School of Medicine, Kalamazoo, Michigan

GUEST EDITORS

MONIKA K. GOYAL, MD, MSCE, Assistant Professor of Pediatrics and Emergency Medicine, Children's National Health System, The George Washington University, Washington, DC

JOHN D. ROWLETT, MD, Director, Pediatric Emergency Medicine, Georgia Emergency Associates, Savannah, Georgia; Professor of Pediatrics, Medical College of Georgia at Georgia Regents University, Augusta, Georgia

DONALD E. GREYDANUS, MD, Dr HC (ATHENS), Professor & Founding Chair, Department of Pediatric & Adolescent Medicine, Western Michigan University Homer Stryker M.D. School of Medicine, Kalamazoo, Michigan

CONTRIBUTORS

DAVID L. BELL, MD, MPH, Columbia University Medical Center, New York, New York

HARSHA CHANDNANI, MD, MBA, MPH, Department of Pediatrics, The University of Nevada School of Medicine, Las Vegas, Nevada

DAVID CHAO, MD, Department of Pediatrics, The University of Nevada School of Medicine, Las Vegas, Nevada; Emergency Medicine Physicians, Canton, Ohio; Division of Emergency Medicine, Rady Children's Hospital and Department of Pediatrics, University of California San Diego, San Diego, California

CAROLINE CRUCE, 2016 Doctoral Candidate, University of Georgia College of Pharmacy, Athens, Georgia

LAWRENCE J. D'ANGELO, MD, MPH, Chief, Division of Adolescent and Young Adult Medicine, Children's National Medical Center, Washington, DC

ERICA DEL GRIPPO, DO, Pediatric Resident, Sidney Kimmel Medical College at Thomas Jefferson University, Nemours/Alfred I. duPont Hospital for Children, Wilmington, Delaware

NADIA DOWSHEN, MD, Assistant Professor of Pediatrics and Director of Adolescent HIV Services, Craig-Dalsimer Division of Adolescent Medicine, Children's Hospital of Philadelphia, Philadelphia, Pennsylvania

WILLIAM EGGLESTON, PharmD, SUNY Upstate Medical University, Upstate New York Poison Center, Syracuse, New York

QUYEN M. EPSTEIN-NGO, PhD, University of Michigan Institute for Research on Women and Gender, Ann Arbor, Michigan; University of Michigan Institute for Clinical and Health Research, Ann Arbor, Michigan; Injury Research Center, University of Michigan, Ann Arbor, Michigan

MONIKA K. GOYAL, MD, MSCE, Assistant Professor of Pediatrics and Emergency Medicine, Children's National Health System, The George Washington University, Washington, DC

ELIZABETH ANNE GREENE, MD, Professor of Pediatrics, University of New Mexico, Pediatric Cardiology Division, Director, Pediatric Electrophysiology and Exercise Testing, Albuquerque, New Mexico

BLAIR P. GRUBB, MD, Professor of Medicine, University of Toledo Medical Center, Toledo, Ohio

ALESSANDRA GUINER, MD, Department of Pediatrics, The University of Nevada School of Medicine, Las Vegas, Nevada

PAULA HILLARD, MD, Professor, Chief of Pediatric and Adolescent Gynecology, Department of Obstetrics and Gynecology, Stanford University School of Medicine, Stanford, California

KHALIL KANJWAL, MD, Assistant Professor of Medicine, Central Michigan University, Staff Cardiac Electrophysiologist, Michigan Cardiovascular Institute, Saginaw, Michigan

JANE LAVELLE, MD, Children's Hospital of Philadelphia, University of Pennsylvania, Perelman School of Medicine, Philadelphia, Pennsylvania

CHRISTINA L. MASTER, MD, Sports Medicine and Performance Center, The Children's Hospital of Philadelphia, Philadelphia, Pennsylvania; Department of Pediatrics, Perelman School of Medicine, University of Pennsylvania, Philadelphia, Pennsylvania

SUNDUS MASUDI, BS, St Mary's of Michigan, Saginaw, Michigan

ZACHARY MCCLAIN, MD, Children's Hospital of Philadelphia, Philadelphia, Pennsylvania

ALEXANDER D. MCGINLEY, BA, Center for Injury Research and Prevention, The Children's Hospital of Philadelphia, Philadelphia, Pennsylvania

KATHERINE A. MITCHELL, MD, MPA, Fellow, Division of Adolescent Health and Medicine, Department of Pediatrics, British Columbia Children's Hospital, University of British Columbia Faculty of Medicine, Vancouver, British Columbia, Canada

CYNTHIA J. MOLLEN, MD, MSCE, Children's Hospital of Philadelphia, University of Pennsylvania, Perelman School of Medicine, Philadelphia, Pennsylvania

EVA M. MOORE, MD, MSPH, Clinical Assistant Professor, Division of Adolescent Health and Medicine, Department of Pediatrics, British Columbia Children's Hospital, University of British Columbia Faculty of Medicine, Vancouver, British Columbia, Canada

ANN PUNNOOSE, MD, Fellow, Pediatric Heart Failure and Heart Transplantation, Lurie Children's Hospital of Chicago, Chicago, Illinois

EMILY ROTHMAN, ScD, School of Public Health, Boston University, Boston, Massachusetts; School of Medicine, Boston University, Boston, Massachusetts

JOHN D. ROWLETT, MD, Director, Pediatric Emergency Medicine, Georgia Emergency Associates, Savannah, Georgia; Professor of Pediatrics, Medical College of Georgia at Georgia Regents University, Augusta, Georgia

CAROLINE SALAS-HUMARA, MD, Adolescent Medicine Fellow, Craig-Dalsimer Division of Adolescent Medicine, Children's Hospital of Philadelphia, Philadelphia, Pennsylvania

PHILIP SCRIBANO, DO, MSCE, Children's Hospital of Philadelphia, University of Pennsylvania, Perelman School of Medicine, Philadelphia, Pennsylvania

STEVEN M. SELBST, MD, Professor of Pediatrics, Sidney Kimmel Medical College at Thomas Jefferson University, Philadelphia, Pennsylvania; Attending Physician, Division of Emergency Medicine, Nemours/Alfred I. duPont Hospital for Children, Wilmington, Delaware; Director, Pediatric Residency Program, Jefferson/duPont Hospital for Children, Wilmington, Delaware

NADINE SMITH, DO, Fellow, Pediatric Emergency Medicine, Sidney Kimmel Medical College at Thomas Jefferson University, Nemours/Alfred I. duPont Hospital for Children, Wilmington, Delaware

CHRISTINE STORK, PharmD, SUNY Upstate Medical University, Upstate New York Poison Center, Syracuse, New York

STEPHEN THACKER, MD, Assistant Professor of Pediatrics, Mercer School of Medicine, Children's Hospital at Memorial Health University Medical Center, Savannah, Georgia

DZUNG X. VO, MD, Clinical Assistant Professor, Division of Adolescent Health and Medicine, Department of Pediatrics, British Columbia Children's Hospital, University of British Columbia Faculty of Medicine, Vancouver, British Columbia, Canada

SARAH M. WOOD, MD, Adolescent Medicine Fellow, Craig-Dalsimer Division of Adolescent Medicine, Children's Hospital of Philadelphia, Philadelphia, Pennsylvania

SOPHIA YEN, MD, MPH, Associate Professor, Division of Adolescent Medicine, Department of Pediatrics, Stanford University School of Medicine, Stanford, California

MARK R. ZONFRILLO, MD, MSCE, Department of Emergency Medicine and Injury Prevention Center, Alpert Medical School of Brown University and Hasbro Children's Hospital, Providence, Rhode Island

CONTENTS

Preface   **xiii**

Adolescent Gynecologic Emergencies   **473**
Sophia Yen, Monika K. Goyal, Paula Hillard

Adolescent females can present to the emergency department with a gynecologic emergency resulting from a variety of possible conditions. In this article we discuss the evaluation and treatment of some of the most serious and common adolescent gynecologic emergencies, including ectopic pregnancy, ovarian torsion, pelvic inflammatory disease, and abnormal uterine bleeding. We also briefly discuss the use of emergency contraception to prevent unplanned pregnancies. We begin by reviewing key elements in conducting confidential sexual histories, which is a critical aspect of the medical evaluation when caring for adolescents, especially when they present with a potential gynecologic emergency.

Adolescent Male Genitourinary Emergencies   **484**
Zachary McClain, David L. Bell

Testicular and scrotal concerns are a common topic for discussion during an adolescent male visit, whether it is in the emergency room or the primary care clinic. Because the spectrum of conditions that affect the testes and scrotum can range from the painless and benign to the painful and emergently devastating, it is paramount that the physician be able to triage these concerns. The objectives of this article are to discuss the clinical evaluation and management of the acute scrotum and to provide physicians with the knowledge needed to differentiate conditions that require patient reassurance from those requiring acute surgical intervention.

Sports-Related Head Injuries in Adolescents: A Comprehensive Update   **491**
Alexander D. McGinley, Christina L. Master, Mark R. Zonfrillo

Sports-related traumatic brain injuries are common, with an estimated incidence of 1.6 to 3.8 million annually. Adolescents represent an at-risk population because of their high rates of participation in sports. Although approximately 90% of these injuries are "mild," they can still result in short- and long-term disability. This article reviews the current state of the rapidly changing field of sports-related head injuries of all severities, with a particular emphasis on mild traumatic brain injury (mTBI) and concussion in adolescents aged 10 to 19 years. The definition, incidence, epidemiology, pathophysiology, diagnosis, management, long-term sequelae, and prevention of these injuries are discussed.

Sports-Related Sudden Cardiac Injury or Death   507
Elizabeth Anne Greene, Ann Punnoose

Some adolescents are at higher risk for sudden cardiac death or cardiac injury because of abnormal cardiac anatomy or cardiac conduction system, and the sports in which they participate. The diagnosis and management of the cardiac etiologies of sudden cardiac death differ based on the specific etiology and have evolved over the years with improvements in diagnostic options.

Approach to the Adolescent with Chest Pain   528
Nadine Smith, Erica Del Grippo, Steven M. Selbst

Adolescents often come to the emergency department (ED) with the complaint of chest pain. This complaint is not as common as abdominal pain or headache, however it is a frequent complaint among teenagers. Many studies have shown that adolescents with chest pain rarely have serious organic pathology and they infrequently present with significant distress that requires immediately resuscitation in the ED. However, the adolescent with chest pain should be taken seriously because underlying heart disease or other serious pathology can sometimes exist.

Approach to the Adolescent Psychiatric and Behavioral Health Emergency   552
Alessandra Guiner, Harsha Chandnani, David Chao

Over the past 2 decades, there has been increased recognition of psychiatric and behavioral health problems in adolescents. These trends have led to a surge in presentations of adolescents with mental health emergencies to acute care settings. The acute care physician is responsible for recognizing and managing these adolescents in crisis. Evaluation of adolescent patients presenting with a psychiatric or behavioral emergency, trends in substance abuse, medical clearance, management of agitated patients, management of suicidal patients, and treatment of homeless and sexual minority youth are discussed.

Generation Z: Adolescent Xenobiotic Abuse in the 21st Century   570
William Eggleston, Christine Stork

Adolescent abuse of illicit xenobiotics has remained consistent over the last decade. The emergence of new synthetic and designer xenobiotics, along with continued use of classic xenobiotics of abuse, has created many challenges for physicians. Understanding the toxicity of these xenobiotics, the symptoms associated with their use, and the appropriate treatment options is necessary for the provision of optimal care in the acutely intoxicated patient.

Emergency Care of Youth with Social and Environmental Vulnerabilities   589
Dzung X. Vo, Katherine A. Mitchell, Eva M. Moore

Adolescents with social and environmental vulnerabilities are disproportionately affected by social determinants of health, and they have special medical and mental health care needs. Emergency care for this population requires a strength-based, trauma-informed, confidential approach to care. This article reviews health concerns and considerations in emergency care and advocacy for 5 populations of vulnerable youth: (1) immigrant and refugee youth; (2) youth in care (foster or juvenile justice); (3) lesbian, gay, bisexual, transgender, and questioning youth; (4) homeless and street-involved youth; and (5) sexually exploited youth.

Human Immunodeficiency Virus: Adolescent Emergencies   619
Caroline Salas-Humara, Sarah M. Wood, Lawrence J. D'Angelo, Nadia Dowshen

Adolescents are at high risk for human immunodeficiency virus (HIV) infection, and often the emergency department setting is where at-risk and HIV-infected adolescents are seen as their sole source of care. It is important to have a high index of suspicion for acute HIV infection and to consider HIV screening during these evaluations. Physicians must make every effort to adhere to state policies on HIV testing and to uphold the adolescent's right for confidential care. If a diagnosis of HIV infection is made, immediate referral and linkage to care with a physician specializing in comprehensive HIV care for adolescents and young adults should be made. Management of the patient infected with HIV should include evaluation for potential opportunistic infections, immune reconstitution inflammatory syndrome, and medication side effects, as well as potential drug interactions in those receiving antiretroviral therapy. Human immunodeficiency virus postexposure prophylaxis may substantially reduce the risk of HIV infection and should be recommended if there is concern for a recent sexual or needlestick exposure. Physicians who see adolescents in acute care settings are well positioned to have an effect on the well-being of adolescents both by preventing new infections and by improving health outcomes for youth living with HIV.

Evaluation and Treatment of the Adolescent Sexual Assault Patient   647
Cynthia J. Mollen, Monika K. Goyal, Jane Lavelle, Philip Scribano

Sexual assault is, unfortunately, a not infrequent occurrence, and emergency department physicians will certainly care for survivors of assault during their careers. Caring for an adolescent patient who has experienced a sexual assault is a complex process that requires cooperation among medical professionals, the patient and family, child protective services, and law enforcement. In order to manage the many aspects of care, including appropriate history taking and physical examination, documentation, forensic evidence collection, treatment, and reporting, an emergency department is most ideally staffed with a multidisciplinary team that can work together to streamline care and minimize stress for the patient. The care providers should understand key aspects of the forensic interview; recognize abnormal and normal physical examination findings; understand the key points of evidence collection; have up-to-date knowledge on treatment and prophylaxis for sexually transmitted infections, human immunodeficiency virus, and pregnancy; and be familiar with local reporting laws. This review highlights each of the aspects of care for these patients, with an emphasis on the multidisciplinary nature of the care team.

Update on Meningitis in Adolescents and Young Adults   658
Stephen Thacker, Caroline Cruce, John D. Rowlett

Bacterial and viral (aseptic) meningitis afflict all age groups, especially adolescents and young adults. New immunizations and therapies are available that have substantially changed the management of both bacterial and viral meningitis. This update will review both new vaccines for preventing bacterial meningitis and new recommendations for older vaccines, and will provide an overview of common forms of viral (aseptic) meningitis. New diagnostic and therapeutic strategies for aseptic meningitis will be reviewed.

Adolescent Dating Violence in the Emergency Department: Presentation, Screening, and Interventions   **675**
Quyen M. Epstein-Ngo, Emily Rothman

> Adolescent dating violence (ADV) is a significant public health concern that is associated with serious consequences, including psychological distress, injury, future intimate partner violence involvement, and mortality. Youth seeking treatment in emergency departments (EDs) report a higher prevalence of ADV than rates reported from national samples of adolescents. Consequently, ED staff have a high likelihood of treating youth involved in ADV. This article provides physicians with relevant background on ADV, associated risks and consequences, presentation in the ED, and the current state of the science in terms of screening and interventions for ADV in the ED.

Syncope in Children and Adolescents   **692**
Khalil Kanjwal, Sundus Masudi, Blair P. Grubb

> Syncope is a common clinical condition. It can result from a wide variety of causes, some of which may result in sudden cardiac death. Thus, syncope produces tremendous social and emotional challenges and often times is a source of anxiety for patients, their parents, teachers, and coaches. Social repercussions of syncope may have more dramatic effects on children than syncope itself.
> As we know children are not merely small adults but differ from adults, and so do the causes of syncope. In this article we attempt to outline the causes, evaluation, and management of syncope in children and adolescents.

Index   **713**

Preface

Acute Emergencies in Adolescents

It has been more than 25 years since an issue of *Adolescent Medicine: State of the Art Reviews* has been devoted to topics on emergency medicine. During that time, emergency department visits in the United States increased approximately 50%, to more than 135 million visits in 2014. Data specific to adolescents are limited. The national datasets have age groups that overlap with both childhood (ages 5-14 years) and adulthood (ages 15-24 years). Previous reports suggest that utilization of emergency services by adolescents was not disproportionately high or low compared to other age groups, although lack of health insurance was more common among adolescents than among children or adults.[1,2] Hard data notwithstanding, there is little reason to believe that adolescent utilization of emergency medical services has diminished.

Adolescents frequently present to the emergency department or to primary care physicians for acute health concerns that range from minor to life-threatening. This issue of *AM:STARs* focuses on many of the more urgent and emergent health problems and concerns that bring adolescents to clinics, private offices, and emergency department settings.

Adolescent medicine physicians are accustomed to evaluating issues related to sex and sexuality. It should come as no surprise that several articles in this issue deal either directly or indirectly with adolescent sexuality. Reviews of adolescent gynecologic emergencies and male genitourinary emergencies cover medical diseases of the reproductive organs. Human immunodeficiency virus (HIV) infection among adolescents is becoming less common, although recent surges remind us that we must be ever vigilant not only in the prevention of HIV transmission but also in the recognition and prompt treatment of new HIV cases and the management of emergencies unique and specific to HIV-infected adolescents. Sexual violence and assault are not uncommon among adolescents. Reviews on the evaluation and treatment of sexual assault survivors and adolescent dating violence provide timely updates on these subjects.

Access to mental health services remains difficult for many youth, and youth presentation to the emergency department for assistance with mental health or behavioral problems is common. This issue includes a review of the initial approach to adolescents with psychiatric and behavioral emergencies and a separate discussion of the emergent care of vulnerable youth. Gone are the days when youth abused just marijuana, alcohol, or the occasional stronger drugs. Today's youth have ready access to an ever-changing collection of new and designer drugs. Although new drugs of abuse are undoubtedly on the horizon, an excellent summary of the newer drugs is included.

More "traditional" emergency medicine topics are also covered. Although rarely serious, chest pain is a frequent reason why adolescents seek emergency services. Physicians will become more comfortable with this presentation after reading about the approach to the adolescent with chest pain. Similarly, the evaluation and management of the not infrequent syncope or near-syncope patient is expertly covered. New vaccines and new indications for old vaccines are highlighted in an update on meningitis. Finally, 2 articles bring the reader up to date on the management of 2 sports-related problems: the much feared but fortunately relatively rare sudden death, and the all too common sports-related head injury.

The broad set of topics in this issue is expertly covered by a talented group of physicians who span the pediatric subspecialties. We thank all of the authors for their contributions and for adhering to the timeline. We especially thank Carrie Peters for her patience, guidance, and expertise in the production of this issue, and the American Academy of Pediatrics for supporting *Adolescent Medicine: State of the Art Reviews*. A special thanks to Dr Donald Greydanus, coeditor in chief of *AM:STARs* and my (JDR) mentor, and Dr Victor Strasburger, his *AM:STARs* coeditor in chief and partner on this project since its inception more than a quarter of a century ago, for entrusting us with this issue of "their baby."

Monika K. Goyal, MD, MSCE
Assistant Professor of Pediatrics
and Emergency Medicine
Children's National Health System
The George Washington University
Washington, DC

John D. Rowlett, MD
Director, Pediatric Emergency Medicine
Georgia Emergency Associates
Savannah, Georgia
Professor of Pediatrics
Medical College of Georgia at Georgia
Regents University
Augusta, Georgia

References

1. Ziv A, Boulet JR, Slap GB. Emergency department utilization by adolescents in the United States. *Pediatrics*. 1998;101:987-994
2. Gindi RM, Jones LI. *Reasons for Emergency Room Use Among U.S. Children: National Health Interview Survey, 2012*. NCHS Data Brief, No. 160. Hyattsville, MD: National Center for Health Statistics; 2014

Adolesc Med 026 (2015) 473–483

Adolescent Gynecologic Emergencies

Sophia Yen, MD, MPH[a]*;
Monika K. Goyal, MD, MSCE[b];
Paula Hillard, MD[c]

[a]Associate Professor, Division of Adolescent Medicine, Department of Pediatrics, Stanford University School of Medicine, Stanford, California; [b]Assistant Professor of Pediatrics and Emergency Medicine, Children's National Health System, The George Washington University, Washington, DC; [c]Professor, Chief of Pediatric and Adolescent Gynecology, Department of Obstetrics and Gynecology, Stanford University School of Medicine, Stanford, California

INTRODUCTION

Adolescent females account for an estimated 8 million emergency department (ED) visits annually, with lower abdominal pain or genitourinary symptoms being the most frequent chief complaints.[1-3] Although these complaints are common, adolescent females presenting with lower abdominal or genitourinary complaints can pose a diagnostic dilemma for the ED clinician (ie, physician, physician assistant, nurse practitioner, or other adolescent medicine provider)because the differential diagnosis is broad and consists of conditions that include surgical emergencies, such as ectopic pregnancy or appendicitis, as well as those that are fairly benign, such as constipation. However, expeditious and accurate diagnosis and treatment of these conditions are essential. In this article, we discuss the evaluation and treatment of some of the most important and serious adolescent gynecologic emergencies that may be encountered in the ED. We also review how to appropriately and confidentially obtain pertinent history when caring for adolescent females.

THE CONFIDENTIAL INTERVIEW

When evaluating adolescents, it is of utmost importance that the patients be interviewed in private because adolescents may not feel comfortable disclosing certain information in the presence of their parents, caregivers, friends, or significant others. In fact, research has demonstrated that concerns about privacy

*Corresponding author
E-mail address: soyen@stanford.edu

may prevent many adolescents from seeking health care and may lead them to withhold information from their clinicians.[4,5] Therefore, addressing confidentiality concerns is particularly important when adolescents present with complaints that may be related to their reproductive or sexual health. Every adolescent, by law, is entitled to confidential care that is related to sexual or mental health. However, the specifics of confidential care vary by state,[6] and it is important for clinicians to be knowledgeable about their state and hospital laws and policies regarding confidential care. The confidential interview should be conducted with only the patient and clinician in the room for accuracy and to obtain full disclosure from the patient. Many clinicians begin with the normalizing statement, "I ask these questions of all my patients because the questions are relevant to your health." Furthermore, before inquiring about sensitive health issues, it is crucial for the clinician to review the limits of confidentiality (eg, "What you say is confidential and will only be shared among the medical team here as needed EXCEPT if you tell us you are hurting yourself or hurting someone or someone is hurting you").[7] Regardless of the clinician's preconceived notions, every adolescent female who presents with pelvic or genitourinary complaints should be confidentially asked about her sexual history.

ECTOPIC PREGNANCY

Ectopic pregnancy, the implantation of a fertilized ovum outside the endometrial cavity, occurs in approximately 2% of pregnancies and is potentially life threatening.[8] Ruptured ectopic pregnancy is the leading cause of morbidity and mortality during the first trimester and accounts for approximately 10% of all maternal deaths.[9] Although ectopic pregnancies are more likely to occur in adults than adolescents, almost 10% of ectopic pregnancies occur in adolescents.[10] Furthermore, ectopic pregnancies have been reported to be diagnosed in up to 16% of females presenting to the ED with first-trimester bleeding or pain.[10]

If the fallopian tube has been damaged and the ovum is unable to travel to the uterus, the ovum can implant outside the uterus, resulting in an ectopic pregnancy. The most common implantation site of an ectopic pregnancy is within a fallopian tube. Damage to the fallopian tubes from pelvic inflammatory disease (PID), previous tubal surgery, or a previous ectopic pregnancy is strongly associated with an increased risk of tubal ectopic pregnancy. However, most adolescents with an ectopic pregnancy present without any known risk factors. Importantly, use of an intrauterine device (IUD) is not associated with increased risk of ectopic pregnancy.[11]

Abdominal pain, amenorrhea, and vaginal bleeding are the classic symptoms of an ectopic pregnancy. These symptoms can occur in both ruptured and unruptured cases. However, only 50% of cases present with this symptom triad.[12] The physical examination findings in an ectopic pregnancy can also be variable. Vitals signs may reveal orthostatic changes and, occasionally, low-grade fever.

Tachycardia is not always present, even with significant hemoperitoneum. However, some patients with a ruptured ectopic pregnancy can present with significant hemodynamic compromise. Other physical examination findings may include abdominal tenderness, cervical motion tenderness or adnexal tenderness, or palpation of an adnexal mass. It is important to note that the physical examination may be unremarkable in a female with a small, unruptured ectopic pregnancy.[13]

Patients with a ruptured ectopic pregnancy present with signs of shock, including hypotension, tachycardia, and rebound tenderness. These patients should have an immediate gynecology or surgical consult and should be taken to the operating room emergently. However, most patients present before rupture, with symptoms that can include vaginal bleeding and crampy abdominal or pelvic pain (which can be unilateral or diffuse). Female patients with abdominal pain and a positive pregnancy test who are hemodynamically stable may have an intrauterine or extrauterine pregnancy. Confirmation of an intrauterine pregnancy can usually be diagnosed rapidly and accurately with the use of ultrasound showing an intrauterine pregnancy and a quantitative serum human chorionic gonadotropin (hCG) test.[14] Although an ectopic tubal pregnancy can sometimes be seen on ultrasound, the combination of the lack of an intrauterine pregnancy with a sufficiently high quantitative hCG measurement strongly suggests an ectopic pregnancy. If the hCG level is not high enough that an intrauterine pregnancy should be visualized, the pregnancy is termed a pregnancy of unknown location. Transvaginal ultrasound has higher sensitivity and specificity than transabdominal ultrasound and, therefore, is the preferred imaging modality.[15] However, some pediatric centers do not have ultrasonographers with expertise in the performance of transvaginal ultrasounds. If an intrauterine pregnancy or an ectopic gestation is visualized on ultrasound, the workup is complete. If, however, as in half of all cases of ectopic pregnancies, the ultrasound is nondiagnostic with no definite gestation visualized either inside or outside the uterus, and the patient is clinically stable, further evaluation with serum hCG is required. An intrauterine gestation is usually visible on a transvaginal ultrasound at an hCG level of 1500 IU/L or more and on a transabdominal ultrasound at an hCG level of greater than 6500 IU/L. Furthermore, the hCG levels can be followed serially, with the levels approximately doubling every 48 hours in a normal intrauterine pregnancy. In an abnormal intrauterine pregnancy or an ectopic pregnancy, the hCG levels can plateau, rise inappropriately, or decline.[16]

If the patient is clinically stable, treatment of an ectopic pregnancy can be surgical or medical. Surgical treatment may involve laparoscopic removal of the ectopic pregnancy with or without removal of the affected fallopian tube. Medical management of ectopic pregnancy with intramuscular administration of methotrexate has become a more commonly used and safe alternative to surgical management in certain situations.[14] These decisions are made by gynecologic consultants. Emergency department management consists of supportive care and emergent transfer to the operating room in cases of ruptured ectopic pregnancies with hemodynamic instability. In the more common cases of unruptured ectopic pregnancies, gynecology should be consulted as soon as the diagnosis is suspected to provide assistance in follow-up and ongoing management decisions.

OVARIAN TORSION

Ovarian torsion is a rare but serious gynecologic emergency that involves the twisting of the ovary around its vascular pedicle (structure containing the arterial and venous supplies to the ovary), causing obstruction of blood flow and resulting in the acute onset of unilateral pain. Ovarian torsion is the fifth most common gynecologic emergency and accounts for almost 3% of all cases of acute abdominal pain in pediatric females, with an estimated incidence of 4.9 per 100,000 in women younger than 20 years.[17-19]

Ovarian torsion almost always occurs in the presence of ovarian cysts and benign tumors, which can serve as a fulcrum for twisting. However, ovarian torsion in adolescents can sometimes occur in the absence of an associated adnexal mass. Initially, the twisting of the vascular pedicle may compromise lymphatic and venous outflow. The arterial supply to the ovary is less affected because arteries are less compressible. Continued arterial perfusion in the setting of blocked outflow leads to marked ovarian engorgement. Ischemia can result in necrosis, infarction, local hemorrhage, and peritonitis, although this is uncommon.[19] Although normal ovarian function can be retained, depending on the duration of torsion, expeditious intervention provides the best chance of ovarian salvage.[20]

Patients with ovarian torsion classically present with sudden onset of severe unilateral abdominal pain. Nausea and vomiting are frequently associated with torsion. Some patients may have a history of prior similar pain episodes that may be caused by torsion and detorsing. The onset of pain may have occurred during strenuous activity, such as exercise, or developed acutely without any inciting factor. Fever can rarely be a late finding as the ovary becomes necrotic. The physical examination may reveal abdominal tenderness with rebound tenderness. A unilaterally tender adnexal mass may be palpated. Therefore, any adolescent female who presents with the onset of acute pelvic pain, particularly if accompanied by signs of peritoneal irritation, such as nausea and vomiting, should be emergently evaluated for ovarian torsion.

Although the diagnosis of ovarian torsion is ultimately made on a clinical basis, the diagnosis is aided by ultrasound. However, ultrasound can be misleading because it sometimes demonstrates ovarian flow even if the ovary is torsed. The absence of flow is diagnostic for torsion. Ultrasound is considered the diagnostic modality of choice because it is quick and readily available in most EDs; it offers appropriate visualization of the pelvic organs; it is not associated with radiation; and Doppler interrogation can quantify blood flow and may increase the sensitivity of ultrasound in diagnosing ovarian torsion. The most common ultrasound finding in ovarian torsion is an enlarged ovary. Free fluid in the pelvis is often detected. Often a coexistent mass within the twisted ovary may be appreciated. Furthermore, in 75% of cases, follicles displaced to the periphery secondary to edema may be seen. Doppler ultrasound may demonstrate a twisted vascular pedicle. Visualization of flow within the vascular pedicle does not rule out ovarian torsion.[19]

Although ultrasound can be a helpful diagnostic tool, it may be misleading; therefore, if ovarian torsion is suspected, a surgical or gynecologic consult should be obtained as soon as possible. If torsion is strongly suspected on clinical grounds, laparoscopy is recommended as the diagnostic and potentially therapeutic tool of choice.[19] Until recently, management of ovarian torsion consisted of oophorectomy. However, over the last 15 years, conservative management, which consists of detorsion, has been found to be almost universally successful in preserving ovarian viability.[21]

Emergency department management should focus on prompt diagnosis and management, and supportive care. Pain control and intravenous fluids should be provided as needed. Furthermore, the evaluation should begin with a pregnancy test. Suspected ovarian torsion is an indication for an emergent ultrasound. A gynecology or surgery consult should be obtained early if ovarian torsion is suspected.

PELVIC INFLAMMATORY DISEASE

Pelvic inflammatory disease is an infection-induced inflammation of the upper female genital tract and includes endometritis, salpingitis, and oophoritis; tubo-ovarian abscess (TOA) and pelvic peritonitis may also occur.[22] Sexually transmitted organisms are implicated in most cases. *Chlamydia trachomatis* is a significant pathogen associated with PID, detected in up to 60% of women with confirmed salpingitis or endometritis. However, anaerobes that compose the vaginal flora are also frequently associated with PID.[23] Pelvic inflammatory disease can result in significant reproductive morbidity, including increased risk of subsequent infertility, ectopic pregnancy, and chronic pelvic pain.

Of the almost 1 million cases of PID diagnosed annually, 20% are estimated to occur in adolescents.[1] Adolescents with PID are more likely to present to EDs than to primary care or obstetrics and gynecology clinics.[24] Because abdominal and genitourinary complaints are the most common reasons for ED visits among adolescent females,[3] PID must be considered when evaluating adolescent females with lower abdominal pain. However, the diagnosis of PID can be difficult because the clinical presentation of PID may mimic other pelvic and abdominal processes. Many episodes of PID go unrecognized and untreated. Although some of these cases are asymptomatic, others are not diagnosed because the clinician fails to recognize the implications of mild or nonspecific symptoms or signs. Women with even mild PID may be at risk for subsequent infertility. Given the difficulty of diagnosis and the morbidity associated with disease, the Centers for Disease Control and Prevention (CDC) recommends that clinicians maintain a low threshold for the diagnosis of PID.[23]

During any ED visit in which a sexually active adolescent female presents with lower abdominal or pelvic pain, PID must be considered in the differential diagnosis. The physical examination should include a bimanual examination for assessment of cervical motion and uterine or adnexal tenderness, as well as palpation for the presence of any pelvic masses. The abdominal examination should include palpation of the right upper quadrant to assess for Fitz-Hugh and Curtis perihepatitis caused by PID. The CDC recommends presumptive treatment of PID in sexually active young women if they are experiencing lower abdominal pain or pelvic pain, if no cause for the illness other than PID is identified, and 1 or more of the following criteria are present: cervical motion tenderness, uterine tenderness, and adnexal tenderness.[23] All patients with suspected PID should undergo testing for gonorrhea and chlamydia, although treatment initiation should not await laboratory confirmation because many patients with PID may test negative for these infections.

Treatment of PID can be either outpatient or inpatient. Indications for inpatient treatment include cases in which surgical emergencies cannot be excluded; presence of a TOA; pregnancy; severe illness, nausea and vomiting, or high fever; inability to follow or tolerate an outpatient oral regimen; or no clinical response to oral antimicrobial therapy. There is no evidence suggesting that adolescents have improved outcomes from hospitalization for treatment of PID, and the clinical response to outpatient treatment is similar among younger and older women.[23] For outpatient treatment, patients should be re-evaluated at 72 hours to assess for improvement. If no improvement is seen at that time, patients should receive intravenous (IV) treatment. Table 1 outlines the 2015 CDC-recommended outpatient and inpatient PID treatment regimens.

Of note, IUDs do not have to be removed in patients with PID per CDC 2015 treatment guidelines. If no clinical improvement occurs within 48 to 72 hours of initiating treatment, clinicians should consider removing the IUD. A systematic review of evidence found that treatment outcomes did not generally differ between women with PID who retained the IUD and those who had the IUD removed, although this finding was for non-hormonal IUDs.[23]

Tubo-ovarian abscess is the most serious acute complication of PID. Although there is no clear way to distinguish TOA from uncomplicated PID on clinical grounds, TOA should be suspected in patients with a palpable adnexal mass,

Table 1
2015 CDC-recommended PID treatment regimens

Parenteral regimens	Intramuscular/oral treatment
Cefotetan 2 g IV every 12 hours and doxycycline 100 mg orally every 12 hours	Ceftriaxone 250 mg IM once and doxycycline 100 mg orally twice per day for 14 days with or without metronidazole 500 mg orally twice per day for 14 days
Cefoxitin 2 g IV every 6 hours and doxycycline 100 mg orally or IV every 12 hours	Cefoxitin 2 g IM once and probenecid 1 g orally administered concurrently in a single dose and doxycycline 100 mg orally twice per day for 14 days with or without metronidazole 500 mg orally twice per day for 14 days
Clindamycin 900 mg IV every 8 hours and gentamycin loading dose IV or IM (2 mg/kg), followed by a maintenance dose (1.5 mg/kg) every 8 hours	
Ampicillin/sulbactam 3 g IV every 6 hours and doxycycline 100 mg orally or IV every 12 hours	

CDC, Centers for Disease Control and Prevention; IM, intramuscular; IV, intravenous; PID, pelvic inflammatory disease.
From Workowski KA, Bolan GA. Sexually transmitted diseases treatment guidelines, 2015. *MMWR Recomm Rep.* 2015;64:1-137.

severe pain or focality, failure to respond to medical therapy, or significant tenderness that precludes the ability to perform an adequate medical examination. A pelvic ultrasound will easily confirm the presence of a TOA. Laboratory data including white blood cell count and erythrocyte sedimentation rate are not useful in differentiating TOA from uncomplicated PID, as studies have found contradictory results. When TOA is suspected, an ultrasound should be obtained for diagnosis. As with uncomplicated PID, complications of TOA include subsequent infertility, chronic pelvic pain, and ectopic pregnancy. Inpatient treatment with 24 to 48 hours of intravenous antibiotic therapy for anaerobic coverage is recommended. If no improvement is seen, interventional radiology should be consulted for potential drainage. Surgical drainage is rarely required.

ABNORMAL UTERINE BLEEDING

Abnormal uterine bleeding (AUB) is a common presenting problem to the ED. Chronic AUB is defined as uterine bleeding that is abnormal in volume, regularity, or timing and has been present for at least 3 of the past 6 months, whereas acute AUB is a clinical term for an episode of heavy bleeding that is of sufficient quantity to require immediate intervention to prevent future blood loss.[25]

The most common cause of AUB in adolescents is anovulatory cycles as a result of an immature hypothalamic-pituitary-ovarian axis. However, anovulation is a diagnosis of exclusion, and heavy bleeding may be a sign of a more serious condition.[26] Table 2 lists a comprehensive differential diagnosis of AUB in the adolescent female. When evaluating an adolescent female with AUB, pregnancy and pregnancy-related complications should first and foremost be ruled out. Sexually transmitted infections are also common causes of acute AUB; therefore, all adolescents should undergo testing for sexually transmitted infections. An underlying bleeding disorder can be a cause of chronically heavy menstrual bleeding in women. Coagulation disorders are the second most common cause of heavy menstrual bleeding in adolescents, with von Willebrand disease being the most common bleeding disorder associated with heavy menstrual bleeding presenting at menarche.[26]

The physical examination should begin with attention to vital signs, including evaluation for postural changes. The skin should be evaluated for signs of anemia as well as underlying bleeding disorders (eg, bruising or petechiae) or androgen excess (eg, acne, hirsutism, or acanthosis nigricans). The thyroid gland should be palpated to assess for enlargement or nodules, a cardiac examination should evaluate for a flow murmur, and the abdomen should be palpated to assess for a uterine fundus suggesting pregnancy. A pelvic examination should be considered if trauma or a foreign body is suspected.

Table 2
Differential diagnosis for an adolescent presenting with vaginal bleeding

Complication of pregnancy
- Ectopic pregnancy
- Threatened, incomplete, completed abortion

Abnormal (excessive) uterine bleeding
- Structural
  - Polyps, adenomyosis, leiomyoma, malignancy/hyperplasia
  - Trauma: high vaginal laceration
  - Sexually transmitted infection/pelvic inflammatory disease
- Non-structural
  - Coagulopathy: von Willebrand disease, acquired bleeding disorders (eg, leukemia and thrombocytopenia), liver disease, kidney disease
  - Ovulatory disorder
    - Hypothalamic: stress, weight loss, exercise, chronic illness
    - Physiologic
    - Hyperandrogenic: polycystic ovarian syndrome, congenital adrenal hyperplasia, adrenal/ovarian tumor
    - Endocrine disorder: hyper/hypothyroidism, diabetes, hyperprolactinemia, primary ovarian insufficiency
  - Endometrial dysfunction
  - Iatrogenic–medications: anticoagulants, hormonal contraceptives, chemotherapy, copper intrauterine device
  - Not otherwise classified

Laboratory evaluation should begin with performance of a pregnancy test by either urine or serum hCG. In a patient with any hemodynamic instability, excessive bleeding, or clinical evidence of anemia, a complete blood count is essential. Coagulation studies, type and cross, and reticulocyte count can also be considered based on the clinical picture. Other laboratory tests, including evaluation for suspected endocrine disorders (eg, thyroid disorder, polycystic ovarian syndrome) or bleeding disorders (eg, von Willebrand disease) may also be helpful and should be obtained before hormonal therapy, although these results will not be available during the ED visit. Testing for gonorrhea and chlamydia should be conducted in a sexually active adolescent. If heavy vaginal bleeding is accompanied by focal abdominal pain or a pelvic mass, a pelvic ultrasound is recommended to assess for ectopic pregnancy, malignancy, or ovarian masses.[26]

Management of AUB depends on hemodynamic stability. In hemodynamically unstable patients, aggressive resuscitation with saline and blood should be instituted emergently, and gynecology or general surgery and adolescent medicine should be consulted. In hemodynamically stable patients, medical management with oral medroxyprogesterone acetate or oral contraceptive pills and iron replacement is typically prescribed.

PREVENTION OF UNPLANNED PREGNANCY: EMERGENCY CONTRACEPTION

More than 750,000 adolescents become pregnant in the United States annually, with most of the pregnancies unintended.[27] Women seeking care in the ED have high rates of unintended pregnancy risk,[28] and more than half of adolescent females presenting to the ED are sexually experienced.[29] If during the ED visit a patient discloses that she was sexually assaulted or had recent unprotected or inadequately protected intercourse and does not desire pregnancy, she may be a candidate for emergency contraception (EC), and the treating clinician should provide the patient the option to receive EC. Many forms of EC are available, including ulipristal acetate, levonorgestrel, the Yuzpe method (combination of estrogen and progestin oral contraceptive pills), and the copper IUD. All methods can be used for up to 5 days after contraceptive failure. Although oral emergency contraceptive pills are the most commonly used forms of EC, the copper IUD is the most effective means of EC and is the only one that provides ongoing contraception. The 2 oral regimens that are currently marketed in the United States are ulipristal acetate (30 mg) and levonorgestrel (1.5 mg). Ulipristal was found to be more effective than levonorgestrel in 2 randomized trials.[30,31] In the United States, levonorgestrel is available without a prescription to men and women of all ages, whereas ulipristal requires a prescription. For women with a Body Mass Index (BMI) of 26 or over who used levonorgestrel EC, pregnancy rates were no different than would be expected if they had not used EC. Ulipristal acetate appears to lose effectiveness at a BMI of 35.[32,33] The most effective form of EC is the copper IUD, which can provide EC and ongoing contraception for up to 10 years.[34]

SUMMARY

Adolescent females frequently present to the ED with complaints that may be caused by a gynecologic emergency. Differentiating and excluding some of the common and most serious gynecologic emergencies reviewed in this article are critical. Timely and effective treatment of these conditions, once diagnosed, can result in better health outcomes.

References

1. Goyal M, Hersh A, Luan X, et al. National trends in pelvic inflammatory disease among adolescents in the emergency department. *J Adolesc Health*. 2013;53:249-252
2. Goyal M, Hersh A, Luan X, et al. Frequency of pregnancy testing among adolescent emergency department visits. *Acad Emerg Medicine*. 2013;20:816-821
3. Ziv A, Boulet JR, Slap GB. Emergency department utilization by adolescents in the United States. *Pediatrics*. 1998;101:987-994
4. Klein JD, Wilson KM, McNulty M, Kapphahn C, Collins KS. Access to medical care for adolescents: results from the 1997 Commonwealth Fund Survey of the Health of Adolescent Girls. *J Adolesc Health*. 1999;25:120-130
5. Reddy DM, Fleming R, Swain C. Effect of mandatory parental notification on adolescent girls' use of sexual health care services. *JAMA*. 2002;288:710-714
6. Guttmacher Institute. An overview of minors' consent law. State Policies in Brief. 2013. Available at: www.guttmacher.org/statecenter/spibs/spib_OMCL.pdf. Accessed February 11, 2015
7. Ford C, English A, Sigman G. Confidential health care for adolescents: position paper for the Society for Adolescent Medicine. *J Adolesc Health*. 2004;35:160-167
8. Chang J, Elam-Evans LD, Berg CJ, et al. Pregnancy-related mortality surveillance—United States, 1991–1999. *MMWR Surveill Summ*. 2003;52:1-8
9. Ectopic pregnancy—United States, 1990–1992. *MMWR Morb Mortal Wkly Rep*. 1995;44:46-48
10. Menon S, Sammel MD, Vichnin M, Barnhart KT. Risk factors for ectopic pregnancy: a comparison between adults and adolescent women. *J Pediatr Adolesc Gynecol*. 2007;20:181-185
11. Xiong X, Buekens P, Wollast E. IUD use and the risk of ectopic pregnancy: a meta-analysis of case-control studies. *Contraception*. 1995;52:23-34
12. Tay JI, Moore J, Walker JJ. Ectopic pregnancy. *BMJ*. 2000;320:916-919
13. Stovall TG, Kellerman AL, Ling FW, Buster JE. Emergency department diagnosis of ectopic pregnancy. *Ann Emerg Med*. 1990;19:1098-1103
14. Barnhart KT. Clinical practice. Ectopic pregnancy. *N Engl J Med*. 2009;361:379-387
15. Brown DL, Doubilet PM. Transvaginal sonography for diagnosing ectopic pregnancy: positivity criteria and performance characteristics. *J Ultrasound Med*. 1994;13:259-266
16. Farquhar CM. Ectopic pregnancy. *Lancet*. 2005;366:583-591
17. Guthrie BD, Adler MD, Powell EC. Incidence and trends of pediatric ovarian torsion hospitalizations in the United States, 2000-2006. *Pediatrics*. 2010;125:532-538
18. Chang HC, Bhatt S, Dogra VS. Pearls and pitfalls in diagnosis of ovarian torsion. *Radiographics*. 2008;28:1355-1368
19. Breech LL, Hillard PJ. Adnexal torsion in pediatric and adolescent girls. *Curr Opin Obstet Gynecol*. 2005;17:483-489
20. Houry D, Abbott JT. Ovarian torsion: a fifteen-year review. *Ann Emerg Med*. 2001;38:156-159
21. Celik A, Ergun O, Aldemir H, et al. Long-term results of conservative management of adnexal torsion in children. *J Pediatr Surg*. 2005;40:704-708
22. Brunham RC, Gottlieb SL, Paavonen J. Pelvic inflammatory disease. *N Engl J Med*. 2015;372:2039-2048
23. Workowski KA, Bolan GA. Sexually transmitted diseases treatment guidelines, 2015. *MMWR Recomm Rep*. 2015;64:1-137

24. Trent M, Ellen JM, Frick KD. Estimating the direct costs of pelvic inflammatory disease in adolescents: a within-system analysis. *Sex Transm Dis.* 2011;38:326-328

25. Munro MG, Critchley HO, Broder MS, Fraser IS. FIGO classification system (PALM-COEIN) for causes of abnormal uterine bleeding in nongravid women of reproductive age. *Int J Gynaecol Obstet.* 2011;113:3-13

26. Bennett AR, Gray SH. What to do when she's bleeding through: the recognition, evaluation, and management of abnormal uterine bleeding in adolescents. *Curr Opin Pediatr.* 2014;26:413-419

27. Finer LB, Zolna MR. Unintended pregnancy in the United States: incidence and disparities, 2006. *Contraception.* 2011;84:478-485

28. Todd CS, Mountvarner G, Lichenstein R. Unintended pregnancy risk in an emergency department population. *Contraception.* 2005;71:35-39

29. Mollen CJ, Miller MK, Hayes KL, Wittink MN, Barg FK. Developing emergency department-based education about emergency contraception: adolescent preferences. *Acad Emerg Med.* 2013;20:1164-1170

30. Creinin MD, Schlaff W, Archer DF, et al. Progesterone receptor modulator for emergency contraception: a randomized controlled trial. *Obstet Gynecol.* 2006;108:1089-1097

31. Glasier AF, Cameron ST, Fine PM, et al. Ulipristal acetate versus levonorgestrel for emergency contraception: a randomised non-inferiority trial and meta-analysis. *Lancet.* 2010;375:555-562

32. Glasier A, Cameron ST, Blithe D, et al. Can we identify women at risk of pregnancy despite using emergency contraception? Data from randomized trials of ulipristal acetate and levonorgestrel. *Contraception.* 2011;84:363-367

33. Moreau C, Trussell J. Results from pooled Phase III studies of ulipristal acetate for emergency contraception. *Contraception.* 2012;86:673-680

34. Cleland K, Zhu H, Goldstuck N, Cheng L, Trussell J. The efficacy of intrauterine devices for emergency contraception: a systematic review of 35 years of experience. *Hum Reprod.* 2012;27:1994-2000

Adolesc Med 026 (2015) 484–490

Adolescent Male Genitourinary Emergencies

Zachary McClain, MD[a]*;
David L. Bell, MD, MPH[b]

*Children's Hospital of Philadelphia, Philadelphia, Pennsylvania;
[b]Columbia University Medical Center, New York, New York*

NORMAL ANATOMY

Given the reports that only 37% of males 15 to 44 years old had undergone a testicular examination in the past year, it is important to review the normal anatomy of the male genitourinary region.[1] The penis is part of the normal anatomy; however, it is the testis, tunica vaginalis, epididymis, spermatic cord, and appendix testis that are structures of particular importance in acute scrotal pathology. The testis (plural testes) is the male gonad responsible for production of androgens (testosterone) and sperm. The tunica vaginalis is a serous covering that surrounds the testis and is a space that may accumulate different types of fluid. The epididymis, located on the posterior pole of the testis, is a tightly coiled tubular structure that matures, stores, and transports spermatozoa, which are produced in the testes. The spermatic cord comprises the testicular blood vessels and the vas deferens, the ductal system that connects the left and right epididymis to the ejaculatory ducts. The appendix testis is a vestigial remnant of the müllerian duct system that is located on the upper pole of the testis.

EVALUATION OF THE ACUTE SCROTUM

The acutely painful scrotum is a common emergency in adolescent males and requires a quick and adept evaluation to identify any pathology that requires immediate surgical intervention. The main objective in the evaluation is preventing testicular loss, which requires a high index of suspicion and prompt surgical intervention.[2] Evaluation of the acute scrotum should start with a thorough history and physical examination. The history should include details on the location, onset, and intensity of the pain, urinary complaints (dysuria, fre-

*Corresponding author
E-mail address: mcclainz@email.chop.edu

quency), presence or absence of a trauma history, and systemic symptoms (fevers, chills). The physical examination should include careful evaluation of the abdomen, inguinal region, spermatic cord, scrotal skin, testes, tunica vaginalis, and epididymis. Special maneuvers should include the eliciting of the cremasteric reflex and transillumination. The cremasteric reflex is contraction of the ipsilateral testis while the skin of the upper thigh is gently stroked. In some studies, an absent reflex in patients with testicular torsion has a sensitivity of 100%.[3] However, the presence of a cremasteric reflex does not definitively rule out testicular torsion. Scrotal pain in adolescents and young adults is often caused by an infection, such as epididymitis, so a urinalysis and urine culture are helpful in determining an infectious cause with presence of pyuria or bacteriuria.[4] Color Doppler ultrasound can be used to rule out testicular torsion in patients in whom it is not clearly evident.

Testicular Torsion

Testicular torsion is a surgical emergency. Rapid diagnosis and detorsion are critical to maximize the likelihood of testicle survival. Acute scrotal pain from testicular torsion occurs after a twisting of the testis, which blocks blood flow to the spermatic cord. There is a bimodal distribution of testicular torsion, with peaks in infancy and early adolescence. Testicular torsion affects 1 in 4000 males younger than age 25 annually.[5] In recent US studies of patients hospitalized for acute scrotal pain, 34% to 51% of cases were the result of testicular torsion, with most occurring in the pubertal group.[2,6,7] Other studies have shown the estimated yearly incidence of testicular torsion in boys 10 to 18 years old ranged from 3.8 to 7.7 per 100,000.[8,9] A congenital malformation, the "bell-clapper deformity," increases susceptibility to induced torsion of the cord and its vessels.[10] In the bell-clapper deformity, the testes are inadequately affixed to the tunica vaginalis, which results in increased mobility on their axis. Most cases (90%) of testicular torsion are caused by a bell-clapper deformity, which allows for the testis to torse on the spermatic cord, resulting in reduced arterial inflow and venous outflow obstruction that ultimately lead to testicular ischemia.

In testicular torsion, the scrotal pain is unilateral and sudden in onset.[3,11] There may be associated nausea and vomiting. The classic finding on physical examination is a high-riding testis on a torsed, shortened spermatic cord. There may be profound testicular swelling. The scrotal skin on the affected side may be erythematous and warm; however, these changes indicate the degree of inflammation and may worsen depending on the length of time the testis has been torsed.[12] The cremasteric reflex should be assessed. Presence of the cremasteric reflex suggests causes of scrotal swelling other than testicular torsion, but there have been case reports of patients with an intact reflex despite torsion.[12,13] If the history and physical examination indicate testicular torsion as the cause of acute scrotal pain, immediate surgical intervention should not be delayed by imaging. However, if history and physical examination are equivocal, color Doppler ultrasonography is the diagnostic test of choice. The sensitivity and specificity of ultrasound in diagnosing torsion approached 100% in most studies.[6,14,15]

The treatment of testicular torsion is prompt surgical exploration with detorsion and fixation of both the involved and contralateral testes. Detorsion restores blood flow to the testis. Historically, there is a 4- to 8-hour window before significant, and possibly irreversible, ischemic damage occurs.[16] A greater than 12-hour delay in surgical intervention may result in prolonged ischemia and lead to orchiectomy.[17] Manual detorsion can be performed if surgery is not immediately available; however, surgical treatment is still required in order to secure the testicle to the scrotal wall and prevent recurrence.[18] Testicular salvage is highly dependent on the time of detorsion from the onset of symptoms, since the majority can be salvaged if detorsed within 12 hours of symptoms.

Epididymitis

Epididymitis is the most common cause of acute scrotal pain, especially in adolescents and young adults. One retrospective study showed a bimodal distribution with peak incidence in men 16 to 30 years of age.[19] Epididymitis refers to inflammation of the epididymis, a coiled tube that connects the vas deferens to the testicle. Approximately 600,000 cases occur annually in the United States.[4]

Epididymitis is most commonly caused by an infectious etiology, particularly sexually transmitted infections, but it can be caused by non-infectious etiologies as well. Epididymitis is divided into 2 categories: acute and chronic. Acute epididymitis is defined as pain, swelling, and inflammation of the epididymis that lasts less than 6 weeks.[20] Chronic epididymitis is defined as scrotal pain and swelling that lasts more than 6 weeks and often is caused by an inflammatory or obstructive process. Although chronic epididymitis can occur in young adults, it is mostly described in middle-aged and older adults.[21]

Patients with acute bacterial epididymitis typically present with gradual, unilateral scrotal pain and swelling. The pain can spread to the adjacent testes and can be accompanied by fever and rigors. Voiding symptoms, such as dysuria, hesitancy, and frequency, can also occur. Of note, these symptoms are typical for epididymitis and orchitis, but not for testicular torsion.[4] Among sexually active men, acute infectious epididymitis is most commonly caused by *Chlamydia trachomatis* or *Neisseria gonorrheae*.[22] Enteric organisms such as *Escherichia coli* and *Pseudomonas* spp may be the cause in males who engage in insertive anal intercourse. Less common organisms include *Ureaplasma urealyticum*, *Corynebacterium* spp, *Mycobacterium* spp, *Brucella* spp, and, in patients with human immunodeficiency virus (HIV) infection, *Cytomegalovirus*, and *Cryptococcus*.[20,22,23]

Acute epididymitis is diagnosed by physical examination in conjunction with urine studies. Examination of the scrotum reveals induration and swelling of the epididymis, with remarkable tenderness to palpation. Because the differential diagnosis of testicular pain includes both epididymitis and testicular torsion, the Prehn sign is sometimes used to help differentiate between the two. A positive Prehn sign consists of pain relief with lifting of the affected testicle, which points toward epididymitis. However, the Prehn sign has been shown to be inferior to Doppler ultrasound in ruling out testicular torsion. In addition to physical examination, a urinalysis and urine culture should be performed; however, without urinary symptoms, the results will likely be negative.[5] A urine nucleic acid amplification test for *N gonorrhoeae* and *C trachomatis* should be sent as well.

Treatment of epididymitis varies depending on the severity of symptoms and the likely organisms involved, with empiric treatment targeted at those pathogens.[4] According to the Centers for Disease Control and Prevention (CDC) treatment guidelines, empiric treatment should include ceftriaxone 250 mg intramuscularly in a single dose plus doxycycline 100 mg orally twice a day for 10 days.[24] If enteric organisms are suspected, treatment with a fluoroquinolone is recommended. For patients who are acutely febrile or dehydrated, hospitalization may be required for intravenous hydration and parental antibiotic therapy. Adjunctive treatments include ice, scrotal elevation, and non-steroidal anti-inflammatory drugs (NSAIDs). An important part of therapy is partner treatment of any culture-positive infections.

As mentioned earlier, chronic epididymitis is usually non-infectious and likely caused by an autoimmune disease (eg, sarcoidosis), trauma, or vasculitis. It has been proposed that idiopathic, non-infectious epididymitis is the result of chemical inflammation from reflux of urine into the vas deferens; however, scant evidence supports this mechanism.[20] In non-infectious epididymitis, there is usually less epididymal inflammation resulting in pain and swelling, and the diagnosis is made after other etiologies are excluded. Treatment is conservative with scrotal elevation, rest from athletic activity, warm baths, and NSAIDs.

Torsion of the Appendix Testis or Appendix Epididymis

As mentioned in the section on normal anatomy, the appendix testis is a vestigial remnant of the müllerian duct system that is located on the upper pole of the testis, and, like the testes, it is also subject to torsion. Although torsion of the appendix testis is less likely to occur in adolescents and young adults given that it most commonly occurs in prepubertal children, it should still be considered in the patient presenting with acute scrotal pain. Most cases occur in patients between the ages of 7 and 14 years.[25] From history alone, it is difficult to differentiate torsion of testis from torsion of the appendix testis, and there is often no difference in presenting symptoms.[26] There is sudden onset of testicular pain. However, physical examination is more helpful in differentiating testicular torsion from torsion of the appendix testis. A tender, hard, 2- to 3-mm nodule may be palpable on the upper part of the testicle, with a visible blue discoloration referred to as the classic "blue dot sign."[27] If the diagnosis of torsion of the appendix testis is unclear after history and physical examination, ultrasonography will demonstrate the torsed appendix testis. Treatment of torsion of the appendix testis is conservative and supportive, including rest, ice, and NSAIDs.

Trauma

In general, trauma to the adolescent male external genitalia during sport activities or accidents is not uncommon. However, such trauma rarely results in severe injuries that necessitate medical attention or surgical intervention. Injuries range from hematocele, blood within the tunica vaginalis, to testicular rupture. In one study, most injuries among adolescents were polytraumatic and secondary to motor vehicle accidents. In addition, this study found that injuries of the scrotum occurred more frequently than did those to the penis.[28] Ultrasound remains the standard imaging study after scrotal trauma. With the exception of testicular rupture or significant hematocele (likely secondary to testicular rupture), which requires surgical intervention, the strategy for treatment of blunt trauma has shifted away from surgical management and toward conservative management with rest, scrotal support, antibiotics, and serial ultrasound.[29]

Incarcerated Inguinal Hernia

An incarcerated inguinal hernia occurs when there is herniation of the bowel through the spermatic cord into the scrotum. Herniation may present with a scrotal mass and pain, whereas hernia cases with a strangulated portion of bowel may present with severe scrotal or abdominal pain. Inguinal hernia pain is likely to present as severe abdomen pain, and must be considered in the differential of abdominal pain, because it is a surgical emergency. The age distribution of inguinal hernias, especially those requiring repair, is bimodal in distribution; it peaks in early childhood and old age, and therefore is less likely to occur in adolescence.[30]

Orchitis

Orchitis occurs when inflammation from a concurrent epididymitis extends to the adjacent testicle.[4] It is uncommon to have an isolated orchitis without epididymitis, with the exception of mumps orchitis. Mumps primarily affects adolescents and young adults, and recent outbreaks and a global resurgence of mumps cases have been reported.[31,32] Adolescents are more likely to be subject to mumps orchitis, which is one of the primary complications of the disease. The incidence of mumps orchitis in postpubertal males is as high as 40%.[33] Unlike the other adolescent scrotal complaints, mumps presents with a prodromal illness of headache, malaise, low-grade fever, and parotid swelling, followed by testicular pain and swelling approximately 10 days later.[34,35] Treatment of mumps orchitis is supportive, with bed rest, ice packs, scrotal support, and pain control. Symptoms resolve in approximately 1 week.[36] Adolescent males who have not been vaccinated should be offered the measles, mumps, and rubella (MMR) vaccine and educated about mumps orchitis and its potential complications, including infertility.[35]

Conclusion

Male genitourinary concerns can be painful, painless, urgent, benign, infectious, or simply an anatomic variation. However, most importantly, for adolescent males, genitourinary concerns are extremely common and it is clear that providers caring for adolescent males be aware of the variety of conditions that affect them.

References

1. Chabot MJ, Lewis C, de Bocanegra HT, Darney P. Correlates of receiving reproductive health care services among U.S. men aged 15 to 44 years. *Am J Mens Health*. 2011;5:358-366
2. Tajchner L, Larkin JO, Bourke MG, et al. Management of the acute scrotum in a district general hospital: 10-year experience. *Sci World J*. 2009;9:281-286
3. Schmitz D, Safranek S. Clinical inquiries. How useful is a physical exam in diagnosing testicular torsion? *J Fam Pract*. 2009;58:433-434
4. Trojian TH, Lishnak TS, Heiman D. Epididymitis and orchitis: an overview. *Am Fam Physician*. 2009;79:583-587
5. Wampler SM, Llanes M. Common scrotal and testicular problems. *Prim Care*. 2010;37:613-626
6. al Mufti RA, Ogedegbe AK, Lafferty K. The use of Doppler ultrasound in the clinical management of acute testicular pain. *Br J Urol*. 1995;76:625-627
7. Molokwu CN, Somani BK, Goodman CM. Outcomes of scrotal exploration for acute scrotal pain suspicious of testicular torsion: a consecutive case series of 173 patients. *BJU Int*. 2011;107: 990-993
8. Huang WY, Chen YF, Chang HC, et al. The incidence rate and characteristics in patients with testicular torsion: a nationwide, population-based study. *Acta Paediatr*. 2013;102:e363-e367
9. Zhao LC, Lautz TB, Meeks JJ, Maizels M. Pediatric testicular torsion epidemiology using a national database: incidence, risk of orchiectomy and possible measures toward improving the quality of care. *J Urol*. 2011;186:2009-2013
10. Sharp VJ, Kieran K, Arlen AM. Testicular torsion: diagnosis, evaluation, and management. *Am Fam Physician*. 2013;88:835-840
11. Ciftci AO, Senocak ME, Taynel FC, Büyükpamukç N. Clinical predictors for differential diagnosis of acute scrotum. *Eur J Pediatr Surg*. 2004;14:333-338
12. Srinivasan A, Cinman N, Feber KM, Gitlin J, Palmer LS. History and physical examination findings predictive of testicular torsion: an attempt to promote clinical diagnosis by house staff. *J Pediatr Urol*. 2011;7:470-474
13. Rabinowitz R. The importance of the cremasteric reflex in acute scrotal swelling in children. *J Urol*. 1984;132:89-90
14. Waldert M, Klatte T, Schmidbauer J, et al. Color Doppler sonography reliably identifies testicular torsion in boys. *Urology*. 2010;75:1170-1174
15. Wilbert DM, Schaerfe CW, Stern WD, et al. Evaluation of the acute scrotum by color-coded Doppler ultrasonography. *J Urol*. 1993;149:1475-1477
16. Bartsch G, Frank S, Marberger H, Mikuz G. Testicular torsion: late results with special regard to fertility and endocrine function. *J Urol*. 1980;124:375-378

17. Dunne PJ, O'Loughlin BS. Testicular torsion: time is the enemy. *Aust N Z J Surg.* 2000;70:441-442
18. Sessions AE, Rabinowitz R, Hulbert WC, et al. Testicular torsion: direction, degree, duration and disinformation. *J Urol.* 2003;169:663-665
19. Kaver I, Matzkin H, Braf ZF. Epididymo-orchitis: a retrospective study of 121 patients. *J Fam Pract.* 1990;30:548-552
20. Tracy CR, Steers WD, Costabile R. Diagnosis and management of epididymitis. *Urol Clin North Am.* 2008;35:101-108, vii
21. Nickel JC, Siemens, DR, Nickel KR, Downey J. The patient with chronic epididymitis: characterization of an enigmatic syndrome. *J Urol.* 2002;167:1701-1704
22. Centers for Disease Control and Prevention. Epididymitis. In: Sexually transmitted diseases treatment guidelines, 2010. *MMWR Recomm Rep.* 2010;59(RR-12):67-69
23. Heidari M, Nazer M, Kheirollahi A, Birjandi M, Zareie H. Frequency of epididymo-orchitis in hospitalized patients with acute scrotum at Shohadaye Ashayer Hospital, Khorramabad, Iran. *J Pak Med Assoc.* 2012;62:44-46
24. Workowski KA, Berman S; Centers for Disease Control and Prevention. Sexually transmitted diseases treatment guidelines, 2010. *MMWR Recomm Rep.* 2010;59(RR-12):1-110
25. Fisher R, Walker J. The acute paediatric scrotum. *Br J Hosp Med.* 1994;51:290-292
26. Mushtaq I, Fung M, Glasson MJ. Retrospective review of paediatric patients with acute scrotum. *ANZ J Surg.* 2003;73:55-58
27. Ringdahl E, Teague L. Testicular torsion. *Am Fam Physician.* 2006;74:1739-1743
28. Widni EE, Hollwarth ME, Saxena AK. Analysis of nonsexual injuries of the male genitals in children and adolescents. *Acta Paediatr.* 2011;100:590-593
29. Cubillos J, Reda EF, Gitlin J, et al. A conservative approach to testicular rupture in adolescent boys. *J Urol.* 2010;184(4 Suppl):1733-1738
30. Burcharth J, Pedersen M, Bisgaard T, et al. Nationwide prevalence of groin hernia repair. *PLoS One.* 2013;8:e54367
31. Gemmill IM. Mumps vaccine: is it time to re-evaluate our approach? *CMAJ.* 2006;175:491-492
32. Centers for Disease Control and Prevention. Update: multistate outbreak of mumps—United States, January 1–May 2, 2006. *MMWR Morb Mortal Wkly Rep.* 2006;55:559-563
33. A retrospective survey of the complications of mumps. *J R Coll Gen Pract.* 1974;24:552-556
34. Beard CM, Benson RC Jr, Kelalis PP, Kurland LT. The incidence and outcome of mumps orchitis in Rochester, Minnesota, 1935 to 1974. *Mayo Clin Proc.* 1977;52:3-7
35. Davis NF, McGuire BB, Mahon JA, et al. The increasing incidence of mumps orchitis: a comprehensive review. *BJU Int.* 2010;105:1060-1065
36. Casella R, Leibundgut B, Lehmann K, Gasser TC. Mumps orchitis: report of a mini-epidemic. *J Urol.* 1997;158:2158-2161

Adolesc Med 026 (2015) 491–506

Sports-Related Head Injuries in Adolescents: A Comprehensive Update

Alexander D. McGinley, BA[a];
Christina L. Master, MD[b,c];
Mark R. Zonfrillo, MD, MSCE[*d]

[a]Center for Injury Research and Prevention, The Children's Hospital of Philadelphia, Philadelphia, Pennsylvania; [b]Sports Medicine and Performance Center, The Children's Hospital of Philadelphia, Philadelphia, Pennsylvania; [c]Department of Pediatrics, Perelman School of Medicine, University of Pennsylvania, Philadelphia, Pennsylvania; [d]Department of Emergency Medicine and Injury Prevention Center, Alpert Medical School of Brown University and Hasbro Children's Hospital, Providence, Rhode Island

DEFINITIONS

Despite the significant effect of traumatic brain injuries (TBIs) on individuals and society, there is a lack of standardization in their definition. The Centers for Disease Control and Prevention (CDC) defines TBI as an injury "caused by a bump, blow, or jolt to the head or a penetrating head injury that disrupts the normal function of the brain."[1] Alternatively, the Department of Veterans Affairs/Department of Defense describe TBI as a "traumatically induced structural injury and/or physiologic disruption of brain function as a result of an external force that is indicated by new onset or worsening of at least one of the following clinical signs, immediately following the event: Any period of loss of or a decreased level of consciousness;…post-traumatic amnesia [PTA]); Any alteration in mental state at the time of the injury…; Neurologic deficits…that may or may not be transient; Intracranial lesion." The Department of Veterans Affairs/Department of Defense describe the trauma as caused by direct, penetrating, or indirect (acceleration/deceleration) forces.[2]

Similarly, concussion is a term that lacks a standard definition but is often used synonymously with mild traumatic brain injury (mTBI). Although there are other mTBIs that are not concussion, for this article the 2 terms will be used interchangeably. A widely accepted definition of concussion comes from the 4th

---

*Corresponding author
E-mail address: zonfrillo@brown.edu

International Conference on Concussion in Sport held in Zurich, Switzerland, in November 2012:

> "Concussion is a brain injury and is defined as a complex pathophysiological process affecting the brain, induced by biomechanical forces. Several common features that incorporate clinical, pathologic and biomechanical injury constructs that may be utilized in defining the nature of a concussive head injury include:
>
> 1. Concussion may be caused either by a direct blow to the head, face, neck or elsewhere on the body with an 'impulsive' force transmitted to the head.
> 2. Concussion typically results in the rapid onset of short-lived impairment of neurological function that resolves spontaneously. However, in some cases, symptoms and signs may evolve over a number of minutes to hours.
> 3. Concussion may result in neuropathological changes, but the acute clinical symptoms largely reflect a functional disturbance, rather than a structural injury and, as such, no abnormality is seen on standard structural neuroimaging studies.
> 4. Concussion results in a graded set of clinical symptoms that may or may not involve loss of consciousness. Resolution of the clinical and cognitive symptoms typically follows a sequential course, [but] symptoms may be prolonged."[3]

The "mild" of mTBI generally refers to the mechanism of injury or to the fact that concussions are generally not life threatening despite the potential for short-term disability and serious ongoing sequelae.[1] A breakdown of the classification of TBI severity is given in Table 1.[2]

Table 1
Classification of traumatic brain injury severity

Criteria	Mild	Moderate	Severe
Structural imaging	Normal	Normal or abnormal	Normal or abnormal
Loss of consciousness	0–30 min	>30 min and <24 hours	>24 hours
Alteration of consciousness/ mental state*	A moment up to 24 hours	>24 hours; severity based on other criteria	
Post-traumatic amnesia (PTA)	0–1 day	>1 and <7 days	> 7 days
Glasgow Coma Scale (best available score in first 24 hours)	13-15	9-12	<9

*Alteration of consciousness/mental state must be immediately related to the trauma to the head. Typical symptoms are looking and feeling dazed and uncertain of what is happening; confusion; difficulty thinking clearly or responding appropriately to mental status questions; and being unable to describe events immediately before or after the trauma event.
Adapted with permission from Institute of Medicine. Report Brief: Sports-Related Concussions in Youth: Improving the Science, Changing the Culture. Available at: www.iom.edu/~/media/Files/Report%20Files/2013/Concussions/concussions-RB.pdf. Accessed September 28, 2014.

Finally, this review will focus on sports-related TBI in adolescents, which for the purposes of this article will be defined as youths 10 to 19 years of age.

EPIDEMIOLOGY

Approximately 1.6 to 3.8 million sports-related TBIs occur annually in the United States, representing a significant public health burden. This encompasses injuries of all severities, including those for which no medical attention is sought.[4] For children 19 years of age and younger, sports-related TBIs resulted in 248,419 visits to the emergency department (ED) in 2009, a 62% increase since 2001. From 2001 to 2009, TBIs of all severities accounted for 6.5% of all sports-related ED visits in that same age group. The highest number of visits was seen in males aged 10 to 19 years and from injuries sustained while participating in bicycling, football, playground, basketball, and soccer.[5]

Most of these injuries are mTBIs/concussions, accounting for approximately 90% of sports- and recreation-related TBIs.[6,7] One study of 12 scholastic sports over 11 years estimated the incidence of concussion at 24 per 100,000 athletic exposures.[8] Another study of high school athletics found that concussions accounted for 13.2% of all sports-related injuries, with most concussions occurring during football, girls' soccer, boys' ice hockey, and boys' lacrosse.[9] Although males account for the largest number of concussions, females have higher rates of concussion in sports with similar playing rules, such as soccer, softball, and baseball.[9]

Although more serious brain injuries are less common, recent estimates of TBI in sports and recreation activities classify 9% to 13% as moderate or severe.[6,7] Additionally, over a 30-year period, 231 deaths occurred from head or neck trauma in athletes aged 21 years and younger, including 138 football players. Second impact syndrome was suspected in 17 of the football deaths because the athletes were reportedly still symptomatic from previous concussion.[10]

MECHANISM AND PATHOPHYSIOLOGY

Mechanism

Traumatic brain injuries of all severities result from the rapid application of force to the head, in the form of linear acceleration, rotational acceleration, or impact deceleration.[11] Recent attempts in high school and collegiate athletes to determine specific acceleration thresholds for concussive injury, using in-helmet devices such as the Head Impact Telemetry system, have had variable success.[12] However, in 1 study using the Head Impact Telemetry system, nearly half of the concussions were the result of impacts to the top of the head, indicating that the location of the impact may play a role in injury potential.[13]

Pathophysiology

A review of concussion/mTBI pathophysiology is necessary to understand the rationale for treatment. At the cellular level, concussive injury begins with the release of excitatory neurotransmitters such as glutamate, resulting in changes to axon membrane permeability leading to ionic imbalance of sodium, potassium, and calcium.[14] Figure 1 shows a more in-depth representation of the ionic imbalance.[15] In addition, diffuse axonal injury-type stretching leads to an influx of calcium, thereby inhibiting production of adenosine triphosphate (ATP), the cellular energy source.[16,17] Axonal attempts to correct the ionic imbalance are hindered by the reduced ability to produce ATP. A compensatory increase in glucose delivery via increased cerebral blood flow would be expected; however, this does not occur because of the response to injury.[18] In this state, in which cerebral blood flow is uncoupled from the metabolic demands of the brain, glucose delivery to the damaged axons may be insufficient to meet the increased cerebral demand for glucose as the result of injury.[15]

Although a detailed discussion of moderate to severe TBI pathophysiology is beyond the scope of this article, several principles that apply to the spectrum of TBI include disruption in cerebral blood flow, glucose metabolism, and axonal architecture. Severity-dependent decreases in cerebral blood flow have been

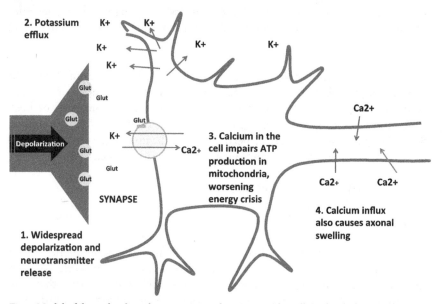

Fig 1. Model of the pathophysiologic processes that occur at the cellular level after a concussion. ATP, adenosine triphosphate. (Adapted with permission from Grady MF, Master CL, Gioia GA. Concussion pathophysiology: rationale for physical and cognitive rest. *Pediatr Ann.* 2012;41: 377-382)

seen in moderate and severe TBI, as well as in mild injury.[14] Cerebral glucose metabolism also shows severity-dependent alterations ranging in duration from days to months.[19] Finally, diffuse axonal injury has been recognized as "one of the most common and important pathological features of traumatic brain injury."[16] Diffuse axonal injury can result from complete breaking to functional disruption of axonal tracts, and it spans the spectrum of TBI presentation from confusion and loss of consciousness (LOC) to cognitive dysfunction and coma.[16] In addition, mass lesion-type moderate and severe TBIs can result in elevated intracranial pressure (ICP), subsequent ischemic injury as a result of insufficient perfusion, or brain herniation.

Finally, it is worth noting that the rare but devastating second impact syndrome, which is thought to result from a second insult before complete recovery from a previous concussion, is believed to be caused by loss of autoregulation of cerebral blood flow, resulting in increased ICP and subsequent herniation.[11,20]

EVALUATION, ASSESSMENT, AND DIAGNOSIS

On-Field Evaluation

The evaluation and proper management of head injuries should begin on the field or sideline after any direct or indirect blow to the head. All athletes suspected of sustaining a concussion or more severe TBI should be immediately removed from play and evaluated by a physician or licensed health care professional on the sideline or at a hospital. Athletes with TBI of any severity, including concussion, should not be allowed to return to play on the same day.[3] Although some concussions can be diagnosed and managed properly on the sideline, the initial priority should be assessment for more severe injuries or potentially life-threatening conditions, including cervical spine and intracranial injuries. Signs indicating a need for immediate transport to an emergency department for further evaluation include LOC of any duration, post-traumatic convulsions, cervical spine tenderness or decreased range of motion, focal neurologic deficits, and deteriorating mental status.[21] After further evaluation in the ED, a subset of these patients may receive a diagnosis of concussion. However, because of the potential for more severe or life-threatening conditions, it is imperative that these injuries be initially managed conservatively.

Concussion and mTBI

Most sports-related TBIs are concussions. The diagnosis of concussion is primarily a clinical one and can be made based on the history and mechanism of the injury, the presence of concomitant signs and symptoms, and the absence of more severe conditions. The clinical features of concussion can be broadly grouped into physical, sleep, thinking/remembering, and mood deficits

(Table 2).[22] Often the most apparent physical signs and symptoms include headache, nausea, vomiting, dizziness and balance deficits, but other signs and symptoms may be present and may cause significant impairment. Loss of consciousness is present in the minority of cases (<10%) and is not thought to be predictive of symptoms or deficits after concussion.[23,24] In fact, a recent article reported that the absence of LOC was actually predictive of a prolonged recovery.[25]

Moderate and Severe TBI

Moderate and severe TBI should be considered when any of the criteria for immediate transport to an ED are met. These injuries include hematomas, contusions, diffuse axonal injuries, skull fractures, and penetrating brain injuries.[11] Athletes with more significant TBI can vary in presentation from no LOC, LOC followed by a lucid interval and subsequent clinical deterioration, to persistent LOC with coma. Athletes may present with significant neurologic deficits or no neurologic deficits at all.[26] Signs on physical examination can include hematomas, lacerations, palpable skull fractures, secondary signs of skull fractures (including hemotympanum, raccoon eyes, otorrhea, or rhinorrhea), or no signs of injury.[19] Because of the variability in presentation, athletes suspected of sustaining a moderate or severe TBI should be brought to medical attention for further evaluation and imaging to evaluate for potential intracranial pathology.

Imaging

Currently standard imaging techniques have little clinical diagnostic value for concussion and mTBI. They are, however, useful for determining the presence of intracranial pathology and the possible need for neurosurgical intervention.

Table 2
Concussion symptoms

Physical	Sleep	Thinking/ remembering	Mood disruption
• Headache	• Sleeping more or	• Difficulty thinking or	• More emotional
• Nausea	less than usual	concentrating	• Irritable
• Vomiting	• Drowsiness or	• Difficulty remembering	• Sad
• Balance	fatigue	• Confusion	• Nervous
• Slowed reaction time	• Trouble falling	• Feeling mentally foggy	• Depressed
• Dizziness	asleep	• Feeling slowed down	
• Sensitivity to light			
• Sensitivity to sound			
• Fuzzy or blurry vision			

Adapted with permission from Master CL, Grady MF. Office-based management of pediatric and adolescent concussion. *Pediatr Ann.* 2012;41:1-6.

Acutely, the imaging modality of choice is non-contrast head computed tomography, although there may be an emerging role for magnetic resonance imaging.[19]

Biomarkers

Although investigations of certain serum biomarkers, such as s100B and neuron-specific enolase, have shown limited clinical utility,[27] and genetic markers such as apolipoprotein E have proven inconclusive to date,[28,29] a recent study has shown some promise in identifying potentially useful biomarkers in the treatment of concussion. In a preliminary study of 13 children aged 11 to 21 years presenting to an ED after concussion, initial glial fibrillary acidic protein levels appeared to correlate with symptom burden 1 month after injury.[30] In addition, recent review articles looking at blood biomarkers for TBIs of all severities have found contradictory evidence supporting the use of biomarkers for diagnostic and prognostic purposes.[31,32] One article called for validation of the assays used in clinical research, as well as investigation of the role of sex and gender in biomarker evaluation,[31] whereas another suggested the use of multibiomarker panels, including clinical scoring, as keys to future biomarker evaluation.[32]

MANAGEMENT

Concussion and mTBI

Most patients with sports-related concussions recover spontaneously in days to weeks.[33] The initial management of concussion focuses on reducing the demands on the body and brain in order to prevent exacerbation of the metabolic mismatch that occurs. The central principles of initial concussion management are cognitive and physical rest until symptoms improve, followed by gradual return to learn and return to play. The concept of return to play is widely accepted. Asymptomatic athletes are progressed in 24-hour increments from no activity, to light aerobic activity, to sport-specific exercises, to non-contact drills, to full-contact practices, and finally to normal game play. If athletes become symptomatic at any point during recovery, they return to the previous asymptomatic step for at least a 24-hour period before advancing further.[3] The analogous concept of return to learn follows a similar stepwise progression from no activity, to gradual reintroduction of cognitive activity, increasing periods of homework at home, re-entry to a partial school day, gradual reintegration into full day school, and finally resumption of full cognitive workload.[34] Conceptually, the intention of this gradual progression is to prevent exacerbation of symptoms from an overload of cognitive activity. Additionally, because the primary "job" of adolescent athletes is school, an emphasis on return to learn before return to play is necessary.

Although time to recovery typically ranges from days to 1 to 2 weeks, a number of known modifiers may affect the length of time an athlete takes to become fully symptomatic and return to full activities.[3,33] Indicators for a potentially protracted recovery include a prior history of concussion and comorbidities such as attention-deficit/hyperactivity disorder, learning disabilities, depression, and migraine headaches.[3,21] Table 3 contains a more complete list.[3] In addition to the number of past concussions, a prior history of concussion should include the timing between concussions, which has been found to affect prognosis.[25] As mentioned previously (see Concussion and mTBI in the section Evaluation, Assessment, and Diagnosis on page 497), the presence of LOC is not in itself predictive of symptoms or deficits; however, prolonged LOC may influence management.[3] Female gender is also a risk factor for concussion and a factor in injury severity.[3] In recent studies, women were found to perform worse than men in 75% of mTBI-related variables and were 2.89 times more likely than men to be symptomatic at 3 months after sports-related concussion.[35,36] A recent consensus statement on future directions of research in emergency medicine calls for the development of surveillance systems to gain more insight into the role of gender in concussion risk and recovery.[37]

Table 3
Concussion modifiers

Factors	Modifier
Symptoms	• Number • Duration (>0 days) • Severity
Signs	• Prolonged loss of consciousness (>1 min) • Amnesia
Sequelae	• Concussive convulsions
Temporal	• Frequency: repeated concussions over time • Timing: injuries close together in time • "Recency": recent concussion or traumatic brain injury
Threshold	• Repeated concussions occurring with progressively less impact force or slower recovery after each successive concussion
Age	• Child and adolescent (<18 years)
Comorbidities and premorbidities	• Migraine, depression, other mental health disorders, attention-deficit/hyperactivity disorder, learning disabilities, sleep disorders
Medication	• Psychoactive drugs, anticoagulants
Behavior	• Dangerous style of play
Sport	• High-risk activity, contact and collision sport, high sporting level

Adapted with permission from McCrory P, Meeuwisse WH, Aubry M, et al. Consensus statement on concussion in sport: the 4th International Conference on Concussion in Sport held in Zurich, November 2012. *Br J Sports Med.* 2013;47:250-258.

Prolonged Recovery

Regardless of the presence of comorbidities, more specifically directed treatment may be necessary in patients who are slow to recover for any reason, which may be the case in as many as 10% to 20% of adolescent concussions.[38] After a period of cognitive and physical rest with symptom improvement, aerobic exercise at a level that does not exacerbate symptoms significantly, as well as vestibular, vision, and psychological therapies, may benefit patients with prolonged recovery from concussion.[39] Physical exertion too early may exacerbate symptoms and slow recovery, but there is emerging evidence that, subacutely, aerobic exercise may help with recovery.[38,40] The same study showed that athletes with prolonged symptoms recovered more quickly than non-athletes when aerobic exercise was added.[40] Oculomotor dysfunction is common after TBI.[41] Short screening tools, such as the vestibular/ocular motor screening assessment, have the potential for rapid clinical identification of deficits,[42] and oculomotor training has been shown to be beneficial for issues with visual tracking.[43] Finally, vestibular rehabilitation can benefit patients with persistent balance, gait, and dizziness deficits.[44] In conclusion, there is evidence supporting a multidisciplinary approach for the treatment of athletes with prolonged recovery from concussion.

Neurocognitive Testing

Neurocognitive testing has become a mainstay of concussion management with the increased availability and ease of use of computerized tests such as ImPACT and CogSport. In addition, a number of sideline evaluation tools, such as the acute concussion evaluation tool, the new sport concussion assessment tool 3, and the King-Devick test, are available. These tests can aid in the removal-from-play decisions, as well as the ongoing monitoring of cognitive recovery after concussion. Normative data exist for some of these tests, but comparison to pre-season baseline testing allows for a more individualized approach. However, none of these tools should be used in isolation to make return-to-school or return-to-play decisions; rather, they should be used in conjunction with a thorough history, physical and clinical evaluation, and monitoring of symptom resolution.[3]

Pharmacologic Therapy

Most concussions can be managed with cognitive and physical rest with a gradual return to activities alone. However, in subset of patients with prolonged or debilitating symptomatology, medications may be a helpful adjunctive therapy. This decision should be left up to the physician experienced in the treatment of complicated concussions. Of note, some the medications used for concussion treatment are off-label. Although the use of non-steroidal anti-inflammatory drugs may help with symptom management early during recovery, they may mask symptoms, thus allowing for premature return-to-learn and play, and prolonged use can lead to rebound headaches. When sleep disturbances are present, melatonin can be safely used to help patients fall asleep.[45] For patients with persistent fogginess and attention difficulties after cognitive and physical rest have been attempted, amantadine may also be useful.[46]

Moderate and Severe TBI

Because of the rarity of moderate and severe TBI in sports and the complexity of their treatment, an in-depth discussion of the principles of management is beyond the scope of this paper. However, several key factors in the management of moderate and severe TBI are worth discussing. Management of these injuries begins on the field with the ABCDE (Airway, Breathing, Circulation, Disability, Exposure/Environment) trauma evaluation, with attention to the possibility of cervical spine injuries and increased ICP from mass effect.[19] Signs of elevated ICP or impending herniation include declining mental status, unilateral dilated pupils, focal neurologic signs or posturing, as well as imaging findings. An emphasis is placed on stepwise progression from non-surgical interventions, including elevation of the head of the bed, sedation, analgesia and neuromuscular block, hyperosmolar intravenous therapeutics, such as mannitol and hypertonic saline, and controlled or mild hyperventilation, to surgical intervention including ventriculostomy. In cases not responding to initial therapies, metabolic suppression, more aggressive hyperventilation, lumbar drain, and decompressive craniectomy may also be indicated.[19]

LONG-TERM SEQUELAE AND COMPLICATIONS

Concussion and mTBI

Most athletes with concussion make a complete recovery in days to weeks and suffer no long-term sequelae. Recently there has been an increased focus on the rare but potential long-term complications of concussion, particularly from repetitive injuries, in both the medical literature and lay press. For concussion/mTBI, these include chronic post-concussion syndrome, second impact syndrome, and chronic traumatic encephalopathy (CTE). The concept that the effects of repeated concussion are cumulative and related to the interval between successive injuries is widely accepted but not entirely conclusive.[47] The concept is supported by animal studies showing that the effects on cognitive performance can be long-lasting or even permanent, especially with a shorter recovery period between injuries.[48] There are no official guidelines for athletes suffering multiple concussions; however, expert opinion has indicated that athletes suffering multiple (3 or more) concussions with increasing recovery times should avoid contact sports for an extended period of time (3-6 months). In addition, those athletes, as well as athletes suffering concussions from less forceful impacts, should consider permanent retirement from contact sports.[24,49]

Infrequently, patients experience symptoms that last more than 1 year after a single concussion. This has been referred to in the medical literature as both "permanent" and "chronic" post-concussion symptoms/syndrome.[11,50] Regardless of the name given, this condition may affect as many 10% to 15% of people in the general population after concussion.[51] Recently there has been evidence that comorbid diagnoses, such as depression, anxiety, and post-traumatic stress disorder, as well as pain, age, and gender, may predispose to this condition.[50,52]

As mentioned in the section Pathophysiology, in the section Mechanism and Pathophysiology on pages 495-496, second impact syndrome, or diffuse cerebral swelling, is a rare but devastating condition resulting from sports. All reported cases of second impact syndrome occurred in male athletes younger than 18 years.[49] Although debate continues as to the exact mechanism of this condition, including the role, if any, of a previous injury,[53] the high mortality rate warrants caution and vigilance in keeping players out of play while they are symptomatic.

CTE is a progressive neurodegenerative disease characterized by the presence of hyperphosphorylated tau protein aggregations on postmortem pathologic studies of brain tissue.[54] The disease has been found in the brains of former athletes, military members, and others with a history of head injuries, and it is believed to be the chronic result of repetitive concussive and subconcussive impacts on the brain.[55] The disease can result in neurocognitive decline, including attention, memory, and executive function deficits, as well as dementia. A recent study used positron emission tomography to look for evidence of tau deposits in the brains of living, retired, former National Football League players having symptoms consistent with CTE. Evidence of deposits was found and, although this requires confirmation at autopsy and in larger studies, may offer a tool for diagnosis of this condition while affected individuals are still alive.[56] Despite a growing body of literature on the topic, a cause-and-effect relationship between CTE and concussion or contact sports has not yet been established; as a result, the most recent Consensus Statement on Concussion in Sport emphasized caution in the interpretation of CTE-related findings and the importance of addressing parent's and athletes' concerns about the condition.[3]

Moderate and Severe TBI

Outcomes after moderate and severe TBI can range from death, to varying degrees of disability, to complete recovery. There is evidence that significant long-term disability occurs in a severity-dependent manner after moderate and severe TBI in children and adolescents.[57,58] However, because of the rarity of these injuries in sports, a complete discussion of outcomes will not be reviewed. Of note, in a recent prospective study of pediatric patients followed for an average of 10 years after moderate and severe TBI, 39% of patients were found to have negative long-term outcomes affecting their ability to function at age-appropriate levels.[59]

PREVENTION

The CDC and others have outlined a sports-related TBI prevention framework that includes primary prevention strategies (coaching of proper and safe techniques, rule changes, adherence to and enforcement of rules to prevent injury mechanisms), secondary prevention strategies (use of protective equipment, including mouth guards, proper strength and conditioning to reduce the likelihood of injuries when injury mechanisms do occur), and tertiary prevention strategies (increased awareness, prompt recognition, and proper treatment to mitigate potential short- and longer-term disability).[3,5,21,47,60]

As a means of primary and tertiary prevention, the CDC Heads Up[61] program and the Children's Hospital of Philadelphia's Minds Matter: Concussion Care for Kids[62] program provide resources aimed at increasing awareness of the risk and proper recognition of concussion. These sites contain resources specifically for athletes, parents, coaches, school staff, and physicians.

Although there is currently no consistent evidence that protective equipment, such as helmets and mouth guards, can prevent concussion,[63] these devices are important in preventing catastrophic brain injuries, such as skull fractures and intracranial bleeds, as well as dental and orofacial injury.[3,21] There is recent evidence that neck strength may correlate with concussion risk, with 1 study finding that a 1-pound increase in neck strength reduced the odds of concussion by 5%.[60]

Finally, proper recognition and treatment of concussion are often impeded by underreporting of these injuries by athletes.[64] When injuries are not reported or recognized, they cannot be treated properly, putting athletes at risk for complications. In 2013, The Institute of Medicine Committee on Sports-Related Concussion in Sports (in youth ages 5-21 years) released a report stating that "the culture of sports negatively influences athletes' self-reporting of concussion symptoms and their adherence to return-to-play guidance" and called for a change to that culture.[65] Other recent work examining the influences on concussion reporting in high school athletes showed that beliefs of social referents, including peers, coaches, and parents, greatly influenced athletes' "intention to report concussion symptoms," adding further weight to the importance of cultural change concerning concussion in sports.[66]

FUTURE DIRECTIONS

The cultural shift in sports discussed here is one of many possible keys to address the head injury crisis in sports. The most recent Consensus Statement on Concussion in Sport stressed the need for concussion education and awareness among athletes, coaches, parents, physicians, and the general public and the value of the backing of professional sports organizations on the conclusions of working groups on concussion to help create this change.[3] A 2014 article on future directions in brain injury research called for investigation in 5 areas: clinical care, rehabilitation, epidemiology, prevention, and biomechanics.[67] Because of the complexity of TBIs in terms of prevention, mechanisms, treatment, and recovery, it is clear that such a multifaceted approach will be needed. Recent successes have shown potential for biomarkers[68] as well as advanced imaging techniques, such as magnetic resonance spectroscopy and diffuse tensor imaging, in the diagnosis of concussion.[69,70] Further validation is needed before these tools would be clinically useful. In addition, biomechanical studies of acceleration thresholds for injury are promising and have the potential to improve injury recognition.[12] Future biomechanical work may also guide the development of helmets and other protective devices designed to reduce the risk of concussion.

References

1. Traumatic Brain Injury in the United States: Fact Sheet. 2014. Available at: www.cdc.gov/traumatic braininjury/get_the_facts.html. Accessed September 30, 2014
2. Department of Veteran Affairs, Department of Defense. Clinical Practice Guideline Summary: Management of concussion/mild traumatic brain injury. Available at: www.dcoe.mil/content/navigation/documents/VA Dod Management of Concussion mild Traumatic Brain Injury Summary.pdf. Accessed September 28, 2014
3. McCrory P, Meeuwisse WH, Aubry M, et al. Consensus statement on concussion in sport: the 4th International Conference on Concussion in Sport held in Zurich, November 2012. *Br J Sports Med.* 2013;47:250-258
4. Langlois JA, Rutland-Brown W, Wald MM. The epidemiology and impact of traumatic brain injury: a brief overview. *J Head Trauma Rehabil.* 2006;21:375-378
5. Centers for Disease Control and Prevention. Nonfatal traumatic brain injuries related to sports and recreation activities among persons aged ≤19 Years—United States, 2001–2009. *MMWR Morb Mortal Wkly Rep.* 2011;60:1337-1342
6. Selassie AW, Wilson DA, Pickelsimer EE, Voronca DC, Williams NR, Edwards JC. Incidence of sport-related traumatic brain injury and risk factors of severity: a population-based epidemiologic study. *Ann Epidemiol.* 2013;23:750-756
7. Crowe LM, Anderson V, Catroppa C, Babl FE. Head injuries related to sports and recreation activities in school-age children and adolescents: data from a referral centre in Victoria, Australia: Paediatric Emergency Medicine. *Emerg Med Australas.* 2010;22:56-61
8. Lincoln AE, Caswell SV, Almquist JL, Dunn RE, Norris JB, Hinton RY. Trends in concussion incidence in high school sports: a prospective 11-year study. *Am J Sports Med.* 2011;39:958-963
9. Marar M, McIlvain NM, Fields SK, Comstock RD. Epidemiology of concussions among united states high school athletes in 20 sports. *Am J Sports Med.* 2012;40:747-755
10. Thomas M, Haas TS, Doerer JJ, et al. Epidemiology of sudden death in young, competitive athletes due to blunt trauma. *Pediatrics.* 2011;128:e1-e8
11. Jordan BD. The clinical spectrum of sport-related traumatic brain injury. *Nat Rev Neurol.* 2013;9:222-230
12. Broglio SP, Surma T, Ashton-Miller JA. High school and collegiate football athlete concussions: a biomechanical review. *Ann Biomed Eng.* 2012;40:37-46
13. Guskiewicz KM, Mihalik JP, Shankar V, et al. Measurement of head impacts in collegiate football players: relationship between head impact biomechanics and acute clinical outcome after concussion. *Neurosurgery.* 2007;61:1244-1252
14. Choe MC, Babikian T, Difiori J, Hovda DA, Giza CC. A pediatric perspective on concussion pathophysiology. *Curr Opin Pediatr.* 2012;24:689-695

15. Grady MF, Master CL, Gioia GA. Concussion pathophysiology: rationale for physical and cognitive rest. *Pediatr Ann.* 2012;41:377-382

16. Johnson VE, Stewart W, Smith DH. Axonal pathology in traumatic brain injury. *Exp Neurol.* 2013;246:35-43

17. Wolf JA, Stys PK, Lusardi T, Meaney D, Smith DH. Traumatic axonal injury induces calcium influx modulated by tetrodotoxin-sensitive sodium channels. *J Neurosci.* 2001;21:1923-1930

18. Udomphorn Y, Armstead WM, Vavilala MS. Cerebral blood flow and autoregulation after pediatric traumatic brain injury. *Pediatr Neurol.* 2008;38:225-234

19. Giza CC. Traumatic brain injury. In: Lisak RP, Truong DD, Carroll WM, Bhidayasiri R, eds. *International Neurology: A Clinical Approach.* Oxford, UK: Wiley-Blackwell; 2009:648-651

20. Cantu RC. Second-impact syndrome. *Clin Sports Med.* 1998;17:37-44

21. Master CL, Balcer L, Collins M, Cotton D, Taichman D, Williams S. In the clinic. Concussion. *Ann Intern Med.* 2014;160:ITC21-ITC216

22. Master CL, Grady MF. Office-based management of pediatric and adolescent concussion. *Pediatr Ann.* 2012;41:1-6

23. Collins MW, Iverson GL, Lovell MR, McKeag DB, Norwig J, Maroon J. On-field predictors of neuropsychological and symptom deficit following sports-related concussion. *Clin J Sport Med.* 2003;13:222-229

24. Grady MF. Concussion in the adolescent athlete. *Curr Probl Pediatr Adolesc Health Care.* 2010;40:154-169

25. Eisenberg MA, Andrea J, Meehan W, Mannix R. Time interval between concussions and symptom duration. *Pediatrics.* 2013;132:8-17

26. Bailes JE, Hudson V. Classification of sport-related head trauma: a spectrum of mild to severe injury. *J Athl Train.* 2001;36:236-243

27. Topolovec-Vranic J, Pollmann-Mudryj MA, Ouchterlony D, et al. The value of serum biomarkers in prediction models of outcome after mild traumatic brain injury. *J Trauma Injury Infect Crit Care.* 2011;71(5 Suppl 1):S478-S486

28. Kristman VL, Tator CH, Kreiger N, et al. Does the apolipoprotein ε4 allele predispose varsity athletes to concussion? A prospective cohort study. *Clin J Sport Med.* 2008;18:322-328

29. Tierney RT, Mansell JL, Higgins M, et al. Apolipoprotein. E genotype and concussion in college athletes. *Clin J Sport Med.* 2010;20:464-468

30. Mannix R, Eisenberg M, Berry M, Meehan WP, Hayes RL. Serum biomarkers predict acute symptom burden in children after concussion: a preliminary study. *J Neurotrauma.* 2014;31:1072-1075

31. Strathmann FG, Schulte S, Goerl K, Petron DJ. Blood-based biomarkers for traumatic brain injury: evaluation of research approaches, available methods and potential utility from the clinician and clinical laboratory perspectives. *Clin Biochem.* 2014;47:876-888

32. Neher MD, Keene CN, Rich MC, Moore HB, Stahel PF. Serum biomarkers for traumatic brain injury. *South Med J.* 2014;107:248-255

33. McCrea M, Guskiewicz K, Randolph C, et al. Incidence, clinical course, and predictors of prolonged recovery time following sport-related concussion in high school and college athletes. *J Int Neuropsychol Soc.* 2013;19:22-33

34. Master CL, Gioia GA, Leddy JJ, Grady MF. Importance of "return-to-learn" in pediatric and adolescent concussion. *Pediatr Ann.* 2012;41:1-6

35. Berz K, Divine J, Foss KB, Heyl R, Ford KR, Myer GD. Sex-specific differences in the severity of symptoms and recovery rate following sports-related concussion in young athletes. *Phys Sportsmed.* 2013;41:58-63

36. Preiss-Farzanegan SJ, Chapman B, Wong TM, Wu J, Bazarian JJ. The relationship between gender and postconcussion symptoms after sport-related mild traumatic brain injury. *PM R.* 2009;1:245-253

37. Raukar N, Zonfrillo MR, Kane K, et al. 2014 Academic Emergency Medicine Consensus Conference on "Gender-Specific Research in Emergency Care: Investigate, Understand and Translate How Gender Affects Patient Outcomes." *Acad Emerg Med.* 2014;21:1370-1379

38. Vidal PG, Goodman AM, Colin A, Leddy JJ, Grady MF. Rehabilitation strategies for prolonged recovery in pediatric and adolescent concussion. *Pediatr Ann.* 2012;41:1-7

39. Makdissi M, Cantu RC, Johnston KM, McCrory P, Meeuwisse WH. The difficult concussion patient: what is the best approach to investigation and management of persistent (>10 days) post-concussive symptoms? *Br J Sports Med.* 2013;47:308-313

40. Leddy JJ, Kozlowski K, Donnelly JP, Pendergast DR, Epstein LH, Willer B. A preliminary study of subsymptom threshold exercise training for refractory post-concussion syndrome. *Clin J Sport Med.* 2010;20:21-27

41. Ciuffreda KJ, Kapoor N, Rutner D, Suchoff IB, Han ME, Craig S. Occurrence of oculomotor dysfunctions in acquired brain injury: a retrospective analysis. *Optometry.* 2007;78:155-161

42. Mucha A, Collins MW, Elbin R, et al. A brief vestibular/ocular motor screening (VOMS) assessment to evaluate concussions: preliminary findings. *Am J Sports Med.* 2014;42:2479-2486

43. Thiagarajan P, Ciuffreda KJ. Versional eye tracking in mild traumatic brain injury (mTBI): effects of oculomotor training (OMT). *Brain Inj.* 2014;28:930-943

44. Alsalaheen BA, Mucha A, Morris LO, et al. Vestibular rehabilitation for dizziness and balance disorders after concussion. *J Neurol Phys Ther.* 2010;34:87-93

45. Meehan WP. Medical therapies for concussion. *Clin Sports Med.* 2011;30:115-124

46. Reddy CC, Collins M, Lovell M, Kontos AP. Efficacy of amantadine treatment on symptoms and neurocognitive performance among adolescents following sports-related concussion. *J Head Trauma Rehabil.* 2013;28:260-265

47. Patel DR, Reddy V. Update on sport-related concussion. *Adolesc Med.* 2013;24:206-224, xiii-xiv

48. Meehan WP 3rd, Zhang J, Mannix R, Whalen MJ. Increasing recovery time between injuries improves cognitive outcome after repetitive mild concussive brain injuries in mice. *Neurosurgery.* 2012;71:885-891

49. Cantu RC. When to disqualify an athlete after a concussion. *Curr Sports Med Rep.* 2009;8:6-7

50. King NS, Kirwilliam S. Permanent post-concussion symptoms after mild head injury. *Brain Inj.* 2011;25:462-470

51. Alexander MP. Mild traumatic brain injury: pathophysiology, natural history, and clinical management. *Neurology.* 1995;45:1253-1260

52. King N. Permanent post concussion symptoms after mild head injury: a systematic review of age and gender factors. *NeuroRehabilitation.* 2014;34:741-748

53. McCrory P, Davis G, Makdissi M. Second impact syndrome or cerebral swelling after sporting head injury. *Curr Sports Med Rep.* 2012;11:21-23

54. McKee AC, Stein TD, Nowinski CJ, et al. The spectrum of disease in chronic traumatic encephalopathy. *Brain.* 2013;136:43-64

55. Baugh CM, Stamm JM, Riley DO, et al. Chronic traumatic encephalopathy: neurodegeneration following repetitive concussive and subconcussive brain trauma. *Brain Imaging Behav.* 2012;6:244-254

56. Small GW, Kepe V, Siddarth P, et al. PET scanning of brain tau in retired national football league players: preliminary findings. *Am J Geriatr Psychiatry.* 2013;21:138-144

57. Babikian T, Asarnow R. Neurocognitive outcomes and recovery after pediatric TBI: meta-analytic review of the literature. *Neuropsychology.* 2009;23:283-296

58. Rivara FP, Koepsell TD, Wang J, et al. Disability 3, 12, and 24 months after traumatic brain injury among children and adolescents. *Pediatrics.* 2011;128:e1129-e1138

59. Shaklai S, Peretz R, Spasser R, Simantov M, Groswasser Z. Long-term functional outcome after moderate-to-severe paediatric traumatic brain injury. *Brain Inj.* 2014;28:915-921

60. Collins CL, Fletcher EN, Fields SK, et al. Neck strength: a protective factor reducing risk for concussion in high school sports. *J Prim Prev.* 2014;35:309-319

61. Centers for Disease Control and Prevention. Heads Up: Concussion. Available at: www.cdc.gov/concussion/HeadsUp. Accessed August 13, 2014

62. The Children's Hospital of Philadelphia. Concussion Care for Kids: Minds Matter. Available at: www.chop.edu/concussion. Accessed August 13, 2014

63. Navarro RR. Protective equipment and the prevention of concussion-what is the evidence? *Curr Sports Med Rep.* 2011;10:27-31

64. Register-Mihalik JK, Guskiewicz KM, McLeod TCV, Linnan LA, Mueller FO, Marshall SW. Knowledge, attitude, and concussion-reporting behaviors among high school athletes: a preliminary study. *J Athl Train.* 2013;48:645-653

65. Institute of Medicine. Report: Sports-related concussions in youth: improving the science, changing the culture. October 30, 2013. Available at: iom.nationalacademies.org/Reports/2013/Sports-Related-Concussions-in-Youth-Improving-the-Science-Changing-the-Culture.aspx?_ga=1.155625147.1624105766.1445371314. Accessed October 20, 2015
66. Register-Mihalik JK, Linnan LA, Marshall SW, McLeod TCV, Mueller FO, Guskiewicz KM. Using theory to understand high school aged athletes' intentions to report sport-related concussion: implications for concussion education initiatives. *Brain Inj.* 2013;27:878-886
67. Gennarelli TA. Future directions in brain injury research. *Prog Neurol Surg.* 2014;28:243-250
68. Zetterberg H, Smith DH, Blennow K. Biomarkers of mild traumatic brain injury in cerebrospinal fluid and blood. *Nat Rev Neurol.* 2013;9:201-210
69. Wilde EA, McCauley SR, Hunter JV, et al. Diffusion tensor imaging of acute mild traumatic brain injury in adolescents. *Neurology.* 2008;70:948-955
70. Gardner A, Iverson GL, Stanwell P. A systematic review of proton magnetic resonance spectroscopy findings in sport-related concussion. *J Neurotrauma.* 2014;31:1-18

Adolesc Med 026 (2015) 507–527

Sports-Related Sudden Cardiac Injury or Death

Elizabeth Anne Greene, MD, FAAP[a]*;
Ann Punnoose, MD[b]

[a]Professor of Pediatrics, University of New Mexico, Pediatric Cardiology Division, Director, Pediatric Electrophysiology and Exercise Testing, Albuquerque, New Mexico; [b]Fellow, Pediatric Heart Failure and Heart Transplantation, Lurie Children's Hospital of Chicago, Chicago, IL

INTRODUCTION

The exact incidence of sudden cardiac death (SCD) in adolescents (ie, children between the ages of 10 and 19 years) during participation in sports is difficult to gauge because of differences across studies in how these deaths are recorded and the definitions of the populations that are investigated.[1] Studies have shown that although there are several non-cardiovascular etiologies for these deaths, a significant proportion of the deaths in this age group can be attributed to cardiac diseases, such as hypertrophic cardiomyopathy (HCM), coronary abnormalities, arrhythmogenic ventricular cardiomyopathy/dysplasia, and ion channelopathies, which result in arrhythmias.[2,3]

A defining feature of SCD is its unexpected nature. In most cases, adolescents who died during sports participation had not been previously diagnosed with cardiac disease.[4] Indeed, SCD can often be a presenting symptom of several genetically inherited cardiac diseases.[5] Studies have suggested that either screening targeted at individuals with a positive family history or symptoms or large-scale screenings could help prevent SCDs. Improved access to defibrillators at sports events and training in cardiopulmonary resuscitation could contribute to improved survival from commotio cordis events.[6]

In addition to the screening that takes place before participation in sports, visits by adolescents to general practitioners for unexplained chest pain, syncope, or

---

*Corresponding author
E-mail address: EGreene@salud.unm.edu

palpitations during physical exertion who have a family history of unexpected death of a family member provide prime opportunities to diagnose patients with cardiac diseases and increased risk of SCD.

Greater awareness of these symptoms by families and general practitioners has led to increased referrals for cardiac evaluation. Concomitantly, recent advances in cardiac diagnostic testing have led to increased diagnosis of cardiac disease that can result in SCD. Improved cardiac diagnostic testing has also facilitated the diagnosis of variants in cardiac anatomy with unknown significance to participation in sports and other activities. In addition to pre-sports participation screening, activity restriction has been a topic fraught with debate and controversy. The 36th Bethesda Conference, a consensus statement based on an expert panel of pediatric and adult cardiologists, attempted to thoughtfully describe the types of activity in which children and adolescents with particular cardiovascular disease could participate, as well as the diseases that necessitated absolutely no participation in competitive sports.[7]

These developments led to changes in the anticipatory guidance provided to these adolescents and their families, as well as the overall management of adolescents with cardiac disease that places them at increased risk for SCD.

SPORTS-RELATED CARDIAC INJURY

Commotio Cordis

Commotio cordis occurs when a child is struck in the chest with a rapidly moving object such as a hard baseball or hockey puck. If the missile strikes the child's chest at just the right moment, during a vulnerable period of the cardiac cycle, an R-on-T phenomenon occurs which can cause ventricular tachycardia or fibrillation. The shape of the missile is crucial to the precision and force of the sudden impact, which is capable of causing an electrical event.[8]

Data show that if the object is less hard or is moving slowly, this phenomenon is much less likely to occur. Safety baseballs with extra padding have been shown to be less likely to cause ventricular arrhythmias, whereas chest protectors have not.[9] The most common age for the occurrence of this phenomenon is 12 years or middle school age.[10] Line drives to third base are a common source of this injury seen in clinical practice because many players are still acquiring fielding skills. If ventricular fibrillation occurs as a result of commotio cordis, the most important thing is to recognize it and provide curative defibrillation and cardiopulmonary resuscitation. In the past, survival has been estimated to be as low as 10%.[10] Programs that provide automatic external defibrillators (AEDs) to schools are important, but these devices must be available on the playing fields, which are often far from the school buildings in which the AEDs are stored. Even lay rescuers using AEDs have been shown to be effective in this setting.[11,12] Public access defibrillation has been a major force in improving the availability of AEDs.[13] Given that the overall incidence of sudden cardiac arrest in high school students was most recently estimated to be 0.63 per 100,000, immediate treatment, regardless of the cause of the injury, is important.[14]

Hypertrophic Cardiomyopathy

In an analysis of 158 sudden deaths in athletes between the ages of 12 and 40 years from 1985 to 1995, Maron et al[15] found that HCM was the most common cause of SCD (36%). Hypertrophic cardiomyopathy can occur as the result of any one of 1400 mutations in several different genes involved in encoding the proteins of the contractile filaments in myocytes. The inheritance pattern is most commonly autosomal dominant. However, HCM can also occur by spontaneous mutations, which are then heritable.[16]

The presentation of HCM on physical examination depends on the degree of left ventricular outflow tract obstruction caused by left ventricular hypertrophy. Patients with little or no obstruction may not have a murmur. In the presence of obstruction with a subaortic gradient, a systolic ejection murmur whose intensity increases with a worsening gradient may be heard.[17,18]

After the family history is obtained and the physical examination performed, the evaluation for HCM begins with the electrocardiogram (ECG), which may show non-specific abnormalities. Increased voltages are indicative of left ventricular hypertrophy and ST-T wave changes. The echocardiogram, which often is obtained concurrently, can be diagnostic by showing asymmetric left ventricular wall thickening without dilation (Figure 1). If the echocardiogram is suggestive of HCM, the next step is genetic testing in order to identify the specific gene mutation, which will allow for targeted testing of other family members. The most recent research has suggested that mutations in any of the 8 genes involved in encoding components of the sarcomere result in HCM.[19,20]

Children with HCM can have a benign course. However, as they reach puberty, they can develop progressive left ventricular hypertrophy that results in mitral valve regurgitation, myocardial ischemia, and impaired ventricular relaxation. As their cardiac function worsens, they are then at risk for life-threatening arrhythmias that can be initiated by physical exertion, resulting in death.[15,16] Determining a patient's risk for SCD is part of the management of HCM. The treatment strategy is based on the patient's history of previous cardiac arrest or sustained ventricular tachycardia and a family history of SCD in a relative with HCM, syncope, or severe left ventricular hypertrophy. In patients in the highest-risk category, placement of implantable cardioverter-defibrillators (ICD) is strongly considered to prevent SCD.[3]

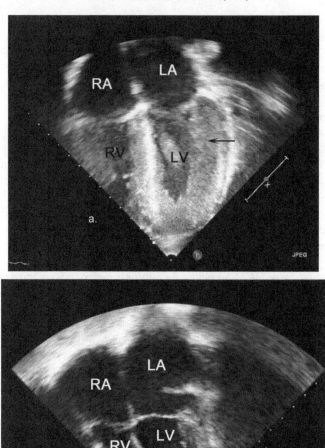

Fig 1. A: Echocardiographic 4-chamber view from a patient with hypertrophic cardiomyopathy. The arrow points to the hypertrophied left ventricular free wall. B: Echocardiographic 4-chamber view from a patient with a normal heart. LA, left atrium; LV, left ventricle; RA, right atrium; RV, right ventricle.

In adolescents who develop symptoms, beta-blocker therapy can be started to control their heart rate and allow for appropriate filling and cardiac output. Other drug classes, such as diuretics and calcium channel blockers, can also be used to control HCM symptoms. Heart transplantation can be considered in patients with heart failure refractory to medical therapy. In patients with significant or worsening left ventricular tract obstruction, surgical septal myectomy or alcohol septal ablation can be performed.

Restricting or allowing patients to participate in activities is an area of great debate. Adolescents with proven HCM can participate in informal, low-intensity aerobic activities, but they should be counseled to avoid competitive, strenuous activities or even low-intensity activities for long durations. It is important to emphasize to adolescents the distinction between competitive and recreational activities.[21]

Coronary Abnormalities

Adolescents with coronary abnormalities are often asymptomatic. However, they can present with chest pain or syncope during exertion, and, as with HCM, SCD during physical exertion can often be the first indication of disease. Adolescents can also present with ventricular arrhythmia.[22]

Coronary artery anomalies that are significant in infants may be associated with other structural heart disease such as Tetralogy of Fallot and Transposition of the Great Arteries. In infants with otherwise normal hearts, coronary abnormalities such as an anomalous left coronary artery from the pulmonary artery can result in irritability and failure to thrive secondary to ischemia, and left ventricular injury. This condition is usually diagnosed during infancy. In contrast, several other coronary abnormalities do not lead to symptoms in young infants. They may be diagnosed incidentally in infancy or early childhood, or with symptoms in later childhood or adolescence. Each of these coronary anomalies has a different risk for SCD.

In the normal ("usual") pattern of coronary arteries, the left main coronary artery arises from the left aortic sinus of Valsalva and, after a short distance, branches into the left circumflex artery, which travels posteriorly in the atrioventricular groove, and the left anterior descending artery, which travels anteriorly to the apex of the heart. The right coronary artery arises from the right aortic sinus of Valsalva and commonly gives rise to the posterior descending artery (Figure 2).[23]

Coronary artery anomalies can follow several patterns. In the most common pattern, the left circumflex coronary artery arises from the right main coronary artery and travels behind the aorta before returning to its normal path. This anomaly does not usually lead to any symptoms. More rarely, the left main coronary artery arises from the right sinus of Valsalva and the path it takes thereafter determines the risk for SCD. If the left main coronary artery travels behind the aorta, over the right ventricular outflow tract, or courses through the ventricular septum, there is no particular association with SCD.[23] However, if after arising from the right sinus of Valsalva, the left main coronary artery travels between the aorta and the pulmonary artery, patients can develop chest pain, syncope, or even SCD with exertion. The angle that the left main coronary artery makes with the coronary ostia, and its position between the great arteries, can lead to a sud-

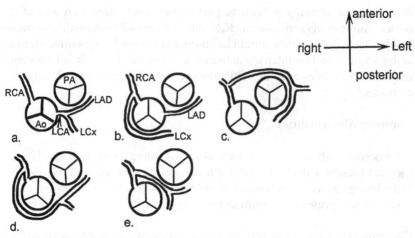

Fig 2. Normal pattern of origin of the coronary arteries as well as pathologic and non-pathologic variants. A: "Usual" pattern. The left coronary artery (LCA) originates from the left coronary sinus and branches into the left anterior descending (LAD) and left circumflex artery (LCx). The right coronary artery (RCA) originates from the right coronary sinus. B: Anomalous circumflex. The LCx originates from the RCA and then travels posterior to the aorta to resume its usual course. C: Anomalous anterior LCA. The LCA originates from the RCA and travels anterior to the pulmonary artery to branch and resume the usual course. D: Anomalous posterior LCA. The LCA originates from the RCA and travels posterior to the aorta to branch into the LCx and the LAD. E: Anomalous interarterial LCA. Pathologic variant that can cause sudden cardiac death. The LCA originates from the RCA and travels between the aorta and the pulmonary arteries before branching. Ao, aortic valve; PA, pulmonary artery.

den decrease in blood flow during exertion and, in turn, myocardial ischemia, which can result in SCD.[24]

Therefore, when patients present with chest pain, syncope, or aborted SCD during exertion, the differential diagnosis should include anomalous origins and the course of the coronary arteries (Table 1). The evaluation starts with an ECG, which will likely be normal but can show evidence of new or previous myocardial injuries with elevated ST segments (Figure 3). The next step in diagnosis is a transthoracic echocardiogram to evaluate coronary artery anatomy, assess for ventricular dysfunction, and eliminate other causes of syncope and chest pain during exertion, such as hypertrophic obstructive cardiomyopathy.[23,24] In patients younger than 50 years, coronary magnetic resonance angiography and computed tomographic angiography are recommended in order to delineate the origin and course of the coronary arteries.[25]

In symptomatic patients, surgical correction is the definitive treatment of left and right coronary arteries that originate from the contralateral sinus and travel between the great arteries. Until the anomalous artery can be reimplanted, patients are usually placed on exercise restrictions. In patients with anomalous

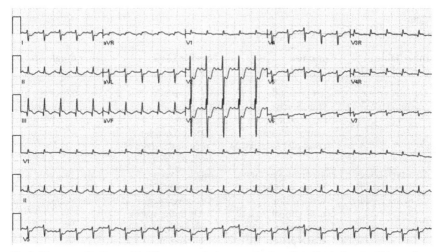

Fig 3. Electrocardiogram with ST-segment changes suggestive of cardiac ischemia. This can be a common pattern in patients with abnormal coronary arteries who had cardiac arrest or aborted sudden death.

right coronary arteries but no symptoms, the management is not obvious, and surgical correction is not always recommended.[22, 25]

Arrhythmogenic Ventricular Cardiomyopathy

With a worldwide prevalence of 1 in 2000, arrhythmogenic ventricular cardio-myopathy (AVC) is a rare disease but is a well-recognized cause of SCD in young adults.[3] Although there are several causative mutations, the most common inheritance pattern for AVC is autosomal dominant.[26]

Recent studies have suggested the "defective desmosome hypothesis," in which disruptions of connections between cardiac myocytes interfere with the proper function of sodium channels. This, in turn, increases the probability of develop-ing ventricular arrhythmias such as ventricular tachycardia and fibrillation, which can result in SCD. The fibro-fatty infiltrates that replace the myocardium and are pathognomonic for AVC are thought to be evidence of inflammation or follow the disruption of the gap junctions and other connections between myo-cytes. In the classic form of AVCC, the myocardium of the right ventricular inflow, outflow tract, and apex is replaced with fibro-fatty infiltrates. In the less common forms of AVC, both ventricles or the left ventricle alone can be affected.[26,27]

Patients with the classic form of AVC—arrhythmogenic right ventricular car-diomyopathy/dysplasia (ARVC/D)—usually present after the age of 10 years. They can present with syncope, dizziness, or palpitations as a result of ventricu-

Table 1
Cardiac diseases with risk for sudden death

Inheritable or congenital lesion	Common symptoms/signs	Possible ECG findings	Other diagnostic tests
Coronary artery anomalies	Chest pain or dizziness with exercise Physical examination consistent with congestive heart failure	May be normal ST depressions or elevations and Q waves may be present as a result of ischemia or infarcts	Echocardiography to show CAA origins
Arrhythmogenic right ventricular cardiomyopathy	Palpitations, shortness of breath, palpitations with exercise Usually normal physical examination if no ectopy present	Epsilon waves on baseline ECG PVCs or ventricular tachycardia may be monomorphic or polymorphic	Cardiac magnetic resonance imaging to show ARVC
Wolff-Parkinson-White syndrome	Palpitations with or without exercise Usually normal physical examination	Delta waves SVT	Stress test, Holter monitoring to evaluate for intermittent preexcitation, electrophysiology study and ablation
Catecholamine-sensitive polymorphic ventricular tachycardia	Palpitations with exercise Usually normal physical examination	May be normal at rest or show polymorphic PVCs	Polymorphic VT on stress test or on Holter monitoring during activity
Hypertrophic cardiomyopathy	Chest pain, shortness of breath, with exercise Outflow tract murmurs	LVH with or without strain pattern Possible PVCs	Echocardiogram shows hypertrophy, outflow tract obstruction
Long QT syndrome	Palpitations or dizziness with exertion/emotion	Prolonged QTc, usually >460 ms in adolescent females or 450 ms in males May see abnormal T-wave morphology	QTc prolongation on stress test Ventricular ectopy on Holter monitoring

ARVC, arrhythmogenic right ventricular cardiomyopathy; CAA, coronary artery anomalies; ECG, electrocardiogram; LVH, left ventricular hypertrophy; PVCs, premature ventricular contractions; SVT, supraventricular tachycardia; VT, ventricular tachycardia.

lar tachyarrhythmias. Unfortunately, as in patients with HCM or coronary abnormalities, SCD can be a presenting symptom.[26]

As with any patients who present to the primary care physician's office with symptoms during exertion, the evaluation for ARVC/D begins with obtaining exhaustive family and personal histories and details about any symptoms that may have been overlooked previously. The diagnosis of ARVC/D can be difficult to make. In 2010, the diagnostic criteria for ARVC were modified from the initial criteria specified in 1994 in order to improve the diagnosis of early ARVC/D and its variants. The criteria detail the findings on ECG, biopsy, echocardiography, and cardiac magnetic resonance imaging that are diagnostic of ARVC/D.[28]

The 12-lead ECG may be suggestive of ARVC/D, showing a prolonged QRS interval, the presence of an epsilon wave (a wave between the QRS complex and the T wave), and an inverted T wave in the right precordial leads. There can also be a left bundle branch block or premature ventricular contractions with an inferior axis.[29] However, these findings are not always present, and if the suspicion for ARVC/D remains, the patients should be referred for an echocardiogram, which may show right atrial and ventricular dilation compared to normal standards for age.[30] If the findings are still equivocal, cardiac magnetic resonance imaging is the next step (Table 1).

As in patients with HCM, adolescents with ARVC/D with the greatest risk for SCD have a previous history of aborted SCD, a family history of SCD, ventricular arrhythmias, and right heart failure. Adolescents with clinical disease are advised to avoid strenuous and competitive sports.[7] Medical management with antiarrhythmic drugs is part of the treatment plan, but ICDs have also been used in patients with previous cardiac arrest or hemodynamically significant ventricular arrhythmias refractory to medical therapies.[27]

Wolff-Parkinson-White Syndrome

To be diagnosed with Wolff-Parkinson-White (WPW) syndrome, a patient would have the ECG pattern of WPW and would have experienced supraventricular tachycardia (SVT) (Table 1). Many patients are discovered to have the ECG pattern for WPW before they are symptomatic. The risk of sudden death in a patient who is asymptomatic is 0.1% per year. If SVT has already occurred, then the risk of sudden death increases to 0.2% per year. The prevalence of WPW syndrome is 1 to 4.5 per 1000 children and adults.[31] In a long-term registry, WPW syndrome accounted for 1% of all sudden deaths in young athletes.[32] The ECG in patients with WPW syndrome shows a distinctive pattern of preexcitation. The QRS is wide and the PR interval is short, at least in some of the leads (Figure 4). These 2 phenomena are caused by premature arrival of the electrical signal from the sinus node to a portion of either the left or right ventricle. This causes early depolarization of a small area of ventricular myocardium while the AV node is conducting the rest of the electrical signal to the His-Purkinje system. In sinus rhythm, this activity just causes an abnormal ECG appearance. In WPW syndrome, because of the 2 connections between the atria and ventricles, there is potential for a reentrant circuit and therefore SVT. This is the cause of symptoms and often requires either medication in infants and young children or ablation in older children and adolescents. The cause of sudden death in patients with WPW syndrome in not SVT, however. Sudden death in WPW syndrome occurs through a combination of circumstances. A child has an accessory path-

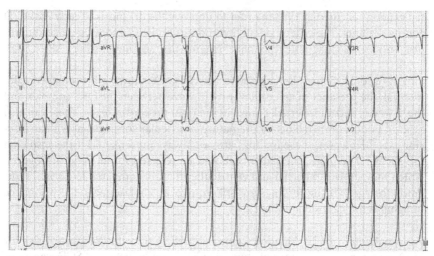

Fig 4. Wolff-Parkinson-White syndrome. Short PR and preexcitation (delta waves).

way that is capable of very rapid conduction and has developed atrial fibrillation. If the pathway is capable of conducting atrial fibrillation, then ventricular fibrillation may occur, which is the mechanism for sudden death in WPW. This may occur in the setting of high catecholamines, as occurs with exercise, or after a child has been in SVT for many hours. Adolescents who have been drinking alcohol may develop atrial fibrillation, called "holiday heart," and if they also have WPW and a rapidly conducting pathway, then they may experience syncope and sudden death. Holter monitoring for arrhythmia screening in children with asymptomatic WPW showed the incidence of atrial fibrillation was 12%.[33] An athlete who has experienced syncope and is found to have the WPW pattern on ECG would ideally be admitted to the hospital and examined by an electrophysiologist so that the accessory pathway can be ablated before another event can occur. A management algorithm for symptomatic patients provided in an expert consensus statement from PACES/HRS includes initial non-invasive investigations to ascertain the presence of intermittent preexcitation on Holter monitoring or loss of preexcitation on stress testing before more invasive electrophysiologic studies and ablation are recommended.[34]

Catecholamine-Sensitive Polymorphic Ventricular Tachycardia

The prevalence of catecholamine-sensitive polymorphic ventricular tachycardia (CPVT) is estimated to be 1 in 10,000. It is a rare cause of sudden death in athletes. The most common presentation is syncope with stress or exercise at age 7 to 9 years.[35] The genetic defect involves errors in intracellular calcium handling regulated by the ryanodine receptor gene *hRyR2* or the calsequestrin gene *CASQ2*.[36] Abnormal release of calcium into the sarcoplasm triggers arrhythmias when catecholamines are present.[37,38] Exercise and emotional stress increase catecholamines and therefore can be triggers for SCD in these patients (Table 1).

The baseline ECG is usually normal, although premature ventricular contractions may be seen (Figures 5 and 6). Important questions to ask patients include the presence of symptoms of syncope or dizziness with exercise, and any family history of sudden death or syncope with exercise or stress. Particularly in patients with exercise-induced symptoms such as syncope, echocardiography is

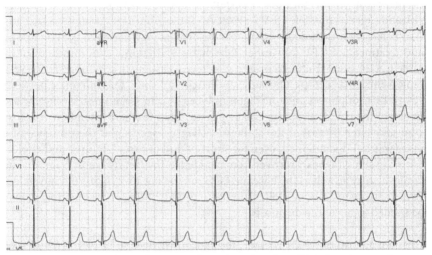

Fig 5. Catecholamine polymorphic ventricular tachycardia. Normal baseline electrocardiogram.

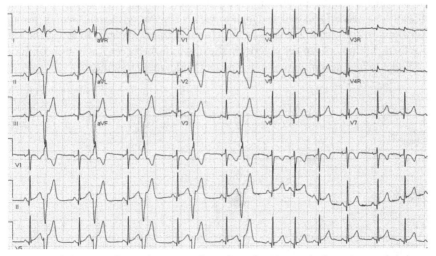

Fig 6. Catecholamine polymorphic ventricular tachycardia. Ventricular bigeminy on electrocardiogram.

needed to rule out structural disease, including HCM and coronary anomalies (see section on coronary abnormalities). If those entities are ruled out, the differential diagnosis then includes inheritable arrhythmias such as CPVT and long QT syndrome (LQTS). Exercise testing is very useful in this setting. Ventricular ectopy that occurs at rest, is unifocal, is not sustained, and has an inferior axis and left bundle branch block pattern consistent with ectopy from the right ventricular outflow tract that suppresses with exercise is much more likely to be benign or not life-threatening. This type of ventricular ectopy may require treatment but is not expected to degenerate into ventricular fibrillation. Ventricular ectopy that is multifocal, sustained, and worsens with exercise is higher risk and suggests possible CPVT or ARVC. If the echocardiogram is normal and ARVC has been excluded by magnetic resonance imaging, then genetic testing and treatment of CPVT or other inheritable arrhythmia syndromes are warranted. A 24-hour Holter recording may reveal sustained, polymorphic, or very rapid ventricular ectopy, and an exercise test can show the difference between ectopy that suppresses and one that is induced by catecholamines. It is important to obtain the details about syncopal episodes from teachers, friends, or coaches who may have witnessed the student's collapse, especially if the presence of a pulse was not documented, even for short period of time. Children and adolescents can spontaneously recover from near lethal rhythms (Figures 7 and 8). The family history as well as the baseline ECG may be negative in this disease state.[39] Exercise testing, 24-hour Holter monitoring, and 30-day event monitoring may be needed to make the diagnosis.

Once a diagnosis of CPVT is made, the patient will need to be placed on exercise restriction. These patients will require ongoing high-dose beta-blocker medication. The addition of verapamil or flecainide has been shown to be an effective adjunct in some patients.[40] If the adolescent has experienced a sudden cardiac arrest, then an ICD will be needed and stellate ganglionectomy considered as well. Genetic testing is helpful to confirm the diagnosis and eventually allow patients to assess the risk for their children. Given the severity of the mutation, however, it is not uncommon to find it to be a new mutation in the patient undergoing treatment.

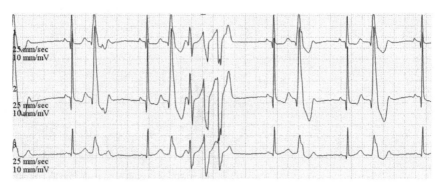

Fig 7. Catecholamine polymorphic ventricular tachycardia with exercise.

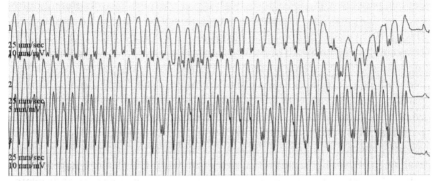

Fig 8. Very fast ventricular tachycardia on Holter monitoring.

Prolonged QT syndrome

Prolonged QT syndrome is another inheritable arrhythmia syndrome. It is estimated that 1 in 2000 people carries a gene for one of the LQTSs.[41] Mutations causing LQTS affect cardiac ion channels and therefore are referred to as channelopathies.

Only 1 copy of an abnormal gene is required to inherit the disease; therefore, every child of an affected individual has a 50% chance of having the disease. It is possible to inherit 2 abnormal genes and thereby have a more severe phenotype.

Currently 13 types of LQTSs have been identified, with types 1, 2, and 3 accounting for most cases.[42,43] Type 1 is classically associated with diving into cold water causing a vagal response as part of the diving reflex. The ECG shows large broad-based T waves.[44] The defect is in the *KCNQ1* gene, and the potassium current I_{Ks} is decreased. A high catecholamine state, as occurs with exercise, is also a common trigger for events in LQTS type 1. Patients with this type of LQTS show QTc prolongation with exercise (Table 1).[45] The more severe form of LQTS type 1 is also associated with congenital deafness (Jervell and Lange-Nielsen syndrome). Type 2 is classically associated with events that occur in bradycardic states, for example, sleep with a sudden rush of catecholamines that accompanies a loud noise (alarm clock, tornado siren). The ECG shows flattened T waves and QT intervals that are difficult to measure. LQTS type 2 is caused by the *HERG* mutation, and the potassium current I_{Kr} is decreased. Type 3 is associated with events that occur in bradycardic states but with no trigger needed for events to occur. The ECG typically shows a flattened ST segment that is prolonged with a large T wave. The mutation is in the *SCN5A* gene and affects the sodium current I_{Na}, causing a gain of function. Pause-dependent ventricular arrhythmias may occur during the patient's sleep. Torsades de pointes is a type of polymorphic ventricular tachycardia seen classically during cardiac arrest in patients with LQTS.[46]

Among patients with LQTS, those with type 1 are most likely to present during exercise or sports. The presenting symptom may be syncope or cardiac arrest (Figure 9). Syncope or loss of consciousness is a common symptom in adolescents and may be the result of dehydration, a vasovagal episode, pregnancy, drug ingestions, or other scenarios such as seizures. The symptom should raise concern until it is explained, especially when the patient is being cleared for sports participation. Patients with LQTS type 2 may experience events when they are emotionally stressed that may be mistaken for vasovagal episodes. A detailed personal history of the student is very important. Any episode of near drowning, seizures, or changes in mental status in the student's past history requires further evaluation. A family history of seizures, sudden infant death syndrome, congenital deafness, syncope (especially with exercise), drowning or near drowning, 1-car accidents, or early death before age 40 are all warning signs that should prompt further investigation for LQTS and increase concern for any athlete who has experienced syncope.

The ECG is the first test used to investigate for LQTS and should be considered in the workup of patients with syncope but no obvious benign explanation. The ECG may be normal in patients with 1 of the LQTS mutations and may vary at different examinations. After puberty the upper limit of normal for the corrected QT interval (QTc) is slightly higher for females, and in both males and females may be slightly greater than 440 ms (which is the usual upper limit of normal). Values can be slightly prolonged after autonomic discharges (eg, syncope, seizures), making the interpretation of the ECG challenging and requiring consideration of the overall clinical picture. If any question remains, then repeat evaluation with more thorough family and personal histories is needed.[47]

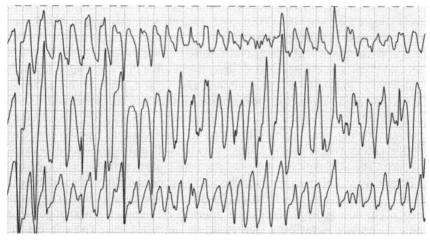

Fig 9. Torsades de pointes in a patient with long QT syndrome.

In terms of risk stratification, a young patient will be at highest risk for a cardiac event if the QTc is greater than 500 ms. This is the case for all patients with LQTS types 1 and 2 and for boys with type 3 (which may not be known unless they already have a positive family history). The lowest risk is seen in patients with QTc less than 500 ms who are type 1 and for boys who have type 2.[48]

Beta-blockade is 95% effective in preventing cardiac events in asymptomatic patients with LQTS type 1. Exercise restriction is advised, especially for students at the high school varsity level, as is avoidance of mediations known to prolong QTc.[49] In patients with LQTS who have experienced syncope (especially if they already are being treated with a beta-blocker) or are found to have significant ventricular arrhythmia on Holter or exercise testing, an ICD or stellate ganglionectomy should be considered. Evaluation is recommended for all first-degree relatives of a patient diagnosed with LQTS (Figures 10, 11, 12, and 13).

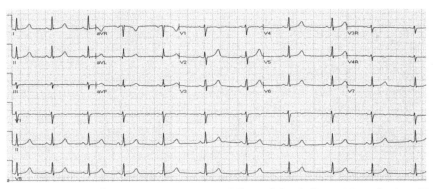

Fig 10. Long QT syndrome, type 1, gene positive. QTc is only borderline at 448 ms, but large T waves are present.

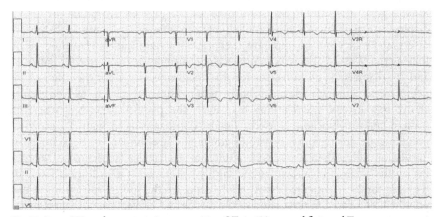

Fig 11. Long QT syndrome, type 2, gene positive. QTc is 498 ms, and flattened T waves are present.

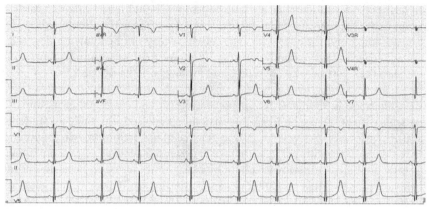

Fig 12. Long QT syndrome, type 3, gene positive. QTc is 485 ms, and flat ST segments are seen.

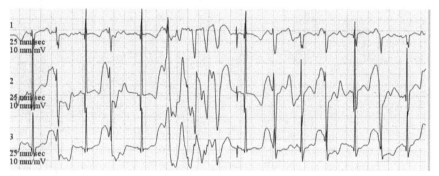

Fig 13. Polymorphic ventricular tachycardia with T-wave alternans in long QT syndrome.

Brugada syndrome is a channelopathy similar to LQTS type 3, but with a loss of function rather than a gain in function in I_{NA} as a result of a mutation in the *SCN5A* gene. The ECG in this syndrome is quite different from that for LQTS, displaying a right bundle branch block pattern in leads V_1-V_3 and ST elevation. This pattern may not be apparent except after a significant arrhythmic event. Raising the V_1 and V_2 leads an interspace may also reveal the pattern (Figures 14 and 15). Exercise is not a trigger for this syndrome as it is for the other channelopathies, although elevated body temperature is related to ventricular arrhythmia events. Medications may elicit the pattern, and challenge with sodium channel blockers is used to make the diagnosis in many cases. Most events occur during sleep in young adults and are thought to be ventricular fibrillation rather than torsades de pointes or ventricular tachycardia. Depending on the other clinical factors and family history, an ICD will most likely be required for these patients in early adolescence, so the sports restrictions at that point will be related to protection of the device and prevention of inappropriate shocks.[50]

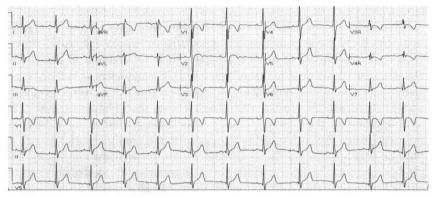

Fig 14. Brugada syndrome. Normal electrocardiogram with usual lead positions for leads V_1 and V_2.

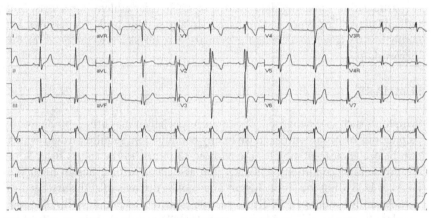

Fig 15. Brugada syndrome unmasked with high V_1 and V_2 leads.

Screening

Prevention of sudden death in young athletes is a universal goal. Several approaches have been taken to accomplish this in the United States and Europe. In Italy, all student athletes are screened, including ECG recordings in middle and high schools. This protocol has been very effective in almost eliminating death from HCM in young athletes[51] and has been recommended by the European Society of Cardiology. Specific parameters for abnormal ECGs were suggested so that a universal standard for all European countries could be adopted.[52] Other investigators have found significant interobserver variability in ECG readings.[53] In the United States, Chandra et al[54] found that 20% of athletes have type 2 (less severe) abnormalities on ECG that would require further evaluation before the athletes were cleared for sports participation. When a computerized ECG reading was added to the preparticipation examination for Stanford athletes, a high percentage of abnormalities was recorded, suggesting false-positive results or minor abnormalities.[55] Hill et al[56] found poor agreement on ECG readings between pediatric cardiologists and pediatric electrophysiologists. Kaltman et al[57] recommended that given the heterogeneity of children in the United States, norms would need to be updated and ECG parameters agreed on (especially with regard to diagnosis of LQTS) before routine ECG screening could be added to the sports clearance process. This view was shared by Maron et al.[58] The writing group for the American Heart Association recommended a 14-point preparticipation evaluation, including personal and family histories as well as physical examination points. In addition to the preparticipation history and physical examination, ECG screening of small cohorts with good quality control and follow-up systems, with the realization that false positive and negative results are likely, was believed to be reasonable in certain circumstances, especially if not limited to athletes. Mandatory universal ECG screening for all US athletes was not recommended. Overall there is controversy regarding the ideal preparticipation screening data needed to safely clear athletes for sports, both individually and on a population basis.[59] In any system, both the personal and family history is key to alerting the primary care physician to the need for further workup.

SUMMARY

Symptoms such as syncope and chest pain, especially if they are accompanied by palpitations or occur with exercise in any combination, require cardiac evaluation before adolescent athletes are allowed to return to the sports field. Some life-threatening conditions will likely be associated with a family history of HCM or LQTS, but the family history may not be discovered at the first medical visit. A family history of CPVT, for example, is hard to elicit unless this diagnosis has already been established in an affected family member. The keys will be the timing of symptoms and the documentation of arrhythmia with exercise. The ECG at baseline in CPVT may be deceptively normal. Hypertrophic cardiomyopathy is progressive, so evaluation during early childhood may be negative. Long QT syndrome may not always result in an abnormal ECG, even in genetically positive individuals. A high index of suspicion is needed to make these diagnoses, especially if the family history is not available.

References

1. Harmon KG, Drezner JA, Wilson MG, et al. Incidence of sudden cardiac death in athletes: a state of the art review. *Heart.* 2014;100:1227-1234
2. Pilmer CM, Krish JA, Hildebrandt D, et al. Sudden cardiac death in children and adolescents between 1 and 19 years of age. *Heart Rhythm.* 2014;11:239-245
3. Maron BJ, Thompson PD, Ackerman MJ, et al. Recommendations and considerations related to preparticipation screening for cardiovascular abnormalities in competitive athletes: 2007 update. A scientific statement from the American Heart Association Council on Nutrition, Physical Activity, and Metabolism. *Circulation.* 2007;115:1643-1655

4. Myerburg RJ, Wellens HJJ. Epidemiology of cardiac arrest. In: Priori SG, Zipes DP, eds. *Sudden Cardiac Death: A Handbook for Clinical Practice*. Malden, MA: Blackwell Publishing; 2006:3-20

5. Mahle WT, Sable CA, Matherne PG, et al. AHA Congenital Heart Defects Committee of the Council of Cardiovascular Disease in the Young. Key concepts in the screening approaches for heart disease in children and adolescents. *Circulation*. 2012;125:2796-2801

6. Maron BJ, Haas TS, Ahluwalia A, et al. Increasing survival rate from commotio cordis. *Heart Rhythm*. 2013;10:219-223

7. Maron BJ, Zipes DP, Ackerman MJ, et al. 36th Bethesda Conference: eligibility recommendations for competitive athletes with cardiovascular abnormalities. *J Am Coll Cardiol*. 2005;45:1312-1333

8. Kalin J, Madias C, Alsheikh-Ali CA, et al. Reduced diameter spheres increases the risk of chest blow-induced ventricular fibrillation (commotio cordis). *Heart Rhythm*. 2011;8:1578-1581

9. Madias C, Maron BJ, Weinstock J, et al. Commotio cordis—sudden cardiac death with chest wall impact. *J Cardiovascular Electrophysiol*. 2007;18:115-122

10. Perron AD, Brady WJ, Erling BF. Commotio cordis: an underappreciated cause of sudden cardiac death in young patients: assessment and management in the ED. *Am J Emerg Med*. 2001;19:406-409

11. Drezner JA, Rao AL, Heistand J, et al. Effectiveness of emergency response planning for sudden cardiac arrest in United States high schools with automated external defibrillators. *Circulation*. 2009;120:518-525

12. Berger S, Utech L, Hazinski MF. Lay rescuer automated external defibrillator programs for children and adolescents. *Pediatr Clin North Am*. 2004;51:1463-1478

13. Hallstrom A, Ornato JP; and the Public Access Defibrillation Trial Investigators. Public-access defibrillation and survival after out-of-hospital cardiac arrest. *N Engl J Med*. 2004;351:637-646

14. Toresdahl BG, Rao AL, Kimberly G, et al. Incidence of sudden cardiac arrest in high school student athletes on school campus. *Heart Rhythm*. 2014;11:1190-1194

15. Maron BJ, Shirani J, Poliac LC, et al. Sudden death in young competitive athletes: clinical, demographic, and pathological profiles. *JAMA*. 1996;276:199-204

16. Roma-Rodriguez C, Fernandez AR. Genetics of hypertrophic cardiomyopathy: advances and pitfalls in molecular diagnosis and therapy. *Appl Clin Genet*. 2014;7:195-208

17. Maron BJ, Maron MS. Hypertrophic cardiomyopathy. *Lancet*. 2013;381:242-255

18. Maron BJ. Hypertrophic cardiomyopathy in childhood. *Pediatr Clin North Am*. 2004;51:1305-1346

19. Maron BJ, Tajik AJ, Ruttenberg HD, et al. Hypertrophic cardiomyopathy in infants: clinical features and natural history. *Circulation*. 1982;65:7-17

20. Gersh BJ, Maron BJ, Bonow RO, et al. 2011 ACCF/AHA guideline for the diagnosis and treatment of hypertrophic cardiomyopathy. *J Am Coll Cardiol*. 2011;58:212-260

21. Maron BJ, Chaitman BR, Ackerman MJ, et al. Recommendations for physical activity and recreational sports participation for young patients with genetic cardiovascular diseases. *Circulation*. 2004;109:2807-2816

22. Graham TP, Driscoll DJ, Gersony WM, et al. Task Force 2: congenital heart disease. *J Am Coll Cardiol*. 2005;45:1326-1333

23. Lim DS, Matherne GP. Congenital anomalies of coronary vessels and the aortic root. In: Allen HD, Driscoll DJ, Shaddy R, et al, eds. *Moss & Adams' Heart Disease in Infants, Children and Adolescents: Including the Fetus and Young Adult*. 8th ed. Philadelphia, PA: Lippincott, Williams & Wilkins; 2013:746-757

24. Basso C, Maron BJ, Corrado D, et al. Clinical profile of congenital coronary artery anomalies with origin from the wrong aortic sinus leading to sudden death in young competitive athletes. *J Am Coll Cardiol*. 2000;35:1493-1501

25. Warnes CA, Williams RG, Bashore T, et al. A Report of the American College of Cardiology/ American Heart Association Task Force on Practice Guidelines (Writing Committee to Develop Guidelines on the Management of Adults with Congenital Heart Disease). *Circulation*. 2008; 118:e714-e833

26. Basso C, Corrado D, Marcus FJ, et al. Arrhythmogenic right ventricular cardiomyopathy. *Lancet*. 2009;373:1289-1300

27. Saguner AM, Brunckhorst C, Duru F. Arrhythmogenic ventricular cardiomyopathy: a paradigm shift from right to biventricular disease. *World J Cardiol.* 2014;6:154-174

28. Marcus FI, McKenna WJ, Sherrill D, et al. Diagnosis of arrhythmogenic right ventricular cardio-myopathy/dysplasia: proposed modification of the task force criteria. *Circulation.* 2010;121: 1533-1541

29. Hoffmayer KS, Bhave PD, Marcus GM, et al. An electrocardiographic scoring system for distin-guishing right ventricular outflow tract arrhythmias in patients with arrhythmogenic right ven-tricular cardiomyopathy from idiopathic ventricular tachycardia. *Heart Rhythm.* 2013;10:477-482

30. Yoerger DM, Marcus F, Sherrill D, et al. Echocardiographic findings in patients meeting task force criteria for arrhythmogenic right ventricular dysplasia: new insights from the Multidisciplinary Study of Right Ventricular Dysplasia. *J Am Coll Cardiol.* 2005;45:860-865

31. Rao AL, Salerno JC, Asif IM, et al. Evaluation and management of Wolff-Parkinson-White in athletes. *Sports Health.* 2014;6:326-332

32. Maron BJ, Doerer JJ, Haas TS, et al. Sudden deaths in young competitive athletes: analysis of 1866 deaths in the United States,1980-2006. *Circulation.* 2009;119:1085-1092

33. Santinelli V, Radinovic A, Manguso F, et al. The natural history of asymptomatic ventricular pre-excitation a long-term prospective follow-up study of 184 asymptomatic children. *J Am Coll Car-diol.* 2009;53:275-280

34. Cohen MI, Triedman JK, Cannon BC, et al. PACES/HRS expert consensus statement on the man-agement of the asymptomatic young patient with a Wolff-Parkinson-White (WPW, ventricular preexcitation) electrocardiographic pattern: developed in partnership between the Pediatric and Congenital Electrophysiology Society (PACES) and the Heart Rhythm Society (HRS). Endorsed by the governing bodies of PACES, HRS, the American College of Cardiology Foundation (ACCF), The American Heart Association (AHA), the American Academy of Pediatrics (AAP), and the Canadian Heart Rhythm Society (CHRS). *Heart Rhythm.* 2012;9:1006-1024

35. Liu N, Ruan Y, Priori SG. Catecholaminergic polymorphic ventricular tachycardia. *Prog Cardio-vasc Dis.* 2008;51:23-30

36. Priori SG; Napolitano C, Tiso N, et al. Mutations in the cardiac ryanodine receptor gene (hRyR2) underlie catecholaminergic polymorphic ventricular tachycardia. *Circulation.* 2001;103:196-200

37. Kontula K, Laitinen P, Lehtonen A, et al. Catecholaminergic polymorphic ventricular tachycardia: recent mechanistic insights. *Cardiovasc Res.* 2005;67:379-387

38. Faggioni M, Kryshtal DO, Knollmann BC. Calsequestrin mutations and catecholaminergic poly-morphic ventricular tachycardia. *Pediatr Cardiol.* 2012;33:959-967

39. Pflaumer A, Davis AM. Guidelines for the diagnosis and management of catecholaminergic poly-morphic ventricular tachycardia. *Heart Lung Circ.* 2012;21:96-100

40. Khoury A, Marai I, Suleiman M, et al. Flecainide therapy suppresses exercise induced ventricular arrhythmias in patients with CASQ2-associated catecholaminergic polymorphic ventricular tachycardia. *Heart Rhythm.* 2013;10:1671-1675

41. Schwartz PJ, Stramba-Badiale M, Crotti L, et al. Prevalence of the congenital long-QT syndrome. *Circulation.* 2009;120:1761-1767

42. Wolf CM, Berul CI. Molecular mechanisms of inherited arrhythmias. *Curr Genomics.* 2008;9: 160-168

43. Webster G, Berul CI. Congenital long-QT syndromes: a clinical and genetic update from infancy through adulthood. *Trends Cardiovasc Med.* 2008;18:216-224

44. Moss AJ, Zareba W, Benhorin J, et al. ECG T-wave patterns in genetically distinct forms of the hereditary long QT syndrome. *Circulation.* 1995;92:2929-2934

45. Wong JA, Gula LJ, Klein GJ, et al. Utility of treadmill testing in identification and genotype predic-tion in long-QT syndrome. *Circ Arrhythm Electrophysiol.* 2010;3:120-125

46. Ackerman MJ. Cardiac channelopathies: it's in the genes. *Nat Med.* 2004;10:463-464

47. Van Dorn CS, Johnson JN, Taggart NW, et al. QTc values among children and adolescents present-ing to the emergency department. *Pediatrics.* 2011;128:1395-1401

48. Priori SG, Schwartz PJ, Napolitano C, et al. Risk stratification in the long-QT syndrome. *N Engl J Med.* 2003;348:1866-1874

49. Postema PG, Neville J, de Jong JS, et al. Safe drug use in long QT syndrome and Brugada syndrome: comparison of website statistics. *Europace.* 2013;15:1042-1049

50. Antselevich C. Brugada Syndrome: overview. In: Antzelevitch C, Brudgada P, Brugada J, et al, eds. *The Brugada Syndrome: From Bench to Bedside.* Malden, MA: Blackwell Publishng; 2005:1-19

51. Pelliccia A, Di Paolo FM, et al. Evidence for efficacy of the Italian national pre-participation screening programme for identification of hypertrophic cardiomyopathy in competitive athletes. *Eur Heart J.* 2006;27:2196-2200

52. Corrado D, Pelliccia A, Bjørnstad HH, et al. Cardiovascular pre-participation screening of young competitive athletes for prevention of sudden death: proposal for a common European protocol. Consensus Statement of the Study Group of Sport Cardiology. *Eur Heart J.* 2005;26:516-524

53. Brosnan M, Gerche AL, Kumar S, et al. Modest agreement in ECG interpretation limits the application of ECG screening in young athletes. *Heart Rhythm.* 2015;12:130-136

54. Chandra N, Bastiaenen R, Papadakis M, et al. Prevalence of electrocardiographic anomalies in young individuals relevance to a nationwide cardiac screening program. *J Am Coll Cardiol.* 2014;63:2028-2034

55. Le VV, Wheeler MT, Mandic S, et al. Addition of the electrocardiogram to the preparticipation examination of college athletes. *Clin J Sport Med.* 2010;20:98-105

56. Hill AC, Miyake CY, Grady S, et al. Accuracy of interpretation of preparticipation screening electrocardiograms. *J Pediatr.* 2011;159:783-788

57. Kaltman JR, Thompson PD, Lantos J, et al. Screening for sudden cardiac death in the young: report from a National Heart, Lung, and Blood Institute Working Group. *Circulation.* 2011;123:1911-1918

58. Maron BJ, Friedman RA, Kligfield P, et al. Assessment of the 12-lead electrocardiogram as a screening test for detection of cardiovascular disease in healthy general populations of young people (12-25 years of age): a scientific statement from the American Heart Association and the American College of Cardiology. *J Am Coll Cardiol.* 2014;64:1479-1514

59. Chaitman BR. An electrocardiogram should not be included in routine preparticipation screening of young athletes. *Circulation.* 2007;116:2610-2615

Adolesc Med 026 (2015) 528–551

Approach to the Adolescent with Chest Pain

Nadine Smith, DO[a], Erica Del Grippo, DO[b],
Steven M. Selbst, MD[c]*

[a]Fellow, Pediatric Emergency Medicine, Sidney Kimmel Medical College at Thomas Jefferson University, Nemours/Alfred I. duPont Hospital for Children, Wilmington, Delaware; [b]Pediatric Resident, Sidney Kimmel Medical College at Thomas Jefferson University, Nemours/Alfred I. duPont Hospital for Children, Wilmington, Delaware; [c]Professor of Pediatrics, Sidney Kimmel Medical College at Thomas Jefferson University, Philadelphia, Pennsylvania; Attending Physician, Division of Emergency Medicine, Nemours/Alfred I. duPont Hospital for Children, Wilmington, Delaware; Director, Pediatric Residency Program, Jefferson/duPont Hospital for Children, Wilmington, Delaware

Chest pain is a common complaint among adolescents and often causes them to seek medical care. Approximately 0.3% to 0.6% of visits to a pediatric emergency department (ED) are for chest pain, and many of these visits involve adolescents.[1,2] Unlike adult patients with chest pain, most studies have shown that teenagers with chest pain rarely have serious organic pathology.[1-8] They rarely present in significant distress such that immediate resuscitation is required. For many, the pain is not acute.[1] Adolescents are more likely than younger children to have chest pain associated with psychogenic disturbance.[1]

Serious, life-threatening heart disease is extremely rare in the adolescent population. However, families come to the ED seeking an explanation and reassurance when their teenager complains of chest pain.[8] It is important to carefully address adolescents with chest pain because underlying heart disease or other serious pathology is sometimes present. Many teenagers and their families associate their chest pain with heart disease or heart attack.[2,7] In one study, more than two-thirds of adolescents with chest pain restricted their activities, and 40% missed school because of pain.[9] Media reports of sudden deaths in young athletes have called attention to chest pain as a sign of serious heart disease. Also, many adolescents are aware of risk factors for cardiac disease because the

*Corresponding author
E-mail address: steven.selbst@nemours.org

medical community has emphasized the prevalence of hypertension and atherosclerotic cardiovascular disease in adults.[7]

DIFFERENTIAL DIAGNOSIS

There are numerous causes of chest pain in adolescents, and it is wise to keep a broad differential diagnosis in mind while assessing the adolescent with this complaint (Table 1).

Table 1
Differential diagnosis of chest pain in adolescents

Non–cardiac-related causes
  Musculoskeletal disorders
    Chest wall strain
    Direct trauma/contusion
    Rib fracture
    Costochondritis
  Respiratory disorders
    Asthma
    Pneumonia
    Pneumothorax/pneumomediastinum
    Pulmonary embolism
  Psychological disorders
    Stress-related pain
  Gastrointestinal disorders
    Esophagitis (reflux or pill-induced)
  Miscellaneous disorders
    Sickle cell crises
    Abdominal aortic aneurysm (Marfan syndrome)
    Pleural effusion (collagen vascular disease)
    Breast tenderness (pregnancy, physiologic)
    Texidor twinge/precordial catch syndrome
    Chest mass
  Idiopathic
Cardiac-related causes
  Coronary artery disease, ischemia/infarction
    Anomalous coronary arteries
    Kawasaki disease (coronary artery aneurysms)
    Diabetes mellitus (longstanding)
  Arrhythmia
    Supraventricular tachycardia
    Ventricular tachycardia
  Structural abnormalities of the heart
    Hypertrophic cardiomyopathy
    Severe pulmonic stenosis
    Aortic valve stenosis
  Infection
    Pericarditis
    Myocarditis

Non-Cardiac Causes of Chest Pain in Adolescents

Idiopathic chest pain is a label given to adolescents when no clear etiology can be found. In 20% to 45% of cases of pediatric chest pain, no diagnosis can be determined with certainty.[1,10] When an etiology for chest pain is identified, *musculoskeletal disorders* are the most common causes of chest pain in the pediatric population.[1,2,11] Active teens frequently strain chest wall muscles while they are exercising, wrestling, or just carrying heavy books. Some develop chest pain after they sustain a direct trauma to the chest, related to a mild contusion of the chest wall. With more significant force, a rib fracture, hemothorax, or pneumothorax is possible. Most often, this diagnosis is straightforward because there is a clear history of trauma. Careful physical examination reveals chest wall tenderness or pain with movement of the torso or upper extremities. Costochondritis is a common musculoskeletal disorder in adolescents. Pain related to this condition is generally sharp, may be bilateral, and is exaggerated by physical activity or breathing. Eliciting tenderness over the costochondral junctions with palpation supports this diagnosis. Pain from costochondritis may persist for several months.[9,10]

Psychogenic disturbances can cause chest pain[1,2,12] and should be considered if the adolescent has experienced a recent major stressful event, such as separation from friends, divorce in the family, or school failure that correlates temporally with the onset of the chest pain, Often, the anxiety or stress that results in somatic complaints is not easily apparent. Hyperventilation and obvious anxiety are not always present.

Gastrointestinal disorders such as reflux esophagitis frequently cause chest pain in adolescents.[1,2] The pain is classically described as burning, substernal in location, and worsened by reclining or eating spicy foods. This condition is diagnosed by history or with a therapeutic trial of antacids.[13] In addition, some adolescents may take medications, such as doxycycline, with little water and then lie down. As the undissolved pill lodges in the esophagus, the adolescent may develop severe "pill esophagitis."[14]

Pulmonary disorders frequently lead to chest pain in adolescents. Those with severe, persistent cough, asthma, or pneumonia may complain of chest pain caused by overuse of chest wall muscles. Diagnosis of these conditions is usually made by history or the presence of rales, wheezes, tachypnea, or decreased breath sounds on physical examination. Consider a spontaneous pneumothorax or pneumomediastinum in adolescents with sudden chest pain, especially if they have respiratory distress. Adolescents at high risk for these conditions are those with asthma, cystic fibrosis, or Marfan syndrome.[15,16] Also, previously healthy teenagers (usually tall, thin males) may develop a pneumothorax by rupture of an unrecognized subpleural bleb with minimal precipitating factors such as coughing or stretching. Adolescents who use marijuana or snort cocaine are also at risk for barotrauma and may complain of severe, sudden chest pain with associated anxiety, hypertension, and tachycardia.[17] Examination often reveals respiratory distress, decreased breath sounds on the affected side (if the pneumothorax is significant), and possibly palpable subcutaneous air. Radiographs of the chest confirm the pneumothorax or pneumomediastinum (pneumomediastinum: Figure 1; bilateral pneumothoraces: Figure 2). Finally, pulmonary embolism (PE) is a rare cause of chest pain in adolescents. Risk factors for PE include obesity (body mass index >25), oral contraceptive use, coagulopathy, deep venous thrombosis, nephrotic syndrome, systemic lupus erythematosis, recent abortion, and recent leg trauma.[18] Patients with PE will experience tachypnea (75%), tachycardia (58%), chest pain (52%), and shortness of breath (44%).[18]

Miscellaneous causes of chest pain include pain related to underlying diseases. For example, patients with sickle cell disease may have pain related to acute chest syndrome.[4] In addition to chest pain, the patient will likely have fever, tachypnea, hypoxemia, and a pulmonary infiltrate on chest radiograph.[19] Adolescents with Marfan syndrome may have chest pain as a result of dissection of an aortic aneurysm. These patients describe sudden, severe, tearing chest pain

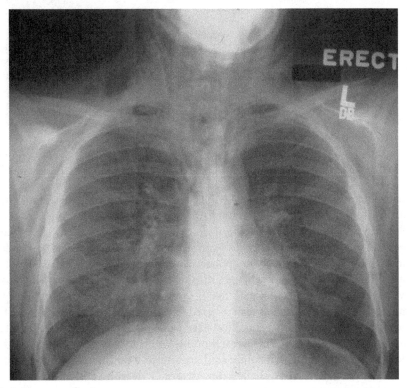

Fig 1. Pneumomediastinum.

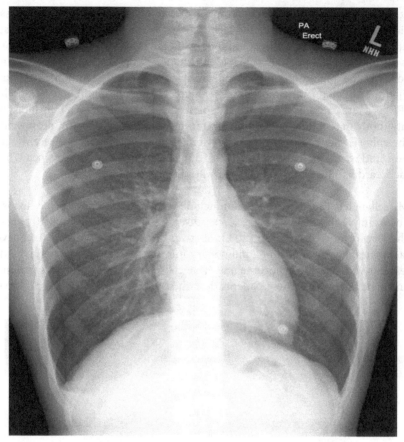

Fig 2. Bilateral pneumothorax.

that radiates to the back or neck.[20] Collagen vascular disorders (eg, lupus) may lead to pleural effusions and chest pain. Coxsackievirus infection may cause pleurodynia with paroxysms of sharp pain in the chest or abdomen. Some young teenagers (boys and girls) may also complain of chest pain with breast tenderness from physiologic changes of puberty. Some teenage girls may note chest or breast pain related to early changes of pregnancy. Finally, Texidor twinge is a syndrome of left-sided chest pain that is brief (>5 minutes' duration) and sporadic. This pain syndrome is also referred to as precordial catch or stitch in the side. Adolescents with this condition have pain that recurs frequently for a few hours and then is absent for several months. The pain is often associated with a slouched posture or bending, unrelated to exercise. Pain is usually relieved when the teenager takes a few shallow breaths, or 1 deep breath, and assumes a straightened posture. The etiology remains unclear.[7,21]

Cardiac Causes of Chest Pain in Adolescents

Cardiac disease (previously undiagnosed) is a rare cause of adolescent chest pain.[1-6] However, this is perhaps the greatest concern of the patient, the family, and the physician when an adolescent complains of acute chest pain. Consider angina or myocardial infarction (MI) if the adolescent has significant, acute chest pain, especially if the patient has an underlying medical condition such as longstanding diabetes mellitus, past history of Kawasaki disease, chronic anemia, thrombophilia, or previous cardiac surgery (transposition repair). Also consider ischemia if the patient has a strong history of familial hypercholesterolemia.[22-25] In many cases, exercise induces the chest pain in those with these disorders because coronary blood flow is limited. Therefore, pain with exertion should be given careful consideration. Syncope may also be reported and is another worrisome associated complaint.[26,27]

Other serious cardiac causes of adolescent chest pain deserve attention. The following cases highlight important considerations and presentations for adolescents with life-threatening chest pain related to cardiac conditions.

Case 1

A 17-year-old female was brought to the ED with the complaint of intermittent chest pain over the past 2 weeks. She had pain localized to the middle of her chest without radiation. She noted her "heart was fluttering," intermittently, with episodes lasting a few seconds. She had no associated dizziness, syncope, or fever. She had a past medical history of anxiety and was taking no medications. On physical examination, her vital signs were weight 55 kg, heart rate 196, blood pressure 104/57, respiratory rate 30, and oxygen saturation was 98% in room air. She was visibly anxious and repetitively asked, "What is happening to me?" She was tachypneic, with clear breath sounds to auscultation. Cardiac examination demonstrated marked tachycardia without a murmur. The patient was warm and well perfused, with brisk capillary refill.

The patient was attached to a cardiac monitor. Electrocardiography (ECG) confirmed marked tachycardia with no discernible P waves (Figure 3). Stable supraventricular tachycardia (SVT) was considered. After intravenous (IV) access was obtained in the left antecubital fossa, vagal maneuvers were attempted but did not improve the patient's rhythm. She was given a dose of IV adenosine (6 mg) with a 2-way stopcock without resolution of SVT. A second dose of IV adenosine 12 mg was administered, and her rhythm converted to sinus tachycardia. She was admitted to the cardiology service for further evaluation.

Supraventricular Tachycardia

Supraventricular tachycardia is the most common symptomatic tachyarrhythmia in the pediatric population.[28] It is defined as any tachycardia that originates above

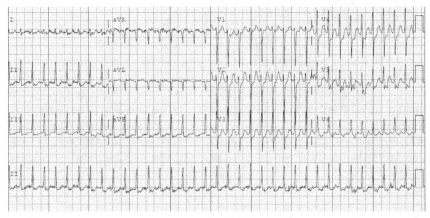

Fig 3. Electrocardiogram showing supraventricular SVT.

the bundle of His within the cardiac electrical pathway.[29] Supraventricular tachycardia is estimated to affect 1 in 250 to 1000 children, with males having a slightly
higher incidence than females.[28,30] Supraventricular tachycardia can occur at any
age. The 3 main classifications of SVT are atrioventricular reentrant tachycardia
(AVRT), atrioventricular nodal reentrant tachycardia, and atrial ectopic tachycar-
dias.[28,29,31] Atrioventricular reentrant tachycardia is the most common type seen in
the early adolescent years, accounting for approximately 75% of SVT cases in pediatric patients.[28,32] Most episodes of SVT have no inciting factor; however, SVT can
occur in the setting of infection, fever, drug exposure (most commonly cold medications or bronchodilator), anxiety, or congenital heart disease.[31,32]

PATHOPHYSIOLOGY
In the normal cardiac conduction system, an impulse begins in the sinoatrial
node and is transmitted by internodal pathways to the atrioventricular node
(AV). From the AV node, signals are conducted through the right and left bundle of His to the Purkinje fibers. This transmission creates depolarization and
repolarization to aid in contraction and relaxation of the heart. With SVT, a
separate impulse originates above the bundle of His, creating irregularity within
the normal conduction pathway.[32] Atrioventricular reentrant tachycardia occurs
as a result of 1 or more accessory conduction pathways that are not a part of the
normal cardiac conduction system.[28,31] With this type of arrhythmia, there can
be both anterograde and retrograde conduction involving the accessory pathway.[28] An example of atrioventricular reentrant tachycardia is Wolff-Parkinson-
White (WPW) syndrome.

CLINICAL FEATURES
Supraventricular tachycardia can be unpredictable, with abrupt onset and termination.[28,31] If a patient is not in sustained SVT, the arrhythmia can often be difficult to diagnose; therefore, in the adolescent population, a detailed history is

imperative. Adolescents often complain of palpitations, chest pain, shortness of breath, and dizziness.[28,33] Depending on their hemodynamics, they may also demonstrate pallor, presyncope or syncope, and diaphoresis.[28,31] Adolescents will have heart rates ranging from 150 to 250 bpm.[28,33,34] Some patients with SVT will present with signs of congestive heart failure if symptoms have been present for more than 24 hours without intervention. This occurs rarely in adolescents because they are able to describe their symptoms promptly.[31-33]

DIAGNOSIS

Supraventricular tachycardia in the adolescent population can mimic other cardiac diseases (congenital heart, myocarditis), psychological disorders (anxiety, stress, panic disorders), endocrine disorders (hyperthyroidism), medication or illicit drug use, or caffeine consumption.[28,31] A 12-lead ECG is the most helpful tool for diagnosing SVT. The QRS complex will be narrow and the P wave will often be difficult to decipher. For those with underlying WPW syndrome, the baseline ECG contains a shortened PR interval and a delta wave. A delta wave is a light upstroke in the initial portion of the QRS complex indicating preexcitation.[28,32] However, this is not always seen in SVT with WPW syndrome. Some patients present with intermittent chest pain and palpitations, but an initial ECG that did not reveal any abnormalities. These patients need an ambulatory ECG monitoring device such as a Holter monitor or an intermittent recorder.[28] After suspicions of SVT are confirmed by ECG, an electrophysiologic study will help to classify the type of SVT. Additional testing may include chest radiography to evaluate for cardiomegaly, serum electrolyte levels to evaluate for abnormalities, thyroid-stimulating hormone level to evaluate for hyperthyroidism, complete blood count to evaluate for anemia and infection, and urine drug screen. If myocarditis or cardiac ischemia is suspected, creatinine kinase and troponin levels should also be obtained.[32]

TREATMENT AND OUTCOME

Treatment of SVT depends on the patient's hemodynamic stability at the time of initial examination. Begin by accessing airway patency, breathing, and circulation (ABCs). Once the ABCs are adequately managed, the goal is to interrupt the reentrant circuit in order regain a normal sinus rhythm. Vagal maneuvers can be attempted first; these stimulate vagal activity and thus slow the heart rate and ultimately terminate SVT. Maneuvers include an ice bag on the face, Valsalva maneuver (bearing down as if having a bowel movement), stimulation of the gag reflex, or breath-holding.[2,17] These maneuvers are effective in approximately 53% of cases,[28,35] and the most successful is the Valsalva maneuver.[28,34,35] Carotid sinus massage is another vagal maneuver used in the adult population but no longer recommended for the pediatric population, especially in those younger than 10 years.[34] Consider pharmacologic interventions for both stable and unstable SVT. Intravenous adenosine is the first-line agent for termination of SVT, as noted in case 1. It works to slow or block the conduction current in the AV node. Adenosine is effective in about 75% of SVT cases.[33] It is initiated at a dose of 0.1 mg/kg (maximum of 6 mg) and may be increased to 0.2 mg/kg (maximum of

12 mg). This medication has a very short half-life, and must be administered intravenously, as close as possible to the heart, with a 5-cc flush of normal saline to be pushed quickly after the medication.[31,36] If the patient has significant hemo-dynamic instability or poor perfusion, synchronized cardioversion (0.5-1 J/kg) should be performed. If this does not improve the rhythm, the dose may be doubled for the second attempt up to 2 J/kg.[34] Mortality from SVT is quite low.[28]

Case 2
A 17-year-old male with a past medical history of mild intermittent asthma pre-sented with chest pain and syncope. The patient was playing basketball when he noted midsternal chest pain. He subsequently fell to the floor and sustained a minor injury to the head. Review of systems was negative for fever, dehydration, jerking movements, and loss of bowel or bladder function. The parents denied a history of any sudden cardiac deaths in the family.

On physical examination, the patient was in no acute distress and had normal vital signs. Cardiac examination revealed a murmur (III/VI) at the left paraster-nal edge, which increased with Valsalva maneuver. No other abnormalities were noted on examination. Chest radiographs were normal. Electrocardiography showed left ventricular hypertrophy with large R waves in lead V_5 and deep S waves in lead V_1.

Because the chest pain was associated with exercise and syncope, hypertrophic cardiomyopathy (HCM) was considered.

Hypertrophic Cardiomyopathy
CLINICAL FEATURES
Hypertrophic cardiomyopathy (HCM), an autosomal dominant disease, occurs in about 0.2% of the general population. Hypertrophic cardiomyopathy is a rare but significant cause of sudden death in adolescents.[37] It can be present in different penetrations and thus display different phenotypes.[38] The arrangement of a hyper-trophied septum with an anterior shift of the mitral valve into the septum creates a left ventricular outflow obstruction. This obstruction can cause symptoms of dyspnea on exertion or syncope secondary to decreased cardiac output as seen in case 2. Fever, tachycardia, dehydration, or exercise can increase clinical symptoms given their potential to decrease preload or increase afterload, worsening the obstruction.[39,40] The patient presented with chest pain during exertion, which is not uncommon. A potential risk of HCM is the concomitant addition of coronary artery abnormalities, which may result in chest pain.[40] Chest pain may also be secondary to inadequate perfusion of the left hypertrophic ventricle.[41]

DIAGNOSIS
Patients with HCM have varying clinical presentations depending on the severity of the left outflow tract obstruction. A heart murmur, similar to aortic stenosis, will have increased intensity with maneuvers that decrease blood volume to the

left ventricle (eg, Valsalva and standing).[39] More than 75% of patients with HCM have ECG changes.[39] Increased voltages in the R waves (V5/V6) and deep S waves (V1/V2) are frequent findings, These findings are seen secondary to left ventricular hypertrophy.[39] The presence of left ventricular hypertrophy on ECG in an adolescent presenting with chest pain and syncope should raise concern for HCM. Electrocardiography may also show cardiac ischemia with T-wave inversion or deep Q waves. Echocardiography is the current gold standard for diagnosis of HCM. Cardiac magnetic resonance imaging can also aid in the evaluation of myocardial scarring and cardiac function.[42] Consult a pediatric cardiologist.

TREATMENT AND OUTCOME

No cure exists for HCM. Management is centered around symptomatic treatment (eg, reducing strenuous exercise). A small subset of patients may be considered for surgical intervention (myectomy). The goal of this treatment is to decrease the obstruction by removing the area of the ventricular muscle that is causing it.[43]

Case 3

A 14-year-old previously healthy female presented to the ED with frequent episodes of vomiting. She complained of substernal chest pain that was not related to vomiting. She denied any radiation or change with breathing, walking, or rest. Review of systems was notable for fever, sore throat, generalized fatigue, malaise, and achy joints.

On arrival to the ED, her initial vital signs were weight 38.2 kg, temperature 38.2°C, pulse 140, blood pressure 83/51, respiratory rate 22, and O_2 saturation 100% on 4-L nasal cannula. She was dehydrated and was given 2 IV saline boluses. She was then noted to be in respiratory distress and had worsening chest pain. Electrocardiography revealed wide complex tachycardia. Other diagnostic testing showed transaminitis (aspartate aminotransferase 483). Venous blood gas showed respiratory acidosis (7.15/51/21/-20). Troponin levels were also elevated (123). Blood cultures were sent. In the ED, her blood pressure decreased to 68/46. She was given IV lidocaine and adenosine. Cardioversion was also attempted. She continued to have wide complex tachycardia with hypotension. She was placed on a dopamine infusion and transferred to a pediatric cardiac intensive care unit (CICU).

In the CICU, she appeared critically ill and pale, and had minimal pulses. She was intermittently moaning. Her skin was cool, and she had prolonged capillary refill. Lungs sounds were clear bilaterally without notable rales. Abdominal examination revealed no hepatomegaly. Her trachea was intubated, and she was placed on mechanical ventilation. Care was escalated to include both epinephrine and vasopressin infusions. Cardiopulmonary resuscitation was initiated after she became bradycardic and a blood pressure reading could not be obtained. She was placed on extracorporeal membrane oxygenation. Myocardial biopsies were eventually obtained. She was diagnosed with cardiogenic shock secondary to myocarditis, and appropriate viral cultures were sent. She was empirically started on IV immunoglobulin.

Myocarditis

CLINICAL FEATURES

Myocarditis is an inflammatory condition of the myocardium with various etiologies ranging from infectious to autoimmune. Viral infection is typically the most common cause (eg, coxsackievirus B, adenovirus, parvovirus, enterovirus), although an underlying etiology is often not identified.[44] Chest pain is the result of ischemia and subsequent myocardial damage from an inciting agent. An inflammatory process ensues secondary to the host's own immune response and cardiac dysfunction occurs. The pain is typically worsened by physical activity given myocardial strain with increased oxygen demands.[44] One study reported an estimated prevalence of 0.5 pediatric myocarditis cases per 10,000 ED visits.[45] The exact incidence of myocarditis is unknown because many cases go undiagnosed; some cases are found at autopsy.

DIAGNOSIS

Consider myocarditis in adolescent patients with fever and chest pain. Adolescents often present with fever, tachypnea, and tachycardia, as did the patient in case 3. Classically, there is a prodrome of a viral illness followed by symptoms of heart failure. Durani et al[46] reported the most common presenting symptoms were respiratory (32%), cardiac (29%), hypoperfusion/shock (23%), Kawasaki-like disease (10%), and gastrointestinal complaints (7%). Electrocardiographic findings are nonspecific for myocarditis and can include sinus tachycardia, abnormal T-wave inversion, ST-segment changes, and arrhythmias. Chest radiography usually shows findings of congestive heart failure, whereas echocardiography demonstrates globally reduced ventricular function.[47] Cardiac magnetic resonance imaging has gained favor in recent years and can detect areas of inflammation in the myocardium.[48] The diagnosis is rarely confirmed by endomyocardial biopsy in the pediatric population, although this is the gold standard.[48] Serum laboratory studies (complete blood count, erythrocyte sedimentation rate [ESR], and C-reactive protein [CRP]) are typically elevated when myocarditis is caused by an infectious etiology. There is no clear research suggesting the usefulness of obtaining cardiac enzymes.

TREATMENT AND OUTCOME

Patients with myocarditis usually have unstable hemodynamics, and treatment should be directed toward stabilizing vital signs. Pediatric cardiology consultation is recommended, and monitoring in an ICU may be necessary. Treat cardiac arrhythmias and give inotropic support for ventricular dysfunction. Consider diuretics, afterload reducers, and aldosterone inhibitors for heart failure. Extracorporeal membrane oxygenation and ventricular assist devices may be needed in more severe cases. Intravenous immunoglobulin is more commonly used in pediatric patients as in case 3 but its value is uncertain.[44,48] Prognosis is variable, with one study reporting a survival rate of 87%.[46]

Case 4

A 16-year-old male with no past medical history presented to the ED with worsening cough for 2 weeks. He had temperatures to 37.7°C with associated chills. At onset of symptoms, he was evaluated by his primary care physician and started on azithromycin for possible atypical pneumonia, but there was no improvement. In the 72 hours before his arrival, he developed worsening cough, chest pain, abdominal pain with cough, night sweats, and continued chills. His appetite was diminished.

On physical examination, vital signs were weight 60 kg, blood pressure 104/54, pulse 110, respiratory rate 20, and temperature 37.7°C. He was pale and ill appearing, but he was interactive and able to answer questions without shortness of breath. He appeared uncomfortable with supine positioning. Neck examination showed non-tender lymphadenopathy. Cardiac examination revealed tachycardia without murmur. He had no reproducible chest pain with palpation. Respiratory examination revealed coarse breath sounds, and no intercostal retractions or accessory muscle use. The remainder of his physical examination was normal.

Chest radiography revealed a widened mediastinum with concern for lymphadenopathy. A complete blood count showed white blood cell count 13,900 K/UL (86% neutrophils), hemoglobin 10.0 g/dL, and platelets 450,000 K/UL. His CRP was 18.0 mg/dL, and ESR was 57 mm/h. Lactate dehydrogenase was 637 U/L. A complete metabolic panel and urinalysis were unremarkable. Computerized tomographic scan of the chest obtained because of concern for malignancy revealed a mediastinal mass with lymphadenopathy and a large pericardial effusion.

Cardiology and cardiothoracic surgery were consulted. Echocardiogram completed at bedside exhibited a large pericardial effusion with findings suggestive of impending tamponade. The patient was taken to the cardiac catheterization laboratory, where a pericardial drain was placed and 650 cc of fluid was drained from the pericardium. He was admitted to the ICU for further management. Culture of the fluid showed no infection. The pericardial effusion was the result of hematogeneous spread from malignancy.

Pericarditis

Acute pericarditis is rare and accounts for about 5% of patients with acute chest pain evaluated in a general ED (the incidence is likely less in the adolescent population).[8,49] Pericarditis is usually benign and self-limiting; however, complications such as a pericardial effusion or recurrent pericarditis can arise, thus increasing morbidity and mortality.[49] A variety of etiologies of pericarditis can be categorized into infectious versus noninfectious. Most cases result from an infectious cause, usually a virus (Coxsackie virus group B and echovirus type 8 in 80%-85%); however, bacterial causes make up about 1% to 5% of cases (*Staphylococcus aureus, Hemophilus influenzae, Streptococcus pneumoniae*).[50]

In these infections there is often hematogeneous or direct spread to the pericardium.[49,51]

Noninfectious causes include collagen vascular diseases, specifically systemic lupus erythematosus, neoplasms, trauma, and postsurgical changes.[49,51] Neoplastic pericarditis generally occurs from tumor invasion or hematologic spread, as seen in case 4. Traumatic pericarditis can occur when there is blunt or penetrating injury to the pericardium. Interventions such as catheterization, pacemaker placement, surgical ablation, and esophageal foreign bodies can cause penetrating pericardial injury.[49] In many cases, an etiology is not found after an extensive workup and pericarditis is considered idiopathic.[8,49-51]

The heart is surrounded by the pericardium, a double-layered fibroserous sac. The 2 layers are approximately 1 to 2 mm in thickness and separated by approximately 15 to 35 mL of pericardial fluid.[49] Pericardial fluid may collect slowly (as much as 2 L have been reported), and this is tolerated better than a rapid accumulation.[8,49] Rapid accumulation can cause constriction, leading to poor cardiac filling during diastole. Left untreated, this can lead to cardiac tamponade or cardiogenic shock.[8,49]

CLINICAL FEATURES

Adolescents with pericarditis often have sharp, stabbing chest pain with radiation to the scapula.[49] The pain is generally relieved when the patient leans forward and worsens when the patients lies supine. Deep inspiration also worsens the pain. Associated symptoms include cough, dyspnea, abdominal pain, and fever.[8,52] On physical examination, patients are usually febrile and in respiratory distress.[51] On cardiac examination, a friction rub is pathognomonic for pericarditis but is present in only 25% of cases.[8,49,51] In fact, in the presence of significant pericardial effusion a friction rub may be absent, and the heart sounds will be distant.[8,49,51] Patients can also have distended neck veins and pulsus paradoxus. If cardiac tamponade is present, patients can demonstrate the Beck triad of hypotension, muffled heart sounds, and raised jugular venous pressure.[49] Additional signs of poor cardiac output with cardiac tamponade include pallor, change in mental status, prolonged capillary refill time, tachycardia, and cool extremities.[8,49]

DIAGNOSIS

An ECG is abnormal in 90% of patients with pericardial disease.[10] Changes on ECG include ST elevation with upright T waves that generally improves over a few days. T waves may become inverted and low-voltage QRS segments can be seen on ECG.[3,4] Chest radiography can be valuable in detecting cardiomegaly if significant pericardial effusion is present.[1,8,49,51] Echocardiography is the most sensitive diagnostic test for pericarditis, specifically if an effusion or constriction is present.[49,51] Echocardiography can help determine the thickness of the pericardium and provide dynamic information of ventricular movement with respiration.[8,49] Computerized tomographic scan and cardiac magnetic resonance imaging can provide additional information.[49,53] Other studies often show evidence of systemic inflammation, including elevated white blood cell count, ESR, and CRP.[49]

Drainage of a pericardial effusion is both diagnostic and therapeutic. Indications for pericardiocentesis include cardiac tamponade, concern for purulent effusion, and malignancy.[8,49] The fluid collected should be tested for cell count, glucose, protein, and lactic dehydrogenase levels, gram stain, bacterial and viral cultures, and polymerase chain reaction for infectious pathogens.[8,49,52]

TREATMENT AND OUTCOMES

For all cases of pericarditis, the main goal is control of pain and inflammation.[4] Non-steroidal anti-inflammatory drugs are the first line of treatment.[49,52] For bacterial pericarditis, drainage alone is not sufficient, and antimicrobial agents are needed.[8,49,51] Corticosteroids are controversial and should be reserved for severe, refractory cases because of the risk of reactivating infection and chronic recurrent pericarditis.[49,50] Acute pericarditis, related to a viral infection, generally has a benign and self-limited course.[49] Purulent pericarditis can have a poor prognosis despite aggressive treatment with antibiotics and drainage.[50]

Case 5

A 16-year-old boy presented to an urban ED with chest pain, shortness of breath, and a jittery feeling for 3 hours.[54] In triage, he was noted to be very agitated and in significant distress. He was extremely anxious and was clutching his chest. He was tachypneic and short of breath. He was unable to respond to questions or to remain stationary. He admitted to using intranasal cocaine 15 minutes before the onset of his chest pain. He denied use of alcohol, tobacco, or medications.

The teenager was immediately placed on supplemental oxygen. Physical examination revealed a heart rate of 140/min, respirations 30/min, and blood pressure 160/98. He was afebrile and acyanotic. He had no nasal flaring. His pupils were equal and reactive. Chest wall movements were symmetric, and breath sounds were equal bilaterally without wheezing. Cardiac examination revealed tachycardia, regular rhythm, and no murmur. He was "hyperalert" and oriented, but he responded to questions only when asked 2 to 3 times. The remainder of his examination was unremarkable.

Chest radiography was normal. The patient's pain improved, and 15 minutes after arrival he was more comfortable and less dyspneic. After a period of observation, he was asymptomatic with normal vital signs, and he was discharged from the ED.

Drugs of Abuse and Chest Pain

Teenagers frequently have chest pain as a result of illicit drug use.[8] It is estimated there were 19.9 million illicit drug users in 2007.[55] After marijuana, cocaine was the second most commonly used illicit drug in the United States. It is estimated that 14% of people in the United States 12 years and older (34 million people) have tried cocaine at least once.[56] Overall, rates of illicit drug use among 12- to 17-year-olds have decreased in the United States, from 11.6% in 2001 to 9.5% of the population in 2007.[55]

Cocaine is the illicit drug that leads to most ED visits.[56] In 2005, almost half a million ED visits in the United States were related to cocaine use (all ages), and most of these were because of chest pain.[56,57] Numerous cases of cocaine-related MI have been reported in young patients with and without coronary artery disease.[58] Cocaine can be consumed by smoking (free-based), nasal insufflation, or IV injection. Smoking (eg, "crack" cocaine) is the most common method of use.[57] Unlike the teenager in case 5, many patients who use cocaine also concomitantly use tobacco, alcohol, or prescription medications.

Chest pain associated with cocaine is often described as "tight" or "pressure-like" rather than "sharp," and it is typically confined to the chest and arm. There is often associated diaphoresis, nausea, vomiting, dyspnea, anxiety, palpitations, or dizziness.[56] Physical examination often reveals elevated blood pressure, tachycardia, and tachypnea, as noted in case 5.[58]

The incidence of acute MI with cocaine use is as high as 6% in adults.[58,59] (The incidence in the adolescent population is unknown.) Cocaine-associated MI occurs soon after ingestion, usually within 3 hours.[56] Chest pain associated with cocaine (even small doses taken intranasally) is commonly related to coronary artery vasospasm. The conduction system may also be affected, leading to cardiac arrhythmias such as torsades de points, atrial fibrillation, supraventricular tachycardia, and ventricular tachycardia.

Some adolescents may also develop spontaneous pneumothorax or pneumomediastinum within 1 to 6 hours of snorting or smoking cocaine.[17] They will complain of pleuritic chest pain, neck pain, sore throat, dysphagia, and dyspnea. Physical examination of these patients will likely reveal tachypnea, tachycardia, subcutaneous emphysema of the chest neck and face, and a crunching sound over the retrosternal area (Hamman crunch). Chest radiography confirms the pneumothorax or pneumomediastinum.

Consider screening for illicit drugs in all teenagers with chest pain. Adolescents are unreliable at self-reporting drug use.[8,60] Cocaine can be detected in urine for 24 to 48 hours after use.[56] An abnormal ECG has been reported in 56% to 84% of patients with cocaine-associated chest pain.[56] Electrocardiography may show findings consistent with acute coronary ischemia, arrhythmias, or pericarditis. Serum cardiac enzymes (troponins) may be elevated in patients with chest pain who use cocaine, indicating evidence of a MI.

Treatment of chest pain associated with ischemia induced by cocaine is similar to that of patients presenting with acute coronary syndrome and should include aspirin and clopidogrel. Use of beta blockers is controversial. Many experts believe these should be avoided, because unopposed alpha-adrenergic stimulation can lead to increased coronary artery vasospasm and worsening cardiac circulation and ischemia.[56] Benzodiazepines should be instituted early because they decrease the central stimulation of cocaine, reduce chest pain, and improve cardiovascular hemodynamics.[61] Nitroglycerine decreases coronary artery vasospasm in cocaine users who present with ischemia.[56]

Methamphetamine, a synthetic central nervous system stimulant, produces a rapid "high" like cocaine. This drug causes chest pain and acute coronary syndrome in young adults.[62] Teenagers may present to the ED with acute severe chest pain after taking Ecstasy (3,4-methylenedioxymethamphetamine [MDMA]) and then dancing for several hours. They usually have tachycardia, hypertension, and palpitations. Chest radiographs and ECG may be normal. Pain is likely related to intercostal muscle spasm rather than cardiac ischemia.[63] However, some patients present with pleuritic chest pain after ecstasy abuse related to spontaneous pneumomediastinum. This may be the result of excessive physical exertion after using this drug.[64]

In addition, crystal methamphetamine (Ice) can cause unstable angina in patients as young as 14 years without significant past medical history or other cardiac risk factors.[8,65] Moreover, amphetamine-based diet pills can lead to chest pain, palpitations, headaches, and insomnia. Although the US Food and Drug Administration has banned most amphetamine-based anorectics, some are still purchased and used illegally.

Finally, adolescents may inhale, ingest, inject, or smoke "bath salts," a powder with amphetamine or cocaine-like effects. These agents contain mephedrone (or other similar chemicals), a chemical analog of amphetamine. They are often labeled as "bath salts," "plant food," or "insect repellent" and are sold in some gas stations, in smoke shops, and on the Internet with names such as Energizing Aromatherapy, Ivory Wave, and Red Dove. In the first 4 months of 2011, 1800 calls about bath salts were made to poison centers nationwide. Some patients using these drugs present with hypertension, tachycardia, and chest pressure or pain so severe they fear that they are dying. They may also have anxiety, extreme paranoia, delusions, hallucinations, and suicidal ideation.[8] On physical examinations, these patients have agitation (53%), tachycardia (40%), hypertension (20%), and seizures (20%).[66]

Adolescents with acute intoxication require urgent management of hypertension, agitation, and hyperthermia. Use IV benzodiazepines to treat severe agitation. Physical restraints are dangerous because patients who struggle against the restraints undergo isometric muscle contractions associated with lactic acidosis, hyperthermia, sudden cardiac collapse, and death.[67]

GENERAL APPROACH TO TEENAGERS WITH CHEST PAIN

The cases described emphasize that adolescent chest pain can be serious and life-threatening. However, most adolescents with chest pain do not need immediate management. There is generally time to take a thorough history and perform a careful physical examination. These will guide the need for laboratory studies, specific treatment, and referral to a specialist for further evaluation.[7]

History

A complete history reveals the etiology of chest pain in most cases. Determine the *onset* of pain. Patients with acute onset of pain (within 48 hours of presentation) are more likely to have an organic etiology for the pain. The etiology is not always serious, but pneumonia, asthma, trauma, pneumothorax, and arrhythmia are more likely if the pain is recent.[1] Adolescents with chronic pain, no specific diagnosis, and no abnormal findings despite months of symptoms are much more likely to be idiopathic or to have a psychogenic etiology.[1,27]

Next, learn what *precipitates* the pain. Chest pain precipitated by running or exercise is very concerning and may relate to cardiac disease or exercise-induced asthma.[3,7,68] Inquire about trauma, rough play, or recent overuse of chest wall muscles (eg, participation in wrestling, football, pushups, weight lifting, or gymnastics). Find out if the teen has recently eaten spicy foods or is taking medications or drugs such as tetracycline, oral contraceptives, or cocaine.[7]

Ask about *associated complaints*. Chest pain associated with syncope or palpitations is more significant and may relate to an arrhythmia or other cardiac disease. Chest pain associated with dizziness when standing suggests dehydration but could also correlate with cardiac insufficiency. Associated fever is highly concerning for an infection such as pneumonia, influenza, myocarditis, or pericarditis. Joint pain or rash associated with chest pain may indicate a collagen vascular disease. Psychogenic chest pain is often associated with other somatic complaints or sleep disturbance. Inquire about recent significant stress (eg, separation from friends, severe illness/death or divorce in the family, school failure.)

Ascertain the *severity* and *frequency* of chest pain. Verify if the pain is so severe that the teen is missing school or work. Constant, frequent severe pain is more likely to be distressing and interrupt daily activity, even if the etiology is not serious.[7]

Ask the patient to *describe the pain*. The location and quality of the pain sometimes point to an etiology. For example, burning pain in the sternal area may indicate esophagitis. Sharp pain in a febrile adolescent, which is relieved by sitting up and leaning forward, implies pericarditis.[7]

Review the *past medical history*. History of asthma places the patient at risk for more serious causes of chest pain, such as pneumonia or pneumothorax. Ask about previously diagnosed heart disease. Previous heart disease or conditions such as longstanding insulin-dependent diabetes mellitus (hyperlipidemia) or Kawasaki disease (coronary artery aneurysms) may increase the risk of cardiac pathology.[7,24,69] Patients who had surgical repair of transposition of the great arteries are at risk for subsequent ischemia and even MI. Most underlying structural cardiac lesions rarely produce chest pain.[7] Consider acute chest syndrome if the patient has sickle cell disease, and aortic dissection or pneumothorax if the patient has Marfan syndrome. Chest pain in an adolescent girl with an underlying collagen vascular disease could be the result of a pleural effusion or pericarditis.

Obtain a *family history* because some cardiac disorders are familial (eg, family history of HCM or sudden death).[37] A negative family history goes against HCM but does not rule it out. Many families/adolescents are understandably concerned about chest pain when there is a family history of serious disease, yet the patient often has a non-organic etiology.[1]

Finally, discover how the pain has been managed at home and ask about their *fears* and *concerns*.

Physical Examination

Perform a careful physical examination (Table 2). Quickly identify the adolescent in severe distress who needs immediate treatment for life-threatening conditions (eg, pneumothorax). Differentiate hyperventilation from respiratory distress. Review the *vital signs*. If the teen has orthostatic changes, consider

Table 2
Important physical examination findings in adolescent chest pain

Severe distress?
Chronically ill appearance?
Skin rash or bruising?
Abdominal pathology?
Arthritis present?
Anxiety apparent?
Chest examination
Inspection: trauma, asymmetry, abnormal breathing pattern?
Auscultation: tachycardia, arrhythmia, murmur, rub, rales, wheezing?
Palpation: tenderness, subcutaneous emphysema?

Adapted from Selbst SM. Evaluation of chest pain in children. *Pediatr Rev.* 1986;8:56-62.

dehydration, but also think about possible cardiac insufficiency (pump failure). If fever is noted, consider pneumonia, influenza infection, myocarditis, or pericarditis.

Note *signs of chronic disease,* such as pallor, poor growth, or a sallow appearance, which suggest the chest pain is a symptom of a more complex problem (eg, Hodgkin lymphoma or lupus). Consider Marfan syndrome if the patient is tall and thin with an upper extremity span that exceeds the patient's height. Look for *signs of anxiety.*[7] Examine the *skin* for rashes (possibly associated with a collagen vascular disease) or bruises (suggesting trauma). Examine the *abdomen* and consider referred pain to the chest. Examine the *joints* (arthritis may point to a collagen vascular disease).

Carefully examine the *chest.* Look for abnormal breathing, signs of trauma, or asymmetry as a result of cardiomegaly, scoliosis, or breast enlargement. Auscultate for rales, wheezes, and decreased breath sounds. Listen for a heart murmur, rub, muffled sounds, and arrhythmia.[7] A murmur that intensifies with a Valsalva maneuver and the standing position is the hallmark of HCM. Examine the heart while the patient is in the upright, supine, and standing positions. *Palpate the chest wall* (including the pectoral muscles) for tenderness. Musculoskeletal chest pain is usually reproduced by palpation or by moving the arms and chest through a variety of positions. Tenderness of the sternum at the costochondral junctions suggests costochondritis. Palpable subcutaneous air implies a pneumothorax or pneumomediastinum.[7,17] Breast tenderness could indicate physiologic changes of adolescence or pregnancy.

Laboratory Studies

Diagnostic studies generally confirm previously known disorders or findings that were suspected clinically but are not always necessary for adolescents with chest pain. If the history and physical examination do not point to a specific diagnosis, laboratory tests are usually not helpful.

Consider chest radiography and electrocardiography when the patient has acute onset of chest pain (began in the past 2 or 3 days) or findings specific for pulmonary problems or cardiac disease. Certainly obtain an ECG and chest radiograph if the chest pain occurs with exertion or syncope or when the patient has a history of heart disease.[1,7,26,70] Obtain a chest radiograph when the patient has fever, respiratory distress, or decreased or abnormal breath sounds. Order an ECG if the patient has an abnormal cardiac examination, including unexplained tachycardia, arrhythmia, murmur, rub, or click.

Laboratory studies are probably not necessary in the adolescent with chronic pain, a normal physical examination, and no history indicating cardiac or pulmonary disease. However, sometimes an ECG is helpful to relieve anxiety about chest pain and to reassure the family. Blood counts and sedimentation rates are of limited value unless sickle cell disease, a collagen vascular disease, infection, or malignancy is suspected. Obtain a drug screen in an adolescent with acute pain that is associated with anxiety, tachycardia, hypertension, or shortness of breath. Cardiac enzymes (troponin) are rarely of value unless there are specific concerns for ischemia based on the history or examination. If PE is suspected, computerized tomographic scan of the chest may be needed because the D-dimer test is not reliable. Refer the patient for Holter monitoring if an arrhythmia is strongly suspected. Consider an echocardiogram to diagnose structural heart disease.[7,26] Table 3 summarizes an approach to the child with chest pain. Table 4 summarizes the indications for diagnostic testing in adolescents with chest pain.

Table 3
Approach to the adolescent with chest pain

---

1. Check the vital signs and general appearance of the patient.
2. Determine whether immediate treatment is needed.
3. Do not assume adolescent chest pain is cardiac in nature.
4. Do not assume adolescent chest pain is always benign.
5. Assess the severity of pain and its effect on the patient's life.
6. Determine whether chest pain is part of a chronic underlying condition.
7. Consider laboratory studies if history is concerning or physical examination is abnormal.
8. Avoid expensive, invasive laboratory studies with chronic pain and normal physical examination, benign history.

Table 4
Indications for diagnostic testing in adolescent chest pain

Worrisome history
  Acute onset of pain
  Pain with exertion
  History of heart disease
  Serious associated medical problems (diabetes mellitus, asthma, Marfan syndrome, Kawasaki disease, anemia, lupus erythematosus)
  Use of drugs (cocaine, oral contraceptives)
  Associated complaints (syncope, dizziness, palpitations)
  Significant trauma
  Fever
Abnormal physical examination
  Respiratory distress
  Palpation of subcutaneous air
  Decreased breath sounds
  Cardiac findings (murmurs, rubs, arrhythmias)
  Fever
  Trauma

Reproduced with permission from Selbst SM. Chest pain and palpitations. In: Wolfson AB, Hendey GW, Ling LJ, et al (eds). *The Clinical Practice of Emergency Medicine*. 6th ed. Philadelphia, PA: Wolters Kluwer; 2014:1141-1145.

MANAGEMENT OF ADOLESCENT CHEST PAIN

Treat specific conditions (eg, pneumonia, asthma) identified as the cause of chest pain. Cardiac pathology needs rapid definitive treatment as noted in the cases discussed here. For most adolescents with musculoskeletal, psychogenic, or idiopathic chest pain, it is best to treat with acetaminophen, non-steroidal anti-inflammatory analgesics, rest, and reassurance. Consider use of heat and relaxation techniques to manage pain. When esophagitis is suspected, begin a therapeutic trial of antacids. For pill-induced esophagitis, discontinue tetracycline medication and treat with sucralfate.[14] Counsel patients with chest pain related to stress and anxiety.[7,26]

DISPOSITION AND REFERRAL

Admit the adolescent who is in distress or has abnormal vital signs to the hospital for monitoring, further diagnostic studies, and extended treatment. Refer all patients who have pain with exertion, syncope, dizziness, or palpitations for further evaluation. They may require a Holter monitor, an echocardiogram, exercise stress tests, or pulmonary function tests to evaluate for an arrhythmia, structural heart disease, or exercise-induced asthma. Refer patients with serious emotional problems to a psychiatrist. Refer patients to a cardiologist if they have known or suspected heart disease, even though the pain may prove to be unrelated.[7] Table 5 summarizes the indications for referring an adolescent with chest pain.

Arrange appropriate follow-up with a primary care physician. Many adolescents with ill-defined chest pain have persistent symptoms for many months. Serious organic pathology is unlikely to be found in the future in such patients.[9,71] However, some of these patients are prevented from participating in their usual activities because of the pain, and some manifest significant psycho-emotional problems or exercise-induced asthma that was not recognized initially.[9,71]

Table 5
When to refer an adolescent with chest pain

- Acute distress
- History of heart disease or related serious medical problem
- Pain with exercise, syncope, palpitations, dizziness
- Pneumothorax, pleural effusion
- Serious emotional disturbance
- Significant trauma

References

1. Selbst SM, Ruddy RM, Clark BJ, et al. Pediatric chest pain: a prospective study. *Pediatrics.* 1988;82:319-323
2. Massin MM, Bourguignont A, Coremans C, et al. Chest pain in pediatric patients presenting to an emergency department or to a cardiac clinic. *Clin Pediatr (Phila).* 2004;43(3):231-238
3. Danduran MJ. Chest pain: characteristics of children and adolescents. *Pediatr Cardiol.* 2008;29: 775-781
4. Drossner DM, Hirsh DA, Sturm JJ, et al. Cardiac disease in pediatric patients presenting to a pediatric ED with chest pain. *Am J Emerg Med.* 2011;29:632-638
5. Friedman KG, Kane DA, Rathod RH, et al. Management of pediatric chest pain using a standardized assessment and management plan. *Pediatrics.* 2011;128:239-245
6. Saleeb SF, Li WY, Warren SZ, et al. Effectiveness of screening for life-threatening chest pain in children. *Pediatrics.* 2011;128:e1062-e1068
7. Selbst SM. Approach to the child with chest pain. *Pediatr Clin North Am.* 2010;57:1221-1234
8. Selbst SM, Palermo R, Durani Y, et al. Adolescent chest pain: is it the heart? *Clin Pediatr Emerg Med.* 2011;12:289-300
9. Selbst, SM, Ruddy R, Clark BJ. Chest pain in children: follow-up of patients previously reported. *Clin Pediatr (Phila).* 1990;29:374-377
10. Driscoll DJ, Glicklich LB, Gallen WJ. Chest pain in children: a prospective study. *Pediatrics.* 1976;57:648-651
11. Eslick GD. Epidemiology and risk factors of pediatric chest pain: a systematic review. *Pediatr Clin North Am.* 2010;57:1211-1219
12. Lipsitz JD, Gur M, Sonnet FM, et al. Psychopathology and disability in children with unexplained chest pain presenting to the pediatric emergency department. *Pediatr Emerg Care.* 2010;26: 830-836
13. Berezin S, Medow MS. Glassman MS, et al. Chest pain of gastrointestinal origin. *Arch Dis Child.* 1988;63:1457
14. Palmer K, Selbst SM, Shaffer S, Proujansky R. Chest pain induced by tetracycline ingestion. *Pediatr Emerg Care.* 1999;15:200-201
15. Dotson K, Johnson LH. Pediatric spontaneous pneumothorax. *Pediatr Emerg Care.* 2012;28: 715-719
16. Bullaro FM, Bartoletti SC. Spontaneous pneumomediastinum in children: a literature review. *Pediatr Emerg Care.* 2007;23:28-30
17. Uva JL. Spontaneous pneumothoraces, pneumomediastinum, and pneumoperitoneum: consequences of smoking crack cocaine. *Pediatr Emerg Care.* 1997;13:24-26
18. Agha BS, Sturm JJ, Simon HK, et al. Pulmonary embolism in the pediatric emergency department. *Pediatrics.* 2013;132:663-667
19. Taylor C, Carter F, Poulose J, et al. Clinical presentation of acute chest syndrome in sickle cell disease. *Postgrad Med J.* 2004;80:346-349
20. Van Karnebeek CDM, Naeff MSJ, Mulder BJM, et al. Natural history of cardiovascular manifestations in Marfan syndrome. *Arch Dis Child.* 2001;84:129-137
21. Miller A, Texidor TA. "Precordial catch" a neglected syndrome of precordial pain. *JAMA.* 1955;159:1364-1365
22. Mahle WT, Campbell RM, Favaloro-Sabatier J. Myocardial infarction in adolescents. *J Pediatr.* 2007;151:150-154
23. Desai A, Patel S, Book W. Myocardial infarction in adolescents: do we have the correct diagnosis? *Pediatr Cardiol.* 2005;26:627-631
24. Madhok AB, Boxer R, Green S. An adolescent with chest pain: sequela of Kawasaki disease. *Pediatr Emerg Care.* 2004;20:765-768
25. Lane JR, Ben-Shachar G. Myocardial infarction in healthy adolescents. *Pediatrics.* 2007;120: e938-e943

26. Gokale J, Selbst SM. Chest pain and chest wall deformity. *Pediatr Clin North Am.* 2009;56:49-65

27. Galioto FM. Child chest pain—a course of action. *Contemp Pediatr.* 2007;24:47-57

28. Schlechte E. Supraventricular tachycardia in the pediatric primary care setting: age-related presentation, diagnosis and management. *J Pediatr Health Care.* 2008;22:289-299

29. Fox DJ, Tschenko A, Krahn D, et al. Supraventricular tachycardia: diagnosis and management. *Mayo Clin Proc.* 2008;83:1400-1411

30. Chun T, Van Hare G. Advances in the approach to treatment of supraventricular tachycardia in the pediatric population. *Curr Cardiol Rep.* 2004;6:322-326

31. Doniger S, Sharieff G. Pediatric dysrhythmias. *Pediatr Clin North Am.* 2006;53:85-105

32. Hanisch D. Pediatric arrhythmias. *J Pediatr Nurs.* 2001;16:351-362

33. Diaz-Para SP, Sanchez-Yanez I, Zabala-Arguelles B, et al. Use of adenosine in the treatment of supraventricular tachycardia in a pediatric emergency department. *Pediatr Emerg Care.* 2014;30:388-393

34. Manole MD, Saladino RA. Emergency department management of the pediatric patient with supraventricular tachycardia. *Pediatr Emerg Care.* 2007;23:176-185

35. Wen ZC, Chen SA, Tai CT, et al. Electophysiological mechanisms and determinants of vagal maneuvers for termination of paroxysmal supraventricular tachycardia. *Circulation.* 1999;98:2716-2733

36. Qureshi A. Optimal dose of adenosine effective for supraventricular tachycardia in children. *J Coll Phys Surg Pak.* 2012;22:648-651

37. Maron BJ, Doerer JJ, Haas TS, et al. Sudden deaths in young competitive athletes: analysis of 1866 deaths in the United States, 1980-2006. *Circulation.* 2009;119:1085-1092

38. Marian AJ. Contemporary treatment of hypertrophic cardiomyopathy. *Tex Heart Inst J.* 2009;36:194-204

39. Cava JR, Sayger PL. Chest pain in children and adolescents. *Pediatr Clin North Am.* 2004;51:1553-1568

40. Elliott PM, Kaski JC, Prasad K, et al. Chest pain during daily life in patients with hypertrophic cardiomyopathy: an ambulatory electrocardiographic study. *Eur Heart J.* 1996;17:1056-1064

41. Maron BJ, McKenna WJ, Danielson GK; American College of Cardiology/European Society of Cardiology clinical expert consensus document on hypertrophic cardiomyopathy. A report of the American College of Cardiology Foundation Task Force on Clinical Expert Consensus Documents and the European Society of Cardiology Committee for Practice Guidelines. *J Am Coll Cardiol.* 2003;42:1687-1713

42. Duarte S, Bogaert J. The role of cardiac magnetic resonance in hypertrophic cardiomyopathy. *Rev Port Cardiol.* 2010;2991:79-93

43. Kasirye Y, Manne JR, Epperla N, et al. Apical hypertrophic cardiomyopathy presenting as recurrent unexplained syncope. *Clin Med Res.* 2011;10:26-31

44. Durani Y, Giordano K, Goudie BW. Myocarditis and pericarditis in children. *Pediatr Clin North Am.* 2010:57:1281-1303

45. Freedman SB, Haladyn JK, Floh A, et al. Pediatric myocarditis: emergency department clinical findings and diagnostic evaluation. *Pediatrics.* 2007;120:1278-1285

46. Durani Y, Egan M, Baffa J, et al. Pediatric myocarditis: presenting clinical characteristics. *Am J Emerg Med.* 2009;27:942-947

47. Levine MC, Klugman D, Teach SJ. Update on myocarditis in children. *Curr Opin Pediatr.* 2010;22:278-283

48. Pettit, MA, Koyfman A, Forman, M, et al. Myocarditis. *Pediatr Emerg Care.* 2014;30:832-838

49. Troughton RW, Asher CR, Klein AL. Pericarditis. *Lancet.* 2004;363:717-727

50. Imazio M, Cecchi E, Demichelis B, et al. Indicators of poor prognosis of acute pericarditis. *Circulation.* 2007;115:2739-2744

51. Roodpeyma S, Sadeghian N. Acute pericarditis in childhood: a 10 year experience. *Pediatr Cardiol.* 2000;21:363-367

52. Blanco CC, Parekh JB, Adam HM. Pericarditis. *Pediatr Rev.* 2010;31:83-84

53. Wang ZJ, Reddy GP, Gotway MB, et al. CT and MRI imaging of pericardial disease. *Radiographics.* 2003;23:S167-S180

54. Woodward GA, Selbst SM. Chest pain secondary to cocaine use. *Pediatr Emerg Care.* 1987;3: 153-154
55. Substance Abuse and Mental Health Services Administration. Results from the 2007 National Survey on Drug Use and Health: National Findings. Office of Applied Studies, NSDUH Series H-34, DHHS Publication No. SMA 08-4343. Rockville, MD: Substance Abuse and Mental Health Services Administration; 2008
56. McCord J, Jneid H, Hollander J, et al. Management of cocaine-associated chest pain and myocardial infarction. A scientific statement from the American Heart Association Acute Cardiac Care Committee of the Council on Clinical Cardiology. *Circulation.* 2008;117;1897-1907
57. Keller KB, Lemberg L. The cocaine-abused heart. *Am J Crit Care.* 2003;12:562-566
58. Hollander J, Hoffman R, Gennis P, et al. Prospective multicenter evaluation of cocaine-associated chest pain. Cocaine Associated Chest Pain (CHOCHPA) Study. *Acad Emerg Med.* 1994;1:330-339
59. Bansal D, Eigenbrodt M, Gupta E, et al. Traditional risk factors and acute myocardial infarction in patients hospitalized with cocaine-associated chest pain. *Clin Cardiol.* 2007;30:290-294
60. Lee M, Vivier P, Diercks D. Is the self-report of recent cocaine or methamphetamine use reliable in illicit stimulant drug users who present to the emergency department with chest pain? *J Emerg Med.* 2009;37:237-241
61. Hollander J. The management of cocaine-associated myocardial ischemia. *N Engl J Med.* 1995;333:1267-1272
62. Turnipseed SD, Richards JR, Kirk JD, et al. Frequency of acute coronary syndrome in patients presenting to the emergency department with chest pain after methamphetamine use. *J Emerg Med.* 2003;24:369-373
63. Ritoo D, Rittoo DB, Rittoo D. Misuse of ecstasy. Letter to the Editor. *BMJ.* 1992;305:309-310
64. Quin GI, McCarthy GM, Harries DK. Spontaneous pneumomediastinum and ecstasy abuse. *J Accid Emerg Med.* 1999;16:382
65. Wijetunga M, Bhan R, Lindsay J, et al. Acute coronary syndrome and crystal methamphetamine use: a case series. *Hawaii Med J.* 2004;63:8-13, 25
66. Wood DM. Clinical pattern of toxicity associated with the novel synthetic cathinone mephedrone. *Emerg Med J.* 2011;28:280-282
67. Boyer EW, Hernon C. *Methamphetamine Intoxication.* Waltham, MA: UpToDate; 2015
68. Weins L, Sabath R, Ewing L, et al. Chest pain in otherwise healthy children and adolescents is frequently caused by exercise induced asthma. *Pediatrics.* 1992;90:350-353
69. Declue TJ, Malone JI, Root AW. Coronary artery disease in diabetic adolescents. *Clin Pediatr.* 1988;27:587-590
70. Swenson JM, Fischer DR, Miller SA. Are chest radiographs and electrocardiograms still valuable in evaluating new pediatric patients with heart murmurs and or chest pain? *Pediatrics.* 1990;29: 374-377
71. Lam JC, Tobias JD. Follow-up survey of children and adolescents with chest pain. *South Med J.* 2001;94:921-924

Adolesc Med 026 (2015) 552–569

Approach to the Adolescent Psychiatric and Behavioral Health Emergency

Alessandra Guiner, MD[a]; Harsha Chandnani, MD, MBA, MPH[a]; David Chao, MD[a,b,c]*

[a]Department of Pediatrics, The University of Nevada School of Medicine, Las Vegas, Nevada; [b]Emergency Medicine Physicians, Canton, Ohio; [c]Division of Emergency Medicine, Rady Children's Hospital and Department of Pediatrics, University of California San Diego, San Diego, California

INTRODUCTION

The Surgeon General of the United States has declared a "crisis in mental health-care for infants, children and adolescents."[1] This crisis is a result of the convergence of a rise in mental health diagnoses among young people and limitations in resources to care for patients with mental health disorders. More than 20% of the adolescent population in the United States suffers from a diagnosable mental or addictive disorder that causes some degree of functional impairment. In approximately half of these young people, the degree of functional impairment is categorized as *severe*.[2] Because of the wide range of factors, such as limitations in access to mental health care and the stigma of mental illness, only 20% to 30% of children and adolescents with identified mental health disorders currently receive mental health services.[3]

Many young people with mental health or behavioral problems present to acute care settings in crisis. It is the responsibility of the acute care physician to assess, stabilize, and determine dispositions for adolescents presenting with psychiatric and behavioral health emergencies safely, appropriately, and efficiently. Psychiatric and behavioral emergencies comprise approximately 3.3% of total pediatric emergency department (ED) visits, an increase from 1.1% of total visits a decade ago.[4,5] These patients place a significant strain on our health care system. They more commonly arrive by ambulance (19.4% vs. 8.2%), stay longer in the ED (3.2 vs. 2.1 hours), and are more often hospitalized (30.5% vs. 11.2%) than patients

*Corresponding author
E-mail address: davidchaomd@yahoo.com

presenting with non-psychiatric complaints.[5] As a result, a tremendous amount of resources are spent on ensuring the proper care of adolescent patients presenting in mental health and behavioral crisis.

EVALUATION OF ADOLESCENTS PRESENTING IN PSYCHIATRIC CRISIS

Goals of Emergency Treatment

A major challenge facing the medical practitioner is the ability to effectively recognize, assess, and manage adolescents presenting to the acute care setting with a range of psychiatric and behavioral symptoms. The most common presenting complaints to the ED for mental health issues among young people are related to substance abuse-related disorders, anxiety disorders, attention deficit and disruptive disorders, mood disorders, and psychotic disorders.[4] In addition to being able to recognize and manage these varied presentations, the physician must be comfortable with crisis intervention and be proficient in coordinating safe dispositions.[6]

The role of the acute care physician is not to make a specific psychiatric *diagnosis,* because that is the responsibility of the mental health physician who ultimately assumes care of the adolescent. Instead, the focus of the acute care physician should be recognizing and managing the adolescent's presenting *symptoms.* In treating an adolescent who presents with an acute mental health or behavioral emergency, several steps must be taken to ultimately ensure a safe disposition. Goals of emergency treatment are listed in Table 1. In order to accomplish these goals, the acute care physician must be able to obtain an adequate history (including a confidential and thorough psychosocial history), perform a complete physical examination (with particular attention to findings related to organic etiologies and manifestations of psychiatric symptoms), and understand how to manage acute psychiatric and behavioral symptoms safely and effectively.

Table 1
Goals of emergency treatment

- Identify psychiatric/behavioral emergency
- Assess for safety and address concerns
- Obtain thorough history and perform complete physical examination
- Identify factors contributing to condition (medical, developmental, social)
- Consider organic etiologies of presenting symptoms
- Stabilize acute symptoms
- Evaluate current level of functioning
- Identify support system
- Enlist help of social and mental health resources
- Formulate safe disposition plan

Patient Assessment

A complete psychosocial evaluation can serve as an informative diagnostic tool as well as the basis for an effective treatment plan for an adolescent presenting with a psychiatric or behavioral emergency. The history of present illness should include details regarding the presenting crisis and identifiable precipitants, a history of past psychiatric or behavioral problems, including similar episodes and previous treatment and hospitalizations, and current mental health treatment and medications. The social history is a critical part of information–gathering from an adolescent, and obtaining a complete social history may prove to be the difference between making a correct diagnosis and being led on a diagnostic misadventure. It is important to remember that an adolescent's physical symptoms may be a somatic manifestation of external stressors. Obtaining a thorough psychosocial history may be challenging in the busy setting of an ED; however, failure to elicit information that may be pertinent to an adolescent's presentation may lead to unnecessary testing, referrals, and future visits, and may compromise the safe discharge of that patient.

When interviewing an adolescent, it is important to first establish rapport as well as a framework for communication. Set the stage by introducing yourself to the adolescent first, and have the adolescent introduce you to the other people in the room. This sends the adolescent a clear message that you are interested in the patient and the presenting symptoms. Inform the caregiver that it is standard procedure for the physician to interview all adolescent patients alone, and then escort caregivers and other family members to an area out of sight and earshot of the patient. Caregivers who fail to comply may raise a red flag that something may be amiss within the family dynamic. When alone with the adolescent, it is critical to initiate the conversation by establishing confidentiality; however, it is important for the physician to be knowledgeable about the laws regarding limits of confidentiality, which vary by locality.[7] Caregivers should also be interviewed in private to ascertain their level of understanding of the adolescent's symptoms and social environment, and to determine the level of support that the family is currently able to provide.

The HEADSS examination is a widely used framework from which to conduct a comprehensive psychosocial interview with an adolescent.[8] It addresses the domains of an adolescent's life and seeks to identify relationships and experiences that may relate to the patient's presenting symptoms. This assessment may also uncover issues that are not related to the adolescent's presenting complaints but that may affect the patient's health and safety. The interview begins with more "benign" topics first and progresses through the following domains: *h*ome, *e*ducation (school), *a*ctivities, *d*rug and alcohol use, *s*exuality, and *s*uicidality/depression. We have adapted the HEADSS examination as described by Cohen et al[8] to include 2 additional topics: *s*afety and *s*trengths ("HEADSSSS"). It is important to assess an adolescent's perception of safety in all environments (home, school, work) and in all interpersonal relationships. It is also important to ask adolescents explicitly whether they are being harmed or feel threatened in any of their relationships. It is our opinion that identification of strengths mollifies the potentially negative tone of the interview. In addition, readiness of an adolescent to identify personal strengths may serve as a basis for an effective disposition plan, whereas difficulties identifying strengths may raise a red flag about the severity of illness and potential for danger.

Conducting a thorough physical examination is crucial in the comprehensive assessment of an adolescent patient presenting with acute psychiatric symptoms. The physician should have a heightened sense of awareness with regard to identifying signs that may point towards possible organic etiologies of psychiatric symptoms. A thorough neurologic, musculoskeletal, and skin examination is important in identifying signs of injury. In addition, if the adolescent is presenting with altered mental status or suspected ingestion, attention should be made to identifying other physical and toxidromic signs. Some common medical causes of altered mental status can be remembered by using the mnemonic "VITAMINS." These causes include: Vascular (eg, stroke, vasculities, atypical migraines), Infections (eg, meningitis, encephalitis, sepsis), Toxins (drugs, poisoning), Accidents/Abuse (eg, head injury), Metabolic (eg, electrolyte abnormalities, vitamin deficiencies, renal or endocrine disease), Intussusception, Neoplasm, and Seizures.[9] Table 2 lists common toxidromes encountered in the acute care setting.[10]

The *mental status examination* is the mental health physician's correlate to the medical physician's physical examination. Clues gathered from this assessment can help the physician formulate a management plan appropriate for the adolescent patient. This examination comprises observations of the adolescent throughout the acute care visit. Features of this examination are listed in Table 3. After the component parts of the mental status examination have been assessed, the physician should organize these components into a comprehensive picture of the mental health of the adolescent, which can serve as the basis of an effective management plan.

CATEGORIES OF ILLNESS

Depression

One in 5 teens experiences clinical depression at some point in adolescence.[11] Adolescents with depression will most commonly present to the acute care setting in a state of crisis, which may take the form of suicidal ideation or a suicide attempt. The primary goals of the acute care physician are to determine whether the mood disturbance is organic or psychiatric in origin, to evaluate the patient for potential suicidality, and to determine a safe disposition plan for the adolescent.[12] Some organic causes of depression include hypothyroidism, infection,

Table 2
Common toxidromes

Physical findings	Adrenergic (decongestant, amphetamine, cocaine)	Anticholinergic (antihistamine, phenothiazine)	Cholinergic/ anticholin-esterase (insecticide)	Opioid toxidrome	Sedative-hypnotic (tranquilizer, barbiturate, ethanol)
Vital signs					
Respiratory rate	Increased	Normal	Normal/ increased	Decreased	Normal/ decreased
Heart rate	Increased	Increased	Decreased	Normal/ decreased	Normal
Temperature	Increased	Increased	No change	Normal/ decreased	Normal
Blood pressure	Increased	Normal/increased	No change	Normal/ decreased	Normal
Physical examination					
Mental status	Alert/ agitated	Depressed/ confused/ hallucinating	Depressed/ confused	Depressed	Depressed
Pupils	Dilated	Dilated	Constricted	Constricted	Normal
Mucous membranes	Wet	Dry	Wet	Normal	Normal
Skin findings	Diaphoretic	Dry	Diaphoretic	Normal	Normal
Reflexes	Increased	Normal	Normal/ decreased	Normal/ decreased	Normal/ decreased
Bowel sounds	Increased	Decreased	Increased	Decreased	Normal
Urinary ability	Increased	Decreased	Increased	Decreased	Normal
Other	Possible seizures	Possible seizures	Muscle fasciculations/ possible seizures/ vomiting		

Adapted with permission from Abbruzzi G, Stork CM. Pediatric toxicologic concerns. *Emerg Med Clin North Am.* 2002;20:223-247.

Table 3
Components of the mental status examination

- Orientation
- Appearance
- Memory
- Cognition
- Behavior
- Relatedness
- Speech
- Affect
- Thought process
- Thought content
- Insight
- Judgment
- Synthesis

anemia, vitamin deficiencies, malignancy, medications, illicit substance abuse, sleep-related disorders, and seizures.

Some characteristics of depression are listed in Table 4. It is important to consider that symptoms of psychiatric illness are influenced by the developmental stage of the child and that many depressed children will not strictly fulfill diagnostic criteria for depression. Depressed adolescents often present with somatic complaints such as headaches and abdominal pain, or nonspecific behavioral symptoms such as irritability and change in school performance. Adolescents may also externalize their feelings by exhibiting harmful behavior, such as sexual promiscuity, physical aggression, and substance abuse. Depressed adolescents should be carefully screened for suicidal ideation because of the strong association between depression and suicidal behavior or deliberate self-harm activity.[13] Medications should not be initiated by the acute care physician unless directed by a mental health specialist who can provide close follow-up in order to monitor for potential side effects.

Psychosis

There is no universally agreed-upon definition of psychosis, although it is characterized by a disruption in thinking often accompanied by delusions or hallucinations.[14] Primary psychotic disorders such as schizophrenia rarely manifest before mid-adolescence, with most diagnoses being made between the ages of 18 to 25 in men and 25 to 35 in women. Given the rarity of primary psychosis in the pediatric population, organic conditions should be strongly considered in adolescents presenting with psychotic symptoms. Some features may aid in differentiating organic and psychiatric etiologies of psychosis. Psychosis secondary to organic cause is usually acute in onset, has a preceding illness or is associated with drug use; if hallucinations are present they are more likely visual or tactile, and the patient may have an altered level of consciousness, abnormal autonomic signs, abnormal laboratory studies, and poor cognitive function. Psychosis because of psychiatric etiology usually has slower onset with hallucinations

Table 4
SIGECAPS mnemonic for characteristics of depression

S	Sleep: early awakenings, sleeping more (or less) than usual, difficulty falling asleep
I	Interest: loss of interest in activities/friends/hobbies
G	Guilt: feelings of fault, constantly apologetic
E	Energy: decreased
C	Concentration: inability to focus or make decisions
A	Appetite: decreased (or increased), weight gain/loss
P	Psychomotor changes: agitation or retardation
S	Suicidality: thoughts or attempts to hurt themselves

being auditory in nature, intact orientation/consciousness, normal cognitive function, and vital signs and laboratory findings that are within normal limits.[15] Organic causes of psychosis are numerous and varied, some of which include conditions of the central nervous system (eg, tumors, stroke, infection, seizure), infections (eg, meningitis, malaria, sepsis, bacterial endocarditis), cerebral hypoxia (eg, anemia, heart failure, carbon monoxide poisoning), metabolic and endocrine conditions (eg, thyroid, electrolyte disturbance, uremia, liver failure), rheumatic disease (eg, lupus), and many other conditions associated with drug ingestion, trauma, and paraneoplastic disorders.[15] Anti–N-methyl-D-aspartate receptor encephalitis is a relatively newly described paraneoplastic syndrome that presents with psychotic symptoms, often seen in young women with undiagnosed ovarian tumors, and should be considered in otherwise healthy young people presenting with acutely progressive psychotic symptoms.[16]

Adolescents with psychosis will usually present with *negative* symptoms, such as social withdrawal and mood changes, which represent a lack of emotions and behaviors that are typically present in healthy individuals. Families and patients with psychosis often will report decline in school grades, loss of interest in activities, and neglect of appearance. Schizophrenic patients are especially at risk for suicidal ideation and comorbidities such as substance abuse, and they should be screened for such behaviors.[17]

Adolescents presenting with psychosis should be admitted for medical reasons if an organic cause is suspected but has not yet been determined. They should be admitted to an inpatient psychiatric hospital if they are at high risk for self-harm, are persistently psychotic, or are newly diagnosed with psychosis in order to stabilize symptoms and initiate treatment.

Substance Abuse

Recent surveys conducted by the US Department of Health and Human Services have revealed encouraging trends reflecting a decrease in substance abuse among youth in the United States.[18,19] They reported decreasing rates of prescription opiate, cigarette, alcohol, methylenedioxymethamphetamine (MDMA; Ecstasy), and inhalant abuse among teens, while rates of marijuana abuse have remained stable. Despite these encouraging trends, drug and alcohol abuse among adolescents continues to be a major public health problem. It is the practitioner's duty to recognize clinical toxidromes and manage intoxicated patients safely and effectively.

Urine toxicology screening tests for drugs of abuse are relatively sensitive in detecting illicit or prescription substances to which an adolescent may have been exposed.[20] These tests are readily available, and turnaround times are typically short enough to make results clinically useful in an acute care setting. The physician must be aware of the time frame for detection of recreational doses as well as the limitations of these tests. For example, opioid screens will not detect synthetic opioids such as oxycodone, amphetamine screens will not detect MDMA, and cannabinoid screens will not detect synthetic cannabinoids. In addition, false-positive results, although uncommon, may mislead practitioners in their management of a patient presenting with altered mental status.

The general approach to treating an intoxicated adolescent is to provide a supportive and safe environment for the patient while the effects of the intoxicant wears off. Verbal reassurance and redirection alone are often effective in the management of the acutely intoxicated patient. If restraints are required to ensure the safety of a patient or staff, the physician must be cautious of potential complications, such as rhabdomyolysis in patients with acute phencyclidine intoxication and interactions between sedative medications and drugs of abuse.

A popular example of emerging drugs of abuse are synthetic cannabinoids (eg, Spice, K2), or synthetic cannabinoid receptor agonists.[21] Adolescents commonly use these substances because they are widely available, they are not detected by routine urine toxicology screening tests, and their legal status is currently evolving. Five of the most commonly used compounds used in these products have been scheduled as controlled substances by the US government, but a number of analogues remain legal and it takes many years for laws against the manufacture and sale of new drugs of abuse to be written and to take effect.[22] Although use among American adolescents is declining, approximately 6% of high school seniors reported using synthetic cannabinoids in the most recent survey conducted by the National Institutes of Health.[18] The effects of synthetic cannabinoids mirror those of natural cannabinoids; however, these substances have the potential to induce additional symptoms such as seizures. These chemicals also have significantly lower safety ratios compared to marijuana. Additionally, as with all of the newly synthesized chemical compounds, the long-term effects of these substances on the body are unknown, a fact that should be emphasized to adolescents who may misperceive these substances as "safer" because, until recently, they were legally obtained. The National Institute of Drug Abuse hosts a Web site that is regularly updated where physicians can access information regarding emerging drugs of abuse (www.drugabuse.gov/drugs-abuse/emerging-trends).

Psychosomatic Disorders

Psychosomatic disorders describe a group of conditions characterized by physical symptoms that cannot be attributed to a medical or neurologic cause. Up to 50% of pediatric patients present to primary care settings with complaints of medically unexplained symptoms that may cause significant functional and emotional impairment.[23,24] This can result in increased utilization of health resources, frequent hospitalizations, consultations, additional investigations and examinations, and unnecessary treatments. The patients usually present with other comorbidities, such as depression, anxiety disorders, social isolation, school problems, and family conflict.

These adolescents commonly present with pain (headaches, back pain, chest pain, abdominal pain), fatigue, loss of appetite, paralysis, abnormal movements, and perceived physical deformities. The diagnosis of psychosomatic disorder in the acute care setting is controversial, as attributing an organic medical condition to psychosomatic disorder is a pitfall. It is important to assess for organic disease while considering psychosomatic disorder as the cause of a patient's symptoms. A reasonable approach to treating an adolescent with suspected psychosomatic disorder is inclusion of referral to mental health services to address the stress-inducing aspects of the adolescent's condition as part of the comprehensive treatment plan.

MANAGEMENT OF ADOLESCENTS PRESENTING IN PSYCHIATRIC CRISIS

Medical Clearance

Acute care physicians are often called on to "medically clear" adolescents before arranging for a mental health assessment. The goals of medical clearance are 2-fold: to stabilize and address acute medical issues, and to assess for possible organic etiologies of psychiatric symptoms. It is important to note that adolescents with acute medical issues such as altered mental status and drug intoxication are not medically clear for psychiatric assessment and disposition until they have been medically stabilized and their mental status has returned to baseline.

The underlying principle behind medical clearance is that the process should be guided by an adolescent's history and physical examination.[25] A detailed history includes previous medical history, medications, allergies, family history, review of symptoms, menstrual history for females, and thorough psychosocial history. Physical examination should also be thorough, with special attention given to vital signs, general appearance, and the neurologic, skin, and mental status examinations.

Obtaining a thorough history and conducting a complete physical examination are sufficient for medical clearance of most adolescents. Any subsequent diagnostic testing should be medically indicated. There is no standard set of tests that is required of all patients presenting with psychiatric or behavioral concerns. In fact, studies have shown that the practice of ordering routine tests yields abnormal results that are often not clinically relevant.[26,27] Tests that may be considered if organic etiologies of psychiatric symptoms are suspected are listed in Table 5. Psychiatric inpatient facilities and detention centers may require the results of tests such as toxicology screens and pregnancy tests before the patients are accepted. Acceding to these requests may facilitate the efficient disposition of patients from busy emergency care settings.

Table 5
Screening tests to consider if medical illness suspected of causing psychiatric symptoms

• Complete blood count	• Lead/heavy metal testing
• Metabolic panel	• Nutritional testing
• Thyroid function tests	• Rapid plasma reagin
• Pregnancy test	• Electrocardiogram
• Urinalysis	• Brain imaging (computerized tomography or magnetic resonance
• Urine and serum	imaging)
toxicology screens	• Lumbar puncture
• Drug levels	• Electroencephalography

Management of the Agitated Adolescent

Many adolescents who are brought to acute care settings for psychiatric or behavioral emergencies present with agitation, or they become agitated during their clinical course. Causes of agitation may be medical, psychiatric, or behavioral in origin, and the etiology of the patient's agitation should be determined because it may affect the management of the patient's symptoms. One goal when restraining a patient should always be to choose the least restrictive modality to maintain the safety of the patient, staff, and others in the patient care setting.

When caring for the agitated adolescent, the safety of the patient and staff is the utmost priority. If all parties are deemed to be safe, the physician and staff should first attempt to verbally de-escalate the adolescent's level of agitation. Seclusion with constant visual observation may be necessary until the adolescent is able to demonstrate acceptable behavioral control.[28] Adolescents who are acutely psychotic should be placed in a space with limited stimuli, such as light and noise, to prevent further agitation. For safety reasons, all personal belongings and other items in the room that are potentially harmful should be removed, and 1:1 observation or video camera monitoring should be used.

When particularly agitated adolescents cannot be calmed with verbal de-escalation techniques or seclusion, it may be necessary to use physical or chemical restraints while they are being assessed and provided treatment. The American Academy of Pediatrics recommendations regarding the use of restraints state that the use of restraints "requires clear indications, safe application, reassessment guidelines, and use only after the consideration of alternative methods."[29] Restraints of any kind should be used as a last resort and should never be used to punish the patient or make management of the patient "easier" for staff.

The decision to physically restrain an adolescent patient should not be made lightly. The use of physical restraints has been shown to lead to significant patient morbidity and death, which include high-profile cases involving pediatric patients.[30,31] The physician should be knowledgeable about both institutional policies as well as standards published by the Joint Commission for Accreditation of Healthcare Organizations (JCAHO) and the Centers for Medicare and Medicaid Services (CMS) regarding physical restraint use (Table 6).[32,33] These protocols include time-restricted physician orders, monitoring of vital signs, and removal of restraints as soon as safety dictates. Only restraint devices designed specifically for use in medical settings should be used. Potential complications of physical restraint use, such as asphyxiation and circulatory compromise, should be a focus of application and reassessment of restrained patients.

The CMS defines a chemical restraint as "a medication used to control behavior or to restrict a patient's freedom of movement and not standard treatment for the patient's medical or psychiatric condition."[33,34] In agitated and violent adolescent patients, the most commonly used medications used for the purposes of restraint are antihistamines, benzodiazepines, and neuroleptics. Use of these medications for the purpose of restraint is not approved by the US Food and Drug Administration; however, off-label use for this purpose is commonly utilized safely in acute care medical settings.[35] It is the responsibility of the medical physician to understand the effects of the medications they choose to use, as well as their potential side effects and complications. When administering medications for the purpose of calming an agitated patient, voluntary administration should always be attempted before administration by force.[36]

High-potency neuroleptics are often used for their sedative properties in restraining a patient in the acute care setting. The most commonly discussed typical neuroleptics reported in the literature are haloperidol and droperidol, although the use of droperidol in practice may be limited secondary to its avail-

Table 6
JCAHO and CMS guidelines on assessment and monitoring of pediatric patients in restraints

Initiation of restraint	Order from a licensed physician or licensed independent practitioner within 1 hour of initiation.
Evaluation by physician or licensed independent practitioner	In-person evaluation within the first 2 hours for patients aged 9-17 years. If patient released before expiration of original order, in-person evaluation within 24 hours of initiation.
Reordering of restraints	Every 2 hours for youth (9-17 years) until released. Reorder can only be completed for 24 hours after initial order.
Reevaluation by physician or licensed independent practitioner	Every 4 hours for youth (<17 years) until child released.
In-person evaluation by nursing or other trained staff	Every 15 minutes to evaluate signs of injury related to restraint, nutrition/hydration, vital signs, circulation in extremities, hygiene/ elimination, physical and psychological status, and readiness to discontinue the restraint or seclusion.

CMS, Centers for Medicare and Medicaid Services; JCAHO, Joint Commission for Accreditation of Healthcare Organizations.

ability and potential association with dysrhythmia.[37] High-potency neuroleptics are associated with extrapyramidal symptoms (EPS), which can occur in approximately 1% of patients receiving a single dose of these medications.[35] Co-administration with antihistamines such as diphenhydramine and benztropine may decrease the risk of EPS and may potentially be more efficacious secondary to the antihistamine's inherent sedative properties. Benzodiazepines such as lorazepam are also commonly used either alone or in conjunction with drugs from other classes. Using a combination of a neuroleptic and a benzodiazepine is more effective and poses less risk of side effects.[38,39] In combative adolescent patients or those refractory to a single medication regimen, rapid tranquilization using a combination of an antihistamine (eg, diphenhydramine), neuroleptic (eg, haloperidol), and benzodiazepine (eg, lorazepam) may be effective.

Atypical neuroleptics are being increasingly used in the management of agitation in pediatric acute care settings. Advantages of using these medications include their improved side effect profile and their use in maintenance therapy for patients with psychotic and behavioral disorders. This subclass of neuroleptic medications is associated with a lower incidence of EPS.[40] Olanzapine is available as an orally disintegrating tablet and can be offered as a non-painful and faster-acting alternative to drugs that can only be given parenterally or are dependent on gastric absorption.[41]

Medications from all of these classes should be used with caution because they can lead to significant sedative effects, resulting in delays in assessment and disposition. Sedated patients should be monitored closely for complications such as respiratory depression. The medications most commonly used for restraining agitated adolescent patients are listed in Table 7.[15]

Management of Suicidal and Other Self-Harm Behaviors

Suicide has risen to become the third leading cause of death in young people aged 15 to 24 years, and the fifth leading cause of death for children aged 5 to 14 years.[42] In a recent survey, approximately 17% of high school students in the United States reported suicidal ideation, and 8% reported at least one suicide attempt within the past year.[19] Risk factors that have been associated with suicidal thoughts and behaviors are listed in Table 8.

Suicidal behavior is a final common pathway undertaken by adolescents who are confronted by stress from a variety of sources, including conflicts in relationships, substance abuse, and primary psychiatric illness. Adolescents are often unequipped to address life stressors in less harmful ways, and feelings of helplessness and hopelessness are almost universally present. An adolescent presenting with suicidal thoughts or behavior is presenting in crisis. It is crucial to help adolescents understand that their life is valuable, and that even the direst crises can be averted by means other than suicide.

Table 7

Medications used to treat acute agitation, doses, time to onset, half-life, and potential adverse effects

Medication	Dose	Onset (min)	Half-life (h)	Adverse effects
Diphenhydramine	1.25 mg/kg	5-15 (IM/IV)	2-8	Paradoxical reaction
	Teen: 50 mg	20-30 (PO)	2-8	
Hydroxyzine	1.25 mg/kg	5-15 (IM/IV)	7-10	Paradoxical reaction
	Teen: 50 mg	20-30 (PO)	7-10	
Lorazepam	0.05-0.1 mg/kg	5-15 (IM/IV)	12	Paradoxical reaction
	Teen: 2-4 mg	20-30 (PO)	12	Respiratory depression
Haloperidol	0.1 mg/kg	15-30 (IM)	21	EPS/NMS
	Teen: 2-5 mg	30-60 (PO)	21	May prolong QTc Transient hypotension
Droperidol	0.03-0.07 mg/kg/dose	3-10 (IM/IV)	2	EPS/NMS
	Teen: 2.5 mg			May prolong QTc Anxiety
Risperidone	<12 years: 0.5 mg	45-60 (PO)	20	EPS/NMS
	Teen: 1 mg			May prolong QTc
Olanzapine	<12 years: 2.5 mg	30-60 (IM)	30	EPS/NMS
	Teen: 5-10 mg	45-60 (PO)	30	May prolong QTc
Quetiapine	25 mg	45-60 (PO)	6	EPS/NMS
				May prolong QTc
Ziprasidone	<12 years: 5 mg	30-60 (IM)	2-5	EPS/NMS
	Teen: 10-20 mg	60 (PO)	7	May prolong QTc

EPS, extrapyramidal symptoms. NMS, neuroleptic malignant syndrome
Adapted with permission from Fleisher GR, Ludwig S, eds. *Textbook of Emergency Medicine.*
Philadelphia, PA: Lippincott Williams & Wilkins; 2010:1709

Table 8

Risk factors associated with suicidal behavior among adolescents

- Previous suicide attempt
- Formulation of plan
- Depression/hopelessness
- Suicide attempt by friend or family member
- Unwillingness to use outside resources, lack of perceived support
- History of substance abuse
- Low social self-competence
- Low social support from friends, including being victim of bullying
- Functional impairment resulting from illness/injury
- Sexual minority status, especially with lack of parental support
- Availability of weapons
- Preoccupation with death

Evaluation of adolescents presenting with suicidal thoughts or behavior should include obtaining a detailed history of the events leading to the thoughts or attempt, expectations regarding the outcome of the attempt, as well as an assessment of impulsivity and potential for future self-harm behavior. Adolescents will not always be forthcoming about suicidal behavior unless directly questioned, and the physician should have a high index suspicion for suicidal thoughts or behaviors when assessing all patients who present with psychiatric or behavioral emergencies, including those presenting with "accidental" overdoses. Physical examination should include a full skin examination to assess for evidence of injury. The concept of "suicidal gesture" should not be used clinically. All attempts at self-harm should be considered potentially lethal because it cannot be assumed that adolescents universally comprehend the potential lethality of their behaviors.

Medication and illicit drug overdose, both intentional and unintentional, should be considered whenever treating an adolescent with altered mental status. In acute overdose, symptoms can vary widely depending on the substance ingested, whether more than one substance was involved, the timing of the overdose, and the quantity of substance ingested. Although the adolescent may report a particular ingested substance, co-ingestion of other substances must always be considered. Diagnostic studies may include a complete blood count, comprehensive metabolic panel, alcohol level, urine toxicology screen, acetaminophen level, salicylate level, and electrocardiogram.[43,44] Specific drug levels and toxic alcohol levels should be considered in the appropriate clinical context. Involvement of the local poison control center and discussion with the clinical toxicologist on duty may help to guide the acute management of an adolescent who presents with drug or medication overdose.

Adolescents who are at high risk for recurrent self-harm behaviors should be admitted to an inpatient psychiatric facility. Relative indications for hospitalization are listed in Table 9. Laws regarding involuntary psychiatric hospitalization differ from state to state, and it is the responsibility of acute care physicians to understand the laws and regulations of their practice locale. In general, there are

Table 9
Indications for hospitalization of suicidal adolescents

- Failure to establish rapport among patient, family, and medical professional
- Poor insight or impulse control
- Serious suicide attempt
- Suicidal ideation involving significantly lethal means
- Active suicidal ideation
- Failure to commit to safety
- Psychiatric comorbidity (including psychosis and severe depression)
- Poor social support
- Prior suicide attempts
- Inability to establish close mental health follow-up

means by which adolescents can be hospitalized against their will if they pose a significant danger to themselves or others.

Discharge to home from an acute care setting may be considered if the adolescent is medically stable and is determined to pose little risk of harm to self. Before discharge, caregivers must commit to removing potentially harmful materials from the home and to closely observing the adolescent at home for safety. Close follow-up with a mental health professional should be arranged before discharge. The use of "no-suicide" contracts has been shown to be unsuccessful in preventing future self-harm behavior, and they pose legal and ethical problems for the physician.[45] However, safety plans that outline steps an adolescent can take if thoughts of self-harm recur should be discussed before any patient who presents with suicidal thoughts or behaviors is discharged.

Adolescents may also present to acute care settings after intentionally harming themselves by exhibiting non-suicidal self-injurious behaviors. Behaviors such as self-cutting are often exhibited by adolescents to self-regulate emotion or seek attention.[46] Most self-cutting behavior is not directly related to an attempt to end one's life but rather a manifestation of poor coping mechanisms. These self-injurious behaviors are often found to be comorbid with other psychiatric conditions such as depression and suicidality. The physician must discern whether patients presenting with self-injurious behaviors are at acute risk for seriously harming themselves by inquiring about the intentions behind the behavior and assessing for other concerning thoughts and behaviors.

SPECIAL POPULATIONS

Homeless Youth

A 1998 national study revealed that the prevalence of homelessness among youths was 7.6%, resulting in a national estimate of 1.6 million youth experiencing homelessness each year, most of whom are males age 13 and older.[47] In 2010, 21.8% of all sheltered individuals in the United States were younger than 18 years.[48] Compared to the general adolescent population, rates of mood disorders, conduct disorder, post-traumatic stress disorder, substance abuse and dependence, and suicide attempts are significantly higher among homeless youth.[49] In addition, homeless youth are at higher risk for medical conditions such as pregnancy and sexually transmitted infections. Evidence reveals that many homeless youth have established a mistrust of medical services as a result of negative past experiences, fear of legal intervention, or involvement of social services department.[50,51]

Sexual Minority Youth

Lesbian, gay, bisexual, transgendered, and questioning (LGBTQ) youth may experience a time of crisis during adolescence as they strive to develop identity while fitting in with their peers. This group of adolescents tends to feel "different" because of their sexual orientation and is often part of a community that does not accept them. As a result, they face not only typical adolescent stressors but also those related to social acceptance of their sexuality. Studies on LGBTQ youth have reported higher rates of mental health problems, such as depression, anxiety, substance abuse, and suicide, and high-risk behaviors, such as truancy, running away, homelessness, pregnancy, and sexually transmitted infections.[52]

Evaluation of Homeless and LGBTQ Youth

The initial evaluation of a homeless and LGBTQ youth should include a thorough assessment of the patient's current living situation, past experiences, and available resources and support. The acute care physician must be aware of the challenges experienced by homeless and LGBT youth and must be ready to address such risk factors. This assessment must include evaluation of circumstances or events that may increase psychiatric risk for the adolescent. Appropriate resources including the patient's family, social services, and mental health professionals should be enlisted to aid in the care for the patient.

CONCLUSION

The epidemic of mental health and behavioral disorders among young people is clearly reflected in trends in emergency care. It is the responsibility of the physician to be prepared to assess and manage the range of psychiatric and behavioral emergencies that may present to acute care settings. As addressing this epidemic becomes a priority for law makers and policymakers, resources should be dedicated to identifying novel ways in which to treat and manage young people presenting in mental health crisis.

References

1. US Department of Health and Human Services, US Department of Education, US Department of Justice. *Report of the Surgeon General's Conference on Children's Mental Health: A National Action Agenda.* Washington, DC: US Department of Health and Human Services; 2000
2. Kessler RC, Berglund P, Demler O. Life-time Prevalence and Age-of-onset Distribution of DSM-IV Disorders in the National Co-morbidity Survey Replication. *Arch Gen Psychiatry.* 2005;62:593-602
3. Kataoka SH, Zhang L, Wells K. Unmet Need for Mental Health Care Among U.S. Children: Variation by Ethnicity and Insurance Status. *Am J Psychiatry.* 2002;159(9):1548-1555
4. Sills MR, Bland SD. Summary statistics for pediatric psychiatric visits to US emergency departments, 1993–1999. *Pediatrics.* 2002;110:e40
5. Mahajan P, Alpern ER, Grupp-Phelan J, et al. Epidemiology of psychiatric-related visits to emergency departments in a multicenter collaborative research pediatric network. *Pediatr Emerg Care.* 2009;25:715-720
6. Kyser JG, Diner BC, Raulston GW, et al. A practical approach to the assessment and management of psychiatric emergencies. *Jefferson J Psychiatry.* 1989;7:81-91
7. Health Insurance Portability and Accountability Act of 1996. Public Law No. 104-191, 110 Stat 1936; 1996

8. Cohen E, MacKenzie RG, Yates GL. HEADSS, a psychosocial risk assessment instrument: implications for designing effective intervention programs for runaway youth. *J Adolesc Health*. 1991;12:539-544

9. Baren JM, Rothrock SG, Brennan JA, et al, eds. *Pediatric Emergency Medicine*. Philadelphia, PA: Elsevier; 2008:119

10. Abbruzzi G, Stork CM. Pediatric toxicologic concerns. *Emerg Med Clin North Am*. 2002;20:223-247

11. Lewinsohn PM, Rohde P, Seeley JR. Major depressive disorder in older adolescents: prevalence, risk factors, and clinical implications. *Clin Psychol Rev*. 1998;18:765-794

12. Birmaher B, Brent D; AACAP Work Group on Quality Issues. Practice parameter for the assessment and treatment of children and adolescents with depressive disorders. *J Am Acad Child Adolesc Psychiatry*. 2007;46:1503-1526

13. Bethell J, Rhodes AE. Identifying deliberate self-harm in emergency department data. *Health Rep*. 2009;20:35-42

14. Volkmar FR. Childhood and adolescent psychosis: a review of the past 10 years. *J Am Acad Child Adolesc Psychiatry*. 1996;35:843-851

15. Katz ER, Chapman LL, Chun TH. Psychiatric emergencies. In: Fleisher GR, Ludwig S, eds. *Textbook of Emergency Medicine*. Philadelphia, PA: Lippincott Williams & Wilkins; 2010:1701-1728

16. Dalmau J, Gleichman AJ, Hughes EG, et al. Anti-NMDA-receptor encephalitis: case series and analysis of the effects of antibodies. *Lancet Neurol*. 2008;7:1091-1098

17. Gut-Fayand, Dervaux A, Olié J, et al. Substance abuse and suicidality in schizophrenia: a common risk factor linked to impulsivity. *Psychiatry Res*. 2001;102:65-72

18. Johnston LD, O'Malley PM, Miech RA, et al. *Monitoring the Future National Survey Results on Drug Use: 1975-2014: Overview, Key Findings on Adolescent Drug Use*. Ann Arbor, MI: Institute for Social Research, The University of Michigan; 2015

19. Centers for Disease Control and Prevention. 2013 Youth risk behavior survey. Available at: www.cdc.gov/yrbs. Accessed March 1, 2015

20. Moeller KE, Lee KC, Kissack JC. Urine drug screening: practical guide for clinicians. *Mayo Clinic Proc*. 2008;83:66-76

21. Harris CR, Brown A. Synthetic cannabinoid intoxication: a case series and review. *J Emerg Med*. 2013;44:360-366

22. Drug Enforcement Administration. Drugs of Abuse: A DEA Resource Guide 2015 Edition. Available at: www.dea.gov/pr/multimedia-library/publications/drug_of_abuse.pdf. Accessed October 6, 2015

23. Ibeziako P, Bujoreanu S. Approach to psychosomatic illness in adolescents. *Curr Opin Pediatr*. 2011;23:384-389

24. Van Ravesteijn H, Wittkampf K, Lucassen P, et al. Detecting somatoform disorders in primary care with the PHQ-15. *Ann Fam Med*. 2009;7:232-238

25. Lukens TW, Wolf SJ, Edlow JA, et al. Clinical policy: critical issues in the diagnosis and management of the adult psychiatric patient in the emergency department. *Ann Emerg Med*. 2006;47:79-99

26. Olshaker, JS, Jerrard, DA, Prendergast H, et al. Medical clearance and screening of psychiatric patients in the emergency department. *Acad Emerg Med*. 1997;4:124-128

27. Santiago LI, Tunik MG, Foltin GL, et al. Children requiring psychiatric consultation in the pediatric emergency department. *Pediatr Emerg Care*. 2006;22:85

28. Dorfman, DH, Mehta, SD. Restraint use for psychiatric patients in the pediatric emergency department. *Pediatr Emerg Care*. 2006;22:7-12

29. American Academy of Pediatrics Committee on Pediatric Emergency Medicine. The use of physical restraint interventions for children and adolescents in the acute care setting. *Pediatrics*. 1997;99:3:497-498

30. Weiss EM. Deadly restraint: a Hartford Courant investigative report. *Hartford Courant*. 1998;Oct:11-15

31. Nunno MA, Holden MJ, Tollar A. Learning from tragedy: a survey of child and adolescent restraint fatalities. *Child Abuse Negl*. 2006;30:1333-1342

32. Joint Commission on Accreditation of Healthcare Organizations. *Comprehensive Accreditation Manual for Hospitals: The Official Handbook.* Oak Brook Terrace, IL: Joint Commission on Accreditation of Health Care Organizations, 1996:TX-47–TX-58

33. United States Code of Federal Regulations. Condition of Participation: Patient's Rights, 42 CFR 482.13; 2014

34. Masters KJ. Practice parameter for the prevention and management of aggressive behavior in child and adolescent psychiatric institutions, with special reference to seclusion and restraint. *J Am Acad Child Adolesc Psychiatry.* 2002;41:4S-25S

35. Sorrentino A. Chemical restraints for the agitated, violent, or psychotic pediatric patient in the emergency department: controversies and recommendations. *Curr Opin Pediatr.* 2004;16:201-205

36. Hill S, Petit J. Psychiatric emergencies: the violent patient. *Emerg Med Clin North Am.* 2000;18:301-315

37. Kao LW, Kirk MA, Evers SJ, et al. Droperidol, QT prolongation, and sudden death: what is the evidence? *Ann Emerg Med.* 2003;41:546-558

38. Bieniek SA, Ownby RL, Penalver A, et al. A double-blind study of lorazepam versus the combination of haloperidol and lorazepam in managing agitation. *Pharmacotherapy.* 1998;18:57–62

39. Battaglia J, Moss S, Rush J et al. Haloperidol, lorazepam, or both for psychotic agitation? A multicenter, prospective, double-blind, emergency department study. *Am J Emerg Med.* 1997;15:335–340

40. Pierre JM. Extrapyramidal symptoms with atypical antipsychotics. *Drug Saf.* 2005;28:191-208

41. Citrone L. Atypical antipsychotics for acute agitation. *Postgrad Med.* 2002;112:85-96

42. Murphy SL, Xu J, Kochanek KD. Deaths: final data for 2010. *Natl Vital Stat Rep.* 2013;61:1-117

43. Zun LS. Evidence-based evaluation of psychiatric patients. *J Emerg Med.* 2005;28:35-39

44. Broderick KB, Lerner B, McCourt JD, et al. Emergency physician practices and requirements regarding the medical screening examination of psychiatric patients. *Acad Emerg Med.* 2002; 9:88-92

45. McMyler C, Pryjmachuk S. Do "no-suicide" contracts work? *J Psychiatr Ment Health Nurs.* 2008;15:512-522

46. Jacobson CM, Gould M. The epidemiology and phenomenology of non-suicidal self-injurious behavior among adolescents: a critical review of the literature. *Arch Suicide Res.* 2007;11:129-147

47. Ringwalt, CL, Greene, JM, Robertson, M, et al. The prevalence of homelessness among adolescents in the United States. *Am J Public Health.* 1998;88:1325-1329

48. US Department of Housing and Urban Development. *The 2010 Annual Homeless Assessment Report to Congress.* Washington, DC: U.S. Department of Housing and Urban Development; 2010

49. Toro, PA, Dworsky, A, Fowler, PJ. Homeless Youth in the United States: Recent Research Findings and Intervention Approaches. *The 2007 National Symposium on Homelessness and Research.* Washington, DC; US Department of Housing and Urban Development and US Department of Health and Human Services; 2007

50. Klein, JD, Woods, AH, Wilson, KM, et al. Homeless and runaway youths' access to health care. *J Adolesc Health.* 2000;27:331-339

51. Garrett SB, Higa DH, Phares MM, et al. Homeless youths' perceptions of services and transitions to stable housing. *Eval Program Plann.* 2008;31:436-444

52. Fergusson DM, Horwood LJ, Beautrais AL. Is sexual orientation related to mental health problems and suicidality in young people? *Arch Gen Psychiatry.* 1999;56:876-880

Adolesc Med 026 (2015) 570–588

Generation Z: Adolescent Xenobiotic Abuse in the 21st Century

William Eggleston, PharmD,
Christine Stork, PharmD, DABAT, FAACT*

SUNY Upstate Medical University, Upstate New York Poison Center, Syracuse, New York

INTRODUCTION

Adolescent abuse of illicit xenobiotics is not a new phenomenon. Reported use of these xenobiotics by grade school and high school students has remained relatively stable over the last decade.[1] However, the emergence of synthetic cannabinoids, designer amphetamines, and novel psychoactive analogs of phencyclidine (PCP) has created a new avenue for adolescent xenobiotic abuse. These newcomers, along with classic hydrocarbons, are readily accessible, inexpensive, easily concealed, and in some cases, legal. The latter factors contribute to the overall appeal of these xenobiotics to adolescent individuals. It is imperative that health care professionals understand the toxicities associated with these xenobiotics, recognize clinical signs of their abuse, and are able to quickly provide appropriate treatments for intoxicated patients.

SYNTHETIC CANNABINOIDS

Introduction

Synthetic cannabinoids (SC), commonly referred to as Spice, K2, synthetic marijuana, and legal marijuana, are cannabinoid receptor agonists that are abused for their psychoactive and mood-altering effects. These xenobiotics were originally developed by pharmaceutical companies and research scientists to study cannabinoid receptors and develop novel therapies. Illicit use of SCs was first reported in the United States in 2009 and has quickly become popular among both seasoned and naïve drug users. Synthetic cannabinoids are obtained by

---

*Corresponding author
E-mail address: storkc@upstate.edu

distributors in liquid form and sprayed onto plant material for use. Typically SCs are smoked by users; however, ingestion is also reported.[2] Initial widespread abuse was partly the result of the marketing of the products as herbal incense and potpourri with the warning "not for human consumption" printed on the packaging. The latter allowed the products to circumvent standard US drug laws and regulations. The xenobiotics were recognized to be a public health threat and the US Drug Enforcement Administration added 5 SCs to the list of schedule I substances in March 2011.[3] Despite continuous efforts to regulate the SC market, the rapid alteration of existing SCs and the development of new SCs have allowed the manufacturers and distributors to remain a step ahead of current legislation.

A survey of students in grades 8, 10, and 12 found that the prevalence of SC use ranked second only to marijuana use among individual illicit xenobiotics reported.[1] Data from the American Association of Poison Control Centers (AAPCC) suggest that use of SCs is increasing in the general population. Surveillance by the AAPCC recorded 6968 SC-related calls to poison control centers during peak use in 2011, which declined to 2668 calls in 2013. Data from 2014 demonstrated a 38% increase to 3682 calls, and data from 2015 (January 1 to May 21) already include 3414 calls related to SC use.[4] Epidemiologic surveys indicate that typical users are in their late teens to early twenties, are predominantly male, and are likely to have abused ethanol or marijuana in their lifetime.[5]

The widespread use of SCs is likely multifactorial and influenced by their legality, lack of detectability, potency, and perceived safety. Currently, new SCs such as MAB-CHMINACA are not nationally scheduled as controlled substances and remain readily available. These xenobiotics are undetectable on standard urine drug assays because of their structural dissimilarity to delta-9-tetrahydrocannabinol (delta-9-THC). Sensitive analytical techniques, such as gas chromatography and mass spectrometry, are needed to detect the presence of SCs in bodily fluids because of product variability and the relatively low concentration of both parent xenobiotic and metabolites.[6] Approximately one-third of overall users and 71% of patients in substance use disorder treatment programs report the lack of detection as their reason for SC use.[5,7]

As a general class, SCs have a significantly higher affinity for cannabinoid receptors than delta-9-THC.[8] Because of their increased receptor affinity, these xenobiotics demonstrate a greater potency and have more profound psychoactive and mood-altering effects than marijuana.[9] The increased potency of SCs is reported to cause a higher incidence of adverse effects, and when surveyed 92.8% of SC users indicate a preference for marijuana. However, users report that they prefer legal xenobiotics of abuse because they consider them less likely to contain adulterants, and users of high school age indicated that they perceived SCs to be safer than other drugs of abuse.[5,10]

Pharmacology

Synthetic cannabinoids function as agonists of the endocannabinoid system and bind to both CB_1 and CB_2 subtype receptors. Both receptors are coupled to $G_{i/o}$ proteins and are found throughout the body. The CB_1 receptors are generally found on presynaptic and postsynaptic nerve terminals in the central nervous system (CNS) but are also found peripherally. These receptors modulate the release of various neurotransmitters. Stimulation of the CB_1 receptor decreases intracellular cyclic adenosine monophosphate, leading to both increased and reduced neurotransmitter release depending on the location of the receptor.[11] The desired and adverse effects of the SCs are postulated to be largely the result of their agonist activity at the CB_1 receptor.[12] The CB_2 receptors are found mainly in immune tissue, spleen, bladder, and liver. Their activation results in immuno-modulatory effects, including inflammation and neuroprotection. They may also play a role in reducing nociception.[13,14] Chronic exposure to cannabimi-metic xenobiotics has been shown to induce receptor downregulation in rats.[15]

Clinical Presentation

Synthetic cannabinoid abuse is associated with a myriad of clinical findings. The most commonly reported manifestations include tachycardia, hypertension, nausea, vomiting, agitation, altered perception, mydriasis, and somnolence.[16,17] Generally, symptoms resolve within 4 to 14 hours after use, without complica-tion. Commonly reported metabolic abnormalities include hypokalemia and hypoglycemia.[17] The incidence of hallucinations and delusions is about 10-fold greater after SC use compared to after marijuana use.[18] Altered mental status and delirium associated with SC use are also reported.[19,20]

Serious adverse events after SC abuse include cardiac complications, cerebral isch-emia, acute kidney injury, and seizures. A case series of 3 otherwise healthy teenage males reported chest pain, ST-segment elevation, and elevated troponin levels asso-ciated with SC use. Two of the patients underwent coronary angiography and were found to have normal coronary arteries.[21] Cerebral ischemia was reported in 3 young patients (19-33 years of age) associated with SC use. All 3 patients had com-puterized tomographic scans that demonstrated an infarct, and 1 patient was treated with tissue plasminogen activator.[22,23] Acute kidney injury was reported in 16 patients (15-33 years of age) after SC use. These patients had elevated serum creatinine (3.3-21 mg/dL), proteinuria, urine casts, urine red blood cells, and urine white blood cells 1 to 6 days after presentation. Approximately one-third of patients required hemodialysis, and one-fourth required treatment with steroids. The impli-cated SCs were reported to be XLR-11 and UR-144.[24,25] Additionally, seizures and fatality have been reported after SC use with confirmatory laboratory testing.[3,26]

Chronic use of SCs causes many of the same adverse consequences as chronic marijuana use. As stated in the section on pharmacology, chronic use of SC xenobiotics has been shown to induce downregulation of CB receptors.[15] Down-regulation is thought to be the cause of cannabinoid hyperemesis syndrome seen after chronic marijuana use. Cannabinoid hyperemesis syndrome has also been reported in a single patient who was chronically using SCs. The patient presented with intractable nausea and vomiting that was relieved only by hot baths and showers. His symptoms resolved with abstinence, consistent with marijuana-associated cannabinoid hyperemesis syndrome.[27] Cessation of SC use is also rarely reported to cause withdrawal in chronic users. Withdrawal symptoms include tachycardia, agitation, irritability, and anxiety.[28,29]

Treatment

Because of the variability in clinical presentation after SC use, treatment is generally symptom based and supportive. Gastrointestinal decontamination is not typically indicated, but a single dose of activated charcoal should be considered after ingestion of an SC in an alert patient or a patient with a protected airway. The most commonly reported interventions include intravenous fluids, benzodiazepines, antiemetic therapy, electrolytes (potassium), and supplemental oxygen.[5,17] Patients presenting with hypotension, a prolonged period of unresponsiveness, or fluid loss from emesis will likely require intravenous fluids. Agitated and combative patients commonly require chemical sedation to prevent excessive hyperthermia, which can result in rhabdomyolysis, seizures, shock, and disseminated intravascular coagulation.[30] Lipophilic benzodiazepines such as midazolam (intravenous/intramuscular) or diazepam (intravenous) should be considered for sedation because of their rapid onset of action. Lorazepam is not an ideal choice because of its delayed time to peak sedation.[31] After initial control is achieved, some patients may require prolonged sedation until their agitation has resolved. Prolonged psychosis is reported after SC use and may be associated with exacerbation or unmasking of an underlying psychiatric condition. Antipsychotics, such as haloperidol, have been successfully used in this patient population.[18,20] Before the administration of antipsychotics, an electrocardiogram should be assessed for conduction abnormalities. The use of antiemetic agents, electrolytes, and supplemental oxygen can be considered based on their standard indications. Because of the wide array of SCs and the lack of rapid testing options, there is no role for confirmatory laboratory testing in the acute setting.

Summary

The term *synthetic cannabinoid* encompasses a broad array of chemicals that act on the endocannabinoid system by CB receptor agonism. They are more potent than standard delta-9-THC and have a higher affinity for the target receptors. These pharmacokinetic differences create more profound mood-altering and psychoactive effects in users. They also result in more adverse outcomes, including tachycardia, hypertension, nausea, vomiting, agitation, altered perception, mydriasis, and somnolence. Case reports of seizures, psychosis, myocardial infarction, cerebral ischemia, acute kidney injury, and death have also been associated with SC use. Treatment is generally symptomatic and supportive. Commonly reported interventions include intravenous fluids, benzodiazepines, antiemetic medications, electrolytes (potassium), and supplemental oxygen.

HYDROCARBONS

Introduction

Hydrocarbons are volatile substances commonly abused for their rapid, short-acting effects on the CNS. These xenobiotics are abused via inhalation of vapors directly from an open container (sniffing), from a soaked rag (huffing), or from a bag in which they are sprayed (bagging). Classically these xenobiotics are divided into 3 groups; solvents, fuels, and anesthetics. Solvents are commercially available in spray paint, paint thinner, glues, nail polish and polish removers, compressed dusting products, and correction fluid. Fuels, such as propane and butane, are available in lighter fluid, hair spray, gas grill fuel, and air freshening products. Because of their differing mechanisms of action, toxicity, and lack of accessibility, anesthetics are not discussed in this review.

Hydrocarbon exposures composed about 1.3% (33,081) of total exposures reported to the AAPCC and accounted for 25 deaths in 2013.[32] Accessibility, ease of concealment, low cost, and legality of solvents and fuels make them ripe for abuse among adolescents. These factors likely contribute to the latter population having the highest prevalence of inhalant abuse.[33] Individuals younger than 18 years compose roughly 75% of the total volatile substance abuse population, and approximately half of users indicate that their first use occurred before 13 years of age.[34,35] When surveyed, students in grade 8 indicated a higher incidence of inhalant abuse than their peers in grades 10 and 12.[1] Adolescents who report use of hydrocarbons are more likely to later abuse ethanol, hallucinogens, nicotine, cocaine, and amphetamines. These individuals also have a higher incidence of suicide, major depression, and conduct disorders.[36] Inhalant abuse typically declines in adulthood, but inhalant use disorder continues to affect 0.1% of Americans between the ages of 18 and 29 years.[37]

Pharmacology

Hydrocarbons enter the bloodstream via absorption through the lungs and rapidly distribute to the CNS and cardiac tissue. They are lipophilic in structure, which allows them to readily cross the blood-brain barrier and accumulate in lipid-rich neurons. A rodent model demonstrated that the peak brain concentration of 1,1-difluoroethane, a commonly abused hydrocarbon, is higher than peak concentrations in other organs.[38] The overall effect of hydrocarbons is CNS depression; however, their precise mechanism of action is multifactorial and involves alteration of dopamine activity, gamma-aminobutyric acid (GABA) receptors, and N-methyl-D-aspartate (NMDA) receptors.[39,40]

The actions of hydrocarbons on dopamine are similar to those of ethanol, 3,4-methylenedioxymethamphetamine (MDMA), and delta-9-THC. Toluene, a hydrocarbon found in spray paints and glues, is shown to augment dopaminergic activity in the ventral tegmental area of the brain in a rodent model.[41] The actions of dopamine in the ventral tegmental area are associated with reward processing, which may explain the euphoric and addictive properties of hydrocarbons.[42] Hydrocarbon-induced CNS depression is a result of enhanced GABA-mediated inhibition. Dose-dependent inhibition of rodent hippocampal neurons is demonstrated to occur by enhanced GABA activity in the presence of various hydrocarbons.[43] Chronic use of hydrocarbons is shown to decrease GABA activity over time, suggesting a mechanism for tolerance and increased frequency of use.[44] Hydrocarbons, similar to ketamine, act as antagonists at NMDA receptors.[45,46] Antagonism at these receptor sites likely contributes to the dissociative and hallucinogenic properties described with inhalant abuse.[47]

Clinical Presentation

Hydrocarbon abuse results in rapid onset of CNS depression. The initial clinical manifestations are similar to those of ethanol intoxication, which include euphoria and disinhibition. These symptoms progress in a dose-dependent manner to headache, blurry vision, ataxia, hallucinations, coma, seizures, and death.[48] The CNS effects tend to resolve rapidly with minimal hangover effect, and redosing is common. Chronic abuse of hydrocarbons results in neuropsychological deficits, leukoencephalopathy evident on magnetic resonance imaging, and impairment of cognitive and motor functions.[49-52] Improvement in neurologic deficits occurs with abstinence; however, complete symptom resolution is not consistently demonstrated, and reversal of magnetic resonance imaging abnormalities is not reported.[53,54] In addition to CNS symptoms, patients may present with burning, frostbite, rhinorrhea, or blistering on the fingers and mouth. Dermal findings are more common after "sniffing" hydrocarbons or directly spraying them from the original container into the mouth or nose.[55,56]

Systemic exposure to hydrocarbons, particularly halogenated hydrocarbons, causes an increased risk for the precipitation of cardiac arrhythmias. Hydrocarbons inhibit cardiac potassium channels responsible for repolarization (I_{Kr}), which results in prolongation of the QT interval on the electrocardiogram.[57] Prolongation of the QT interval increases the risk for ventricular dysrhythmias, specifically torsades de pointes.[58] In addition to their direct arrhythmogenic effect, halogenated hydrocarbons decrease conduction velocity in the presence of epinephrine. Slowed conduction velocity, likely as a result of gap junction inhibition, further increases the risk for development of fatal dysrhythmias.[59] Ventricular dysrhythmias are thought to be the cause of sudden sniffing death syndrome, which accounts for approximately 50% of hydrocarbon-related deaths.[60-64] Fatality may also occur from asphyxiation, vagal inhibition, respiratory depression, or trauma as a result of dangerous behavior.[65] Aspiration of hydrocarbons causes direct pulmonary toxicity through surfactant degradation and edema.[39] Angioedema is also reported after 1,1-difluoroethane use.[66]

Specific solvents are linked to unique toxicologic manifestations in addition to the general toxicities described. Chronic toluene abuse is associated with leukoencephalopathy, which causes dementia, visuospatial dysfunction, and impaired attention.[67] Additionally, chronic toluene exposure causes a distal renal tubular acidosis characterized by hyperchloremia, a non-anion gap metabolic acidosis, hypokalemia, elevated urine hippuric acid, and decreased urine citrate.[68,69] A case report of first-degree atrioventricular block also occurred after toluene abuse, although the etiology of the conduction abnormality was undetermined.[70,71] 2,5-Hexanedione, a metabolite of n-hexane and 2-hexanone (methyl-n-butyl ketone), causes retrograde demyelination of nerve fibers and slowing of conduction.[72-74] The resulting clinical effects include sensory dysfunction (stocking glove neuropathy) and muscle weakness. Exposure to methylene chloride causes systemic toxicity after hepatic conversion of the parent xenobiotic to carbon monoxide.[75,76] Lastly, the development of trigeminal neuralgia has been demonstrated after exposure to trichloroethylene.[77]

Treatment

In general, treatment of acute hydrocarbon toxicity involves symptomatic and supportive care, cardiac and respiratory support, and correction of electrolyte abnormalities. There is no role for gastrointestinal decontamination after inhalational exposure. Beta blockers can be administered for treatment of tachydysrhythmias, although limited evidence supporting this practice exists.[78,79] Additionally, because of the sensitized state of the myocardium, use of epinephrine or other catecholamines may be harmful in patients who are acutely intoxicated. Treatment of chemical pneumonitis is supportive.[80] Agitation can be managed using benzodiazepines, with midazolam and diazepam providing the most rapid sedation.[31] Derangements in volume status, electrolyte disturbances, and acidosis should be monitored and corrected as needed.[81] There is no role for obtaining serum or urine concentrations of hydrocarbons in the acute setting because of their rapid metabolism and the delayed reporting time of test results. Both urine hippuric acid and citrate can be used in conjunction with clinical findings to assess patients for toluene abuse.[68,69]

Summary

Hydrocarbons are ubiquitous xenobiotics found in numerous consumer products as solvents and fuels. Their low cost, legality, ease of concealment, and accessibility make them a common xenobiotic of choice for adolescents. Inhalation of these xenobiotics results in CNS depression, euphoria, and disinhibition. Their abuse can precipitate CNS toxicity, respiratory depression, and cardiac dysrhythmias. Chronic abuse causes neuropsychological deficits that may improve with abstinence. Specific hydrocarbons, such as toluene, methylene chloride, and trichloroethylene, are associated with specific toxicologic manifestations. Treatment is largely supportive, and beta blockers can be considered in patients with tachydysrhythmias.

PHENYLETHYLAMINE DERIVATIVES

Introduction

Phenylethylamine derivatives are a broad class of xenobiotics synthesized by the addition of chemical substitutions to the phenylethylamine base structure in order to enhance the hallucinogenic or stimulatory properties of the xenobiotic. This class includes club drugs such as MDMA (Ecstasy), prescription medications such as methylphenidate and dextroamphetamine, and stimulants such as methamphetamine, 2C compounds (25C-NBOMe), and cathinones (alpha-PVP, MDPV, "bath salts"). These xenobiotics exert their sympathomimetic and hallucinogenic effects by modulating the actions of dopamine, norepinephrine, and serotonin to varying degrees through differing mechanisms. The overall prevalence of abuse is difficult to interpret because of the variety of xenobiotics and degree of legality. Excited delirium, cardiovascular complications, and neurologic findings are commonly encountered adverse reactions associated with phenylethylamine derivative use.[82]

In general, xenobiotics belonging to the class of substituted phenylethylamines are not commonly abused by adolescents in the United States because of their high cost, lack of availability, and legal status. However, the misuse of prescription amphetamines (methylphenidate, amphetamine salts) and MDMA were reported in 5.6% and 2.2% of surveyed students in grades 8, 10, and 12 during 2014.[1] Both methylphenidate and amphetamine salts are abused for their stimulant properties, and abuse liability is increased when they are taken differently than prescribed or for non-medical reasons.[83,84] Non-medical use of these medications was reported by 23% of adolescents referred for substance abuse treatment and 20% of students on a college campus.[85,86] Furthermore, 1 of 5 adolescent patients taking methylphenidate reported being approached to sell, give away, or trade their medication.[87,88] Among 12 million adolescents and young adults who reported using these drugs at least once, MDMA was the most popular club drug. Abuse of MDMA is often coupled with the use of marijuana and other illicit xenobiotics.[89]

Pharmacology

Phenylethylamine derivatives exert their desired and adverse effects by augmenting the action of monoamine neurotransmitters. Hallucinogenic xenobiotics, such as MDMA, are designed to enhance the activity of serotonin to a greater degree than dopamine or norepinephrine. The latter is accomplished by enhanced release of intracellular serotonin and inhibition of reuptake by the serotonin transporter (SERT).[90,91] Additionally, MDMA inhibits tyrosine hydroxylase, which results in persistently decreased serotonin levels after discontinuation of use.[92] Methylphenidate exerts its effects by increasing the extracellular concentration of dopamine in the striatal structures of the forebrain.[93] Stimulants, such as methamphetamine and cathinones, increase extracellular concentrations of catecholamines and serotonin. These xenobiotics enhance the activity of monoamines by causing their direct release from storage vesicles and neuronal bodies into the extracellular space, inhibiting their reuptake, decreasing their metabolism, and increasing their production.[94-98] Neurotransmitter selectivity is generally lost when higher doses of phenylethylamine derivatives are used, and patients exhibit clinical manifestations of excess serotonin, norepinephrine, and dopamine neurotransmission.

Clinical Presentation

Phenylethylamine toxicity manifests as heightened neurologic and sympathomimetic effects from catecholamine excess. The most commonly encountered neurologic findings include agitation, paranoia, hallucinations, and psychosis. Sympathomimetic effects include hypertension, tachycardia, tremor, diaphoresis, and chest pain.[99-101] MDMA can cause hyponatremia as a result of increased vasopressin secretion and increased oral intake of fluids.[102] It also causes transient urinary retention.[103] Severe toxicity can precipitate hepatotoxicity, hyperthermia, acute kidney injury, rhabdomyolysis, seizures, and death. Serotonin intoxication has been reported, especially when these xenobiotics are abused in combination with other serotonergic agents.[95,104] The onset and duration of symptoms vary depending on the xenobiotic involved, route of administration, and rate of metabolism. Common routes of abuse include insufflation, ingestion, and sublingual administration. Intravenous and inhalational administration are less common but do result in a more rapid onset of action.[82,95]

Chronic exposure to phenylethylamine xenobiotics may result in neurotoxicity and prolonged clinical effects. Patients who report abusing MDMA have deficits in both episodic memory and learning ability compared to non-using control subjects.[105,106] Positron emission tomography scans demonstrate a reduction in the distribution of SERT in MDMA users compared to controls. These findings persisted after 4.6 months in one study; however, subsequent studies found a reversal at 17.2 and 29 months.[107,108] The imaging results suggest that MDMA's effect on SERT is reversible but do not indicate whether the neurons are functioning appropriately. Additionally, chronic abuse of phenylethylamine derivatives results in tolerance, craving, and withdrawal on cessation of use.[91,100,109] Both parent xenobiotic and metabolites can be detected in urine, although lack of testing availability, variable metabolism, unclear clinical correlation of quantitative levels, and delayed results limit the clinical utility of confirmatory testing.[110-113] The rapid development of new phenylethylamine derivatives adds a complication to the testing process. As of 2013, 44 unique cathinones had been encountered, and comprehensive analysis of seized products demonstrated a wide variability in intraproduct and interproduct content and concentration.[114,115]

Treatment

As discussed in the clinical presentation section, patients may present with a variety of clinical findings after abuse of a phenylethylamine derivative. Treatment of this population is largely symptom based and supportive. Patients presenting with sympathomimetic manifestations such as agitation, tachycardia, and seizures should be managed with rapid-acting benzodiazepines.[31] In addition to benzodiazepines, aggressive cooling measures should be initiated in patients presenting with hyperthermia.[82] In patients with asymptomatic hyponatremia after MDMA use, consider fluid restriction. In patients with acute symptomatic hyponatremia (seizures or decreased level of consciousness), hypertonic saline can be used to correct the serum sodium.[100] Prolonged psychosis is reported and is likely caused by aggravation or precipitation of an underlying psychiatric disorder rather than acute xenobiotic effect. Standard psychiatric management principles should guide treatment of prolonged psychotic manifestations. Because of the extensive number of products available and the lack of rapid testing options, there is no role for serum or urine analysis in the acute management of phenylethylamine derivative intoxicated patients.

Summary

Phenylethylamine derivatives are a broad class of chemicals that include club drugs, prescription medications, and stimulants. The xenobiotics in this class most commonly abused by adolescents include MDMA, methylphenidate, and dextroamphetamine. These xenobiotics produce their clinical manifestations by augmenting the activity of dopamine, norepinephrine, and serotonin to varying degrees. Abuse of phenylethylamine xenobiotics typically results in sympathomimetic and neurologic manifestations. Common findings include agitation, hallucinations, psychosis, hypertension, tachycardia, tremor, and diaphoresis. Severe toxicity can result in seizures, acute kidney injury, rhabdomyolysis, hyperthermia, and death. Care is symptom based and involves the use of benzodiazepines, fluids, and electrolytes (sodium).

N-METHYL-D-ASPARTATE RECEPTOR ANTAGONISTS

Introduction

N-methyl-D-aspartate receptor antagonists are a class of xenobiotics that produce their dissociative effects by opposing the actions of glutamate at the NMDA receptor. Phencyclidine, which was originally developed as a general anesthetic, was the first NMDA receptor antagonist widely abused for its dissociative properties. Ketamine, a less potent and shorter-acting analog of PCP, was developed after PCP was removed from the market because of the high rate of adverse events seen with clinical use.[116] New psychoactive xenobiotics such as methoxetamine (MXE), methoxphenidine (MXP), and diphenidine are illicit derivatives of PCP that are becoming popular as drugs of abuse in the 21st century. Recreational use of MXE was first reported in 2010, and like SCs, the xenobiotic circumvented existing legislation with the warning "not for human consumption." The development and emergence of these xenobiotics are increasing at more rapid rates than the legislation banning their use. According to the European Monitoring Center for Drugs and Drug Addiction (EMCDDA), approximately 2 new psychoactive xenobiotics were detected per month in 2009 and per week in 2014.[117] These xenobiotics are typically insufflated or ingested, although intravenous and intramuscular administration have been reported.[118]

Dextromethorphan (DXM), an over-the-counter (OTC) antitussive, and its active metabolite dextrorphan (DOR), also inhibit NMDA receptors at supratherapeutic serum concentrations. Dextromethorphan is available in numerous preparations both alone and in combination cold products. Users also report abuse of purified free-base DXM or "Crystal Dex." Free-base preparations allow users to abuse higher doses of DXM without the unwanted toxicity associated with added medications (in combination products) or excipients.[119] The high prevalence of DXM abuse among adolescents is likely a result of its low cost, ease of accessibility as an OTC medication, lack of stigma associated with its use, and absence of a rapid screening method on standard urine drug screen kits.[120]

Ketamine abuse was reported by 1.5% of high school seniors in 2014, and this same group of students reported a 4.1% incidence of OTC cough and cold medication abuse.[1] Abuse of PCP-dipped marijuana cigarettes, referred to as "wet" or "fry," is also described.[121] According to the California Poison Control System (CPCS), there was a 15-fold increase in calls regarding adolescent abuse of DXM from 1999 to 2004. Over the 6-year period, 74.5% of the DXM abuse cases reported to the CPCS involved patients between 9 and 17 years of age, with the highest frequency occurring between 15 and 16 years of age.[122] Epidemiologic data regarding adolescent abuse of new psychoactive PCP derivatives are lacking.

Pharmacology

N-methyl-D-aspartate receptor antagonists exert their primary clinical effects by non-competitively inhibiting glutamate's activity at the NMDA receptor. This action blocks the influx of cations, primarily calcium, and prevents depolarization of the neuron.[123] Ketamine has approximately 5% to 10% the potency of PCP at the NMDA receptor, and its receptor inhibition occurs in a dose-dependent manner.[116] Methoxetamine also binds to the PCP site on the NMDA receptor, and its receptor affinity is similar to ketamine.[118] At supratherapeutic concentrations, DMX is also capable of inhibiting glutamate's activity at the NMDA receptor. Users report clinical effects similar to those achieved with PCP and ketamine at doses greater than 300 mg or approximately greater than 2 mg/kg.[124,125] Dextromethorphan is metabolized via cytochrome P450 2D6 enzymes (CYP2D6) to DOR, a more potent NMDA receptor antagonist than DXM.[126,127] The NMDA receptor antagonists also act as opioid receptor agonists, inhibit nitric oxide synthase, and modulate the effects of dopamine, norepinephrine, and serotonin.[124,128]

Clinical Presentation

Abuse of NMDA receptor antagonists typically results in neuropsychiatric and sympathomimetic clinical manifestations. Patients presenting after ketamine abuse complain of anxiety and palpitations. Common physical examination findings include tachycardia, hypertension, mydriasis, altered mental status, nystagmus (horizontal, vertical, and rotary), respiratory depression, and slurred speech.[129] A retrospective review demonstrated that 48% of ketamine users presented with transient neurologic features, including confusion, dizziness, and an impaired level of consciousness.[130] Reports of MXE, MXP, and diphenidine abuse also demonstrate hypertension, tachycardia, anxiety, nystagmus, and altered consciousness.[117,131-133] Abuse of DXM produces diaphoresis, tachycardia, nausea, vomiting, dyskinesia, slurred speech, hallucinations, altered mental status, and rarely respiratory depression.[134] Patients presenting after abuse of NMDA receptor antagonists exhibit horizontal, vertical, and rotary nystagmus. This unique physical examination finding strongly suggests recent use of a NMDA receptor antagonist in a clinically intoxicated patient. Seizures, cerebellar toxicity, and death have also been reported with severe NMDA receptor antagonist toxicity.[135-137]

Ketamine abuse is associated with the development of lower urinary tract symptoms and cystitis.[138-140] These findings have not been reported in humans after MXE, MXP, or diphenidine use. Ketamine abuse causes chronic abdominal pain and is reported to cause dilation of the common bile ducts.[129,130] Dextromethorphan transiently inhibits micturition, likely secondary to a direct effect on the cholinergic neurons innervating the bladder.[141] Serotonin toxicity has been reported with DXM use in combination with other serotonergic medications.[142] Dependence and withdrawal have been reported with both chronic ketamine and DXM abuse.[143,144]

Treatment

Treatment, as with many other xenobiotics of abuse, is largely symptomatic and supportive. Tachycardia, hypertension, anxiety, agitation, and seizures can be managed with GABAergic medications such as benzodiazepines or propofol.[117,118] Fluids, antiemetics, and respiratory support should be given based on standard indications. Hyperthermia requires aggressive cooling measures in addition to sedative medications. Treatment of serotonin toxicity as a result of DXM use does not differ from standard serotonin toxicity management. Cessation of ketamine use has been reported to improve the subjective findings and voiding function parameters in patients with ketamine-induced lower urinary tract symptoms and cystitis.[145] The emergence of substituted products, lack of rapid qualitative serum or urine analyses, and numerous false-positives and false-negatives associated with urine drug screens makes testing acutely intoxicated patients impractical. Instead, management is based on clinical presentation and standard laboratory assessment.

Summary

NMDA receptor antagonists include the prescription medication ketamine, the illicit xenobiotics PCP, MXE, and other novel PCP analogs, and the OTC medication DXM. The NMDA receptor antagonist most commonly abused by adolescents in the United States is DXM. These xenobiotics cause dissociative effects by non-competitively inhibiting the action of glutamate at the NMDA receptor. Additionally, these agents modulate the actions of monoamine neurotransmitters, agonize opioid receptors, and inhibit nitric oxide synthase. Patients typically present with sympathomimetic and neuropsychiatric clinical manifestations after abuse of NMDA receptor antagonists. Treatment is generally symptomatic and supportive. Interventions include benzodiazepines, propofol, fluids, antiemetics, aggressive cooling, and respiratory support.

References

1. Johnston LD, O'Malley PM, Miech RA, Bachman JG, Schulenberg JE. *Monitoring the Future national Survey Results on Drug Use: 1975-2014: Overview, Key Findings on Adolescent Drug Use.* Ann Arbor, MI: Institute for Social Research, The University of Michigan; 2015
2. Lapoint J, James LP, Moran CL, et al. Severe toxicity following synthetic cannabinoid ingestion. *Clin Toxicol (Phila)*. 2011;49:760-764
3. Schneir AB, Baumbacher T. Convulsions associated with the use of a synthetic cannabinoid product. *J Med Toxicol*. 2012;8:62-64
4. American Association of Poison Control Centers. Synthetic marijuana data. May 21, 2015. Available at: aapcc.s3.amazonaws.com/files/library/Syn_Marijuana_Web_Data_through_5.21.15.pdf. Accessed May 23, 2015
5. Castaneto MS, Gorelick DA, Desrosiers NA, et al. Synthetic cannabinoids: epidemiology, pharmacodynamics, and clinical implications. *Drug Alcohol Depend*. 2014;144:12-41
6. Kronstrand R, Roman M, Andersson M, Eklund A. Toxicological findings of synthetic cannabinoids in recreational users. *J Anal Toxicol*. 2013;37:534-541
7. Bonar EE, Ashrafioun L, Ilgen MA. Synthetic cannabinoid use among patients in residential substance use disorder treatment: prevalence, motives, and correlates. *Drug Alcohol Depend*. 2014;143:268-271
8. Gurney SM, Scott KS, Kacinko SL, Presley BC, Logan BK. Pharmacology, toxicology, and adverse effects of synthetic cannabinoid drugs. *Forensic Sci Rev*. 2014;26:53-71

9. Harris CR, Brown A. Synthetic cannabinoid intoxication: a case series and review. *J Emerg Med.* 2013;44:360-366
10. McElrath K, Van Hout MC. A preference for mephedrone: drug markets, drugs of choice, and the emerging "legal high" scene. *J Drug Issues.* 2011;41:487-508
11. Govaerts SJ, Muccioli GG, Hermans E, Lambert DM. Characterization of the pharmacology of imidazolidinedione derivatives at cannabinoid CB1 and CB2 receptors. *Eur J Pharmacol.* 2004;495:43-53
12. Pertwee RG. Pharmacology of cannabinoid CB1 and CB2 receptors. *Pharmacol Ther.* 1997;74: 129-180
13. Atwood BK, Mackie K. CB2: a cannabinoid receptor with an identity crisis. *Br J Pharmacol.* 2010;160:467-479
14. Tambaro S, Casu MA, Mastinu A, Lazzari P. Evaluation of selective cannabinoid CB(1) and CB(2) receptor agonists in a mouse model of lipopolysaccharide-induced interstitial cystitis. *Eur J Pharmacol.* 2014;729:67-74
15. Breivogel CS, Childers SR, Deadwyler SA, et al. Chronic Δ9-tetrahydrocannabinol treatment produces a time-dependent loss of cannabinoid receptors and cannabinoid receptor-activated G proteins in rat brain. *J Neurochem.* 1999;73:2447-2459
16. Centers for Disease Control and Prevention (CDC). Notes from the field: severe illness associated with synthetic cannabinoid use—Brunswick, Georgia, 2013. *MMWR Morb Mortal Wkly Rep.* 2013;62:939
17. Hermanns-Clausen M, Kneisel S, Szabo B, Auwärter V. Acute toxicity due to the confirmed consumption of synthetic cannabinoids: clinical and laboratory findings. *Addict Abingdon Engl.* 2013;108:534-544
18. Papanti D, Schifano F, Botteon G, et al. "Spiceophrenia": a systematic overview of "spice"-related psychopathological issues and a case report. *Hum Psychopharmacol.* 2013;28:379-389
19. Centers for Disease Control and Prevention (CDC). Notes from the field: severe illness associated with reported use of synthetic marijuana—Colorado, August–September 2013. *MMWR Morb Mortal Wkly Rep.* 2013;62:1016-1017
20. Schwartz MD, Trecki J, Edison LA, et al. A common source outbreak of severe delirium associated with exposure to the novel synthetic cannabinoid ADB-PINACA. *J Emerg Med.* 2015;48:573-580
21. Mir A, Obafemi A, Young A, Kane C. Myocardial infarction associated with use of the synthetic cannabinoid K2. *Pediatrics.* 2011;128:e1622-e1627
22. Freeman MJ, Rose DZ, Myers MA, et al. Ischemic stroke after use of the synthetic marijuana "spice." *Neurology.* 2013;81:2090-2093
23. Takematsu M, Hoffman RS, Nelson LS, et al. A case of acute cerebral ischemia following inhalation of a synthetic cannabinoid. *Clin Toxicol.* 2014;52:973-975
24. Buser GL, Gerona RR, Horowitz BZ, et al. Acute kidney injury associated with smoking synthetic cannabinoid. *Clin Toxicol.* 2014;52:664-673
25. Centers for Disease Control and Prevention (CDC). Acute kidney injury associated with synthetic cannabinoid use—multiple states, 2012. *MMWR Morb Mortal Wkly Rep.* 2013;62:93-98
26. Patton AL, Chimalakonda KC, Moran CL, et al. K2 toxicity: fatal case of psychiatric complications following AM-2201 exposure. *J Forensic Sci.* 2013;58:1676-1680
27. Hopkins CY, Gilchrist BL. A case of cannabinoid hyperemesis syndrome caused by synthetic cannabinoids. *J Emerg Med.* 2013;45:544-546
28. Nacca N, Vatti D, Sullivan R, et al. The synthetic cannabinoid withdrawal syndrome. *J Addict Med.* 2013;7:296-298
29. Macfarlane V, Christie G. Synthetic cannabinoid withdrawal: a new demand on detoxification services. *Drug Alcohol Rev.* 2015;34:147-153
30. Sithinamsuwan P, Piyavechviratana K, Kitthaweesin T, et al. Exertional heatstroke: early recognition and outcome with aggressive combined cooling—a 12-year experience. *Mil Med.* 2009;174:496-502
31. Barr J, Zomorodi K, Bertaccini EJ, Shafer SL, Geller E. A double-blind, randomized comparison of i.v. lorazepam versus midazolam for sedation of ICU patients via a pharmacologic model. *Anesthesiology.* 2001;95:286-298

32. Mowry JB, Spyker DA, Cantilena LR, McMillan N, Ford M. 2013 Annual Report of the American Association of Poison Control Centers' National Poison Data System (NPDS): 31st Annual Report. *Clin Toxicol (Phila)*. 2014;52:1032-1283

33. Muller AA, Muller GF. Inhalant abuse. *J Emerg Nurs*. 2006;32:447-448

34. Williams JF, Storck M; American Academy of Pediatrics Committee on Substance Abuse, American Academy of Pediatrics Committee on Native American Child Health. Inhalant abuse. *Pediatrics*. 2007;119:1009-1017

35. Wu LT, Pilowsky DJ, Schlenger WE. Inhalant abuse and dependence among adolescents in the United States. *J Am Acad Child Adolesc Psychiatry*. 2004;43:1206-1214

36. Sakai JT, Hall SK, Mikulich-Gilbertson SK, Crowley TJ. Inhalant use, abuse, and dependence among adolescent patients: commonly comorbid problems. *J Am Acad Child Adolesc Psychiatry*. 2004;43:1080-1088

37. Substance-related and addictive disorders. In: *Diagnostic and Statistical Manual of Mental Disorders*. 5th ed. Arlington, VA: American Psychiatric Association; 2013: 533-540

38. Avella J, Kunaparaju N, Kumar S, et al. Uptake and distribution of the abused inhalant 1,1-difluoroethane in the rat. *J Anal Toxicol*. 2010;34:381-388

39. Tormoehlen LM, Tekulve KJ, Nañagas KA. Hydrocarbon toxicity: a review. *Clin Toxicol*. 2014;52:479-489

40. Duncan JR, Lawrence AJ. Conventional concepts and new perspectives for understanding the addictive properties of inhalants. *J Pharmacol Sci*. 2013;122:237-243

41. Perit KE, Gmaz JM, Caleb Browne JD, et al. Distribution of c-Fos immunoreactivity in the rat brain following abuse-like toluene vapor inhalation. *Neurotoxicol Teratol*. 2012;34:37-46

42. Gessa GL, Muntoni F, Collu M, Vargiu L, Mereu G. Low doses of ethanol activate dopaminergic neurons in the ventral tegmental area. *Brain Res*. 1985;348:201-203

43. MacIver MB. Abused inhalants enhance GABA-mediated synaptic inhibition. *Neuropsychopharmacology*. 2009;34:2296-2304

44. Bowen SE, Batis JC, Paez-Martinez N, Cruz SL. The last decade of solvent research in animal models of abuse: mechanistic and behavioral studies. *Neurotoxicol Teratol*. 2006;28:636-647

45. Chen H-H, Lin Y-R, Chan M-H. Toluene exposure during brain growth spurt and adolescence produces differential effects on N-methyl-D-aspartate receptor-mediated currents in rat hippocampus. *Toxicol Lett*. 2011;205:336-340

46. Cruz SL, Balster RL, Woodward JJ. Effects of volatile solvents on recombinant N-methyl-D-aspartate receptors expressed in Xenopus oocytes. *Br J Pharmacol*. 2000;131:1303-1308

47. Cruz SL, Domínguez M. Misusing volatile substances for their hallucinatory effects: a qualitative pilot study with Mexican teenagers and a pharmacological discussion of their hallucinations. *Subst Use Misuse*. 2011;46(Suppl 1):84-94

48. Kurtzman TL, Otsuka KN, Wahl RA. Inhalant abuse by adolescents. *J Adolesc Health*. 2001;28:170-180

49. Beauvais F, Jumper-Thurman P, Plested B, Helm H. A survey of attitudes among drug user treatment providers toward the treatment of inhalant users. *Subst Use Misuse*. 2002;37:1391-1410

50. Takagi M, Lubman DI, Yücel M. Solvent-induced leukoencephalopathy: a disorder of adolescence? *Subst Use Misuse*. 2011;46(Suppl 1):95-98

51. Meyer-Baron M, Blaszkewicz M, Henke H, et al. The impact of solvent mixtures on neurobehavioral performance: conclusions from epidemiological data. *Neurotoxicology*. 2008;29:349-360

52. Caplan JP, Pope AE, Boric CA, Benford DA. Air conditioner refrigerant inhalation: a habit with chilling consequences. *Psychosomatics*. 2012;53:273-276

53. Cairney S, Maruff P, Burns CB, Currie J, Currie BJ. Neurological and cognitive recovery following abstinence from petrol sniffing. *Neuropsychopharmacology*. 2005;30:1019-1027

54. Demarest C, Torgovnick J, Sethi NK, Arsura E, Sethi PK. Acute reversible neurotoxicity associated with inhalation of ethyl chloride: a case report. *Clin Neurol Neurosurg*. 2011;113:909-910

55. Phatak DR, Walterscheid J. Huffing air conditioner fluid: a cool way to die? *Am J Forensic Med Pathol*. 2012;33:64-67

56. Anderson CE, Loomis GA. Recognition and prevention of inhalant abuse. *Am Fam Physician*. 2003;68:869-874

57. Himmel HM. Mechanisms involved in cardiac sensitization by volatile anesthetics: general applicability to halogenated hydrocarbons? *Crit Rev Toxicol.* 2008;38:773-803

58. Fossa AA, Wisialowski T, Magnano A, et al. Dynamic beat-to-beat modeling of the QT-RR interval relationship: analysis of QT prolongation during alterations of autonomic state versus human ether a-go-go-related gene inhibition. *J Pharmacol Exp Ther.* 2005;312:1-11

59. Jiao Z, De Jesús VR, Iravanian S, et al. A possible mechanism of halocarbon-induced cardiac sensitization arrhythmias. *J Mol Cell Cardiol.* 2006;41:698-705

60. Vance C, Swalwell C, McIntyre IM. Deaths involving 1,1-difluoroethane at the San Diego County Medical Examiner's Office. *J Anal Toxicol.* 2012;36:626-633

61. Avella J, Wilson JC, Lehrer M. Fatal cardiac arrhythmia after repeated exposure to 1,1-difluoroethane (DFE). *Am J Forensic Med Pathol.* 2006;27:58-60

62. Peyravi M, Mirzayan MJ, Krauss JK. Fatal outcome despite bilateral decompressive craniectomy for refractory intracranial pressure increase in butane intoxication. *Clin Neurol Neurosurg.* 2012;114:392-393

63. Xiong Z, Avella J, Wetli CV. Sudden death caused by 1,1-difluoroethane inhalation. *J Forensic Sci.* 2004;49:627-629

64. Sakai K, Maruyama-Maebashi K, Takatsu A, et al. Sudden death involving inhalation of 1,1-difluoroethane (HFC-152a) with spray cleaner: three case reports. *Forensic Sci Int.* 2011; 206:e58-e61

65. Novosel I, Kovačić Z, Gusić S, et al. Immunohistochemical detection of early myocardial damage in two sudden deaths due to intentional butane inhalation. Two case reports with review of literature. *J Forensic Leg Med.* 2011;18:125-131

66. Kurniali PC, Henry L, Kurl R, Meharg JV. Inhalant abuse of computer cleaner manifested as angioedema. *Am J Emerg Med.* 2012;30:265.e3-e5

67. Filley CM. Toluene abuse and white matter: a model of toxic leukoencephalopathy. *Psychiatr Clin North Am.* 2013;36:293-302

68. Cámara-Lemarroy CR, Gónzalez-Moreno EI, Rodriguez-Gutierrez R, González-González JG. Clinical presentation and management in acute toluene intoxication: a case series. *Inhal Toxicol.* 2012;24:434-438

69. Kwon B, Kim S, Kim S, et al. 1H NMR spectroscopic identification of a glue sniffing biomarker. *Forensic Sci Int.* 2011;209:120-125

70. Tsao J-H, Hu Y-H, How C-K, et al. Atrioventricular conduction abnormality and hyperchloremic metabolic acidosis in toluene sniffing. *J Formos Med Assoc.* 2011;110:652-654

71. Pan S-Y, Lin S-L. Toluene intoxication-atrioventricular block due to hypokalemia? *J Formos Med Assoc.* 2012;111:523

72. Couri D, Milks M. Toxicity and metabolism of the neurotoxic hexacarbons n-hexane, 2-hexanone, and 2,5-hexanedione. *Annu Rev Pharmacol Toxicol.* 1982;22:145-166

73. Hashizume A, Koike H, Kawagashira Y, et al. Central nervous system involvement in n-hexane polyneuropathy demonstrated by MRI and proton MR spectroscopy. *Clin Neurol Neurosurg.* 2011;113:493-495

74. Spencer PS, Schaumburg HH. Experimental neuropathy produced by 2,5-hexanedione: a major metabolite of the neurotoxic industrial solvent methyl n-butyl ketone. *J Neurol Neurosurg Psychiatry.* 1975;38:771-775

75. Horowitz BZ. Carboxyhemoglobinemia caused by inhalation of methylene chloride. *Am J Emerg Med.* 1986;4:48-51

76. Leikin JB, Kaufman D, Lipscomb JW, Burda AM, Hryhorczuk DO. Methylene chloride: report of five exposures and two deaths. *Am J Emerg Med.* 1990;8:534-537

77. Feldman RG, Mayer RM, Taub A. Evidence for peripheral neurotoxic effect of trichloroethylene. *Neurology.* 1970;20:599-606

78. Zahedi A, Grant MH, Wong DT. Successful treatment of chloral hydrate cardiac toxicity with propranolol. *Am J Emerg Med.* 1999;17:490-491

79. Mortiz F, de La Chapelle A, Bauer F, et al. Esmolol in the treatment of severe arrhythmia after acute trichloroethylene poisoning. *Intensive Care Med.* 2000;26:256

80. Joundi RA, Wong BM, Leis JA. Antibiotics "just-in-case" in a patient with aspiration pneumonitis. *JAMA Intern Med.* 2015;175:489-490

81. Broussard LA. The role of the laboratory in detecting inhalant abuse. *Clin Lab Sci J Am Soc Med Technol.* 2000;13:205-209

82. Dean BV, Stellpflug SJ, Burnett AM, Engebretsen KM. 2C or not 2C: phenethylamine designer drug review. *J Med Toxicol.* 2013;9:172-178

83. Bogle KE, Smith BH. Illicit methylphenidate use: a review of prevalence, availability, pharmacology, and consequences. *Curr Drug Abuse Rev.* 2009;2:157-176

84. Kollins SH. Comparing the abuse potential of methylphenidate versus other stimulants: a review of available evidence and relevance to the ADHD patient. *J Clin Psychiatry.* 2003;64(Suppl 11):14-18

85. Varga MD. Adderall abuse on college campuses: a comprehensive literature review. *J Evid Based Soc Work.* 2012;9:293-313

86. Williams RJ, Goodale LA, Shay-Fiddler MA, Gloster SP, Chang SY. Methylphenidate and dextroamphetamine abuse in substance-abusing adolescents. *Am J Addict.* 2004;13:381-389

87. Kollins SH. Abuse liability of medications used to treat attention-deficit/hyperactivity disorder (ADHD). *Am J Addict.* 2007;16(Suppl 1):35-42

88. Wilens TE, Adler LA, Adams J, et al. Misuse and diversion of stimulants prescribed for ADHD: a systematic review of the literature. *J Am Acad Child Adolesc Psychiatry.* 2008;47:21-31

89. Nanda S, Konnur N. Adolescent drug & alcohol use in the 21st century. *Pediatr Ann.* 2006;35:193-199

90. Verrico CD, Miller GM, Madras BK. MDMA (Ecstasy) and human dopamine, norepinephrine, and serotonin transporters: implications for MDMA-induced neurotoxicity and treatment. *Psychopharmacology (Berl).* 2007;189:489-503

91. Nakagawa T, Kaneko S. Neuropsychotoxicity of abused drugs: molecular and neural mechanisms of neuropsychotoxicity induced by methamphetamine, 3,4-methylenedioxymethamphetamine (ecstasy), and 5-methoxy-N,N-diisopropyltryptamine (foxy). *J Pharmacol Sci.* 2008;106:2-8

92. Seger D. Cocaine, metamfetamine, and MDMA abuse: the role and clinical importance of neuroadaptation. *Clin Toxicol (Phila).* 2010;48:695-708

93. Markowitz JS, Patrick KS. Differential pharmacokinetics and pharmacodynamics of methylphenidate enantiomers: does chirality matter? *J Clin Psychopharmacol.* 2008;28(3 Suppl 2):S54-S61

94. Coppola M, Mondola R. 3,4-methylenedioxypyrovalerone (MDPV): chemistry, pharmacology and toxicology of a new designer drug of abuse marketed online. *Toxicol Lett.* 2012;208:12-15

95. Bersani FS, Corazza O, Albano G, et al. 25C-NBOMe: preliminary data on pharmacology, psychoactive effects, and toxicity of a new potent and dangerous hallucinogenic drug. *Biomed Res Int.* 2014;2014:734749

96. Cameron K, Kolanos R, Vekariya R, et al. Mephedrone and methylenedioxypyrovalerone (MDPV), major constituents of "bath salts," produce opposite effects at the human dopamine transporter. *Psychopharmacology (Berl).* 2013;227:493-499

97. Kolanos R, Solis E, Sakloth F, De Felice LJ, Glennon RA. "Deconstruction" of the abused synthetic cathinone methylenedioxypyrovalerone (MDPV) and an examination of effects at the human dopamine transporter. *ACS Chem Neurosci.* 2013;4:1524-1529

98. Baumann MH, Partilla JS, Lehner KR, et al. Powerful cocaine-like actions of 3,4-methylenedioxypyrovalerone (MDPV), a principal constituent of psychoactive "bath salts" products. *Neuropsychopharmacology.* 2013;38:552-562

99. Thornton SL, Gerona RR, Tomaszewski CA. Psychosis from a bath salt product containing flephedrone and MDPV with serum, urine, and product quantification. *J Med Toxicol.* 2012;8:310-313

100. Coppola M, Mondola R. Synthetic cathinones: chemistry, pharmacology and toxicology of a new class of designer drugs of abuse marketed as "bath salts" or "plant food." *Toxicol Lett.* 2012;211:144-149

101. Gregg RA, Rawls SM. Behavioral pharmacology of designer cathinones: a review of the preclinical literature. *Life Sci.* 2014;97:27-30

102. Giorgi FS, Lazzeri G, Natale G, et al. MDMA and seizures: a dangerous liaison? *Ann N Y Acad Sci.* 2006;1074:357-364

103. Beuerle JR, Barrueto F. Neurogenic bladder and chronic urinary retention associated with MDMA abuse. *J Med Toxicol.* 2008;4:106-108
104. German CL, Fleckenstein AE, Hanson GR. Bath salts and synthetic cathinones: an emerging designer drug phenomenon. *Life Sci.* 2014;97:2-8
105. Gouzoulis-Mayfrank E, Daumann J. Neurotoxicity of drugs of abuse: the case of methylenedioxy amphetamines (MDMA, ecstasy), and amphetamines. *Dialogues Clin Neurosci.* 2009;11:305-317
106. Verdejo-García AJ, López-Torrecillas F, Aguilar de Arcos F, Pérez-García M. Differential effects of MDMA, cocaine, and cannabis use severity on distinctive components of the executive functions in polysubstance users: a multiple regression analysis. *Addict Behav.* 2005;30:89-101
107. Thomasius R, Petersen K, Buchert R, et al. Mood, cognition and serotonin transporter availability in current and former ecstasy (MDMA) users. *Psychopharmacology (Berl).* 2003;167:85-96
108. Buchert R, Thomasius R, Nebeling B, et al. Long-term effects of "ecstasy" use on serotonin transporters of the brain investigated by PET. *J Nucl Med.* 2003;44:375-384
109. Prosser JM, Nelson LS. The toxicology of bath salts: a review of synthetic cathinones. *J Med Toxicol.* 2012;8:33-42
110. Kanamori T, Tsujikawa K, Ohmae Y, et al. A study of the metabolism of methamphetamine and 4-bromo-2,5-dimethoxyphenethylamine (2C-B) in isolated rat hepatocytes. *Forensic Sci Int.* 2005;148:131-137
111. Theobald DS, Maurer HH. Identification of monoamine oxidase and cytochrome P450 isoenzymes involved in the deamination of phenethylamine-derived designer drugs (2C-series). *Biochem Pharmacol.* 2007;73:287-297
112. Carmo H, Hengstler JG, de Boer D, et al. Metabolic pathways of 4-bromo-2,5-dimethoxyphenethylamine (2C-B): analysis of phase I metabolism with hepatocytes of six species including human. *Toxicology.* 2005;206:75-89
113. Theobald DS, Fritschi G, Maurer HH. Studies on the toxicological detection of the designer drug 4-bromo-2,5-dimethoxy-β-phenethylamine (2C-B) in rat urine using gas chromatography–mass spectrometry. *J Chromatogr B.* 2007;846:374-377
114. Schneir A, Ly BT, Casagrande K, et al. Comprehensive analysis of "bath salts" purchased from California stores and the internet. *Clin Toxicol (Phila).* 2014;52:651-658
115. De Felice LJ, Glennon RA, Negus SS. Synthetic cathinones: chemical phylogeny, physiology, and neuropharmacology. *Life Sci.* 2014;97:20-26
116. Hofer KE, Grager B, Müller DM, et al. Ketamine-like effects after recreational use of methoxetamine. *Ann Emerg Med.* 2012;60:97-99
117. Helander A, Beck O, Bäckberg M. Intoxications by the dissociative new psychoactive substances diphenidine and methoxphenidine. *Clin Toxicol (Phila).* 2015;53:446-453
118. Zawilska JB. Methoxetamine: a novel recreational drug with potent hallucinogenic properties. *Toxicol Lett.* 2014;230:402-407
119. Hendrickson RG, Cloutier RL. "Crystal Dex:" free-base dextromethorphan. *J Emerg Med.* 2007;32:393-396
120. Miller SC. Coricidin HBP cough and cold addiction. *J Am Acad Child Adolesc Psychiatry.* 2005;44:509-510
121. Gilbert CR, Baram M, Cavarocchi NC. "Smoking Wet." *Tex Heart Inst J.* 2013;40:64-67
122. Bryner JK, Wang UK, Hui JW, et al. Dextromethorphan abuse in adolescence: an increasing trend: 1999-2004. *Arch Pediatr Adolesc Med.* 2006;160:1217-1222
123. Zarantonello P, Bettini E, Paio A, et al. Novel analogues of ketamine and phencyclidine as NMDA receptor antagonists. *Bioorg Med Chem Lett.* 2011;21:2059-2063
124. Antoniou T, Juurlink DN. Dextromethorphan abuse. *CMAJ.* 2014;186:E631-E631
125. Schwartz RH. Adolescent abuse of dextromethorphan. *Clin Pediatr (Phila).* 2005;44:565-568
126. Miller SC. Dextromethorphan psychosis, dependence and physical withdrawal. *Addict Biol.* 2005;10:325-327
127. Roberge RJ, Hirani KH, Rowland III PL, Berkeley R, Krenzelok EP. Dextromethorphan- and pseudoephedrine-induced agitated psychosis and ataxia: case report. *J Emerg Med.* 1999;17:285-288
128. Corazza O, Assi S, Schifano F. From "Special K" to "Special M": the evolution of the recreational use of ketamine and methoxetamine. *CNS Neurosci Ther.* 2013;19:454-460

129. Ng SH, Tse ML, Ng HW, Lau FL. Emergency department presentation of ketamine abusers in Hong Kong: a review of 233 cases. *Hong Kong Med J.* 2010;16:6-11

130. Yiu-Cheung C. Acute and chronic toxicity pattern in ketamine abusers in Hong Kong. *J Med Toxicol.* 2012;8:267-270

131. Wood DM, Davies S, Puchnarewicz M, Johnston A, Dargan PI. Acute toxicity associated with the recreational use of the ketamine derivative methoxetamine. *Eur J Clin Pharmacol.* 2012;68:853-856

132. Hofer KE, Degrandi C, Müller DM, et al. Acute toxicity associated with the recreational use of the novel dissociative psychoactive substance methoxphenidine. *Clin Toxicol (Phila).* 2014;52:1288-1291

133. Hill SL, Harbon SCD, Coulson J, et al. Methoxetamine toxicity reported to the National Poisons Information Service: clinical characteristics and patterns of enquiries (including the period of the introduction of the UK's first Temporary Class Drug Order). *Emerg Med J.* 2014;31:45-47

134. Ziaee V, Akbari Hamed E, Hoshmand A, et al. Side effects of dextromethorphan abuse, a case series. *Addict Behav.* 2005;30:1607-1613

135. Imbert L, Boucher A, Delhome G, et al. Analytical findings of an acute intoxication after inhalation of methoxetamine. *J Anal Toxicol.* 2014;38:410-415

136. Shields JE, Dargan PI, Wood DM, et al. Methoxetamine associated reversible cerebellar toxicity: three cases with analytical confirmation. *Clin Toxicol (Phila).* 2012;50:438-440

137. Wikström M, Thelander G, Dahlgren M, Kronstrand R. An accidental fatal intoxication with methoxetamine. *J Anal Toxicol.* 2013;37:43-46

138. Chen Y-C, Chen Y-L, Huang G-S, Wu C-J. Ketamine-associated vesicopathy. *QJM.* 2012;105:1023-1024

139. Wu S, Lai Y, He Y, Li X, Guan Z, Cai Z. Lower urinary tract destruction due to ketamine: a report of 4 cases and review of literature. *J Addict Med.* 2012;6:85-88

140. Gray T, Dass M. Ketamine cystitis: an emerging diagnostic and therapeutic challenge. *Br J Hosp Med (Lond).* 2012;73:576-579

141. Levin RM, Whitbeck C, Sourial MW, Tadrous M, Millington WR. Effects of dextromethorphan on in vitro contractile responses of mouse and rat urinary bladders. *Neurourol Urodyn.* 2006;25:802-807

142. Navarro A, Perry C, Bobo WV. A case of serotonin syndrome precipitated by abuse of the anti-cough remedy dextromethorphan in a bipolar patient treated with fluoxetine and lithium. *Gen Hosp Psychiatry.* 2006;28:78-80

143. Morgan CJA, Rees H, Curran HV. Attentional bias to incentive stimuli in frequent ketamine users. *Psychol Med.* 2008;38:1331-1340

144. Mutschler J, Koopmann A, Grosshans M, et al. Dextromethorphan withdrawal and dependence syndrome. *Dtsch Arztebl Int.* 2010;107:537-540

145. Tam Y-H, Ng C-F, Pang KK-Y, et al. One-stop clinic for ketamine-associated uropathy: report on service delivery model, patients' characteristics and non-invasive investigations at baseline by a cross-sectional study in a prospective cohort of 318 teenagers and young adults. *BJU Int.* 2014;114:754-760

Adolesc Med 026 (2015) 589–618

Emergency Care of Youth with Social and Environmental Vulnerabilities

Dzung X. Vo, MD[a]*; Katherine A. Mitchell, MD, MPA[b];
Eva M. Moore, MD, MSPH[c]

[a]Clinical Assistant Professor, Division of Adolescent Health and Medicine, Department of Pediatrics, British Columbia Children's Hospital, University of British Columbia Faculty of Medicine, Vancouver, British Columbia, Canada; [b]Fellow, Division of Adolescent Health and Medicine, Department of Pediatrics, British Columbia Children's Hospital, University of British Columbia Faculty of Medicine, Vancouver, British Columbia, Canada; [c]Clinical Assistant Professor, Division of Adolescent Health and Medicine, Department of Pediatrics, British Columbia Children's Hospital, University of British Columbia Faculty of Medicine, Vancouver, British Columbia, Canada

INTRODUCTION

Caring for vulnerable and marginalized adolescents requires a strong appreciation of social determinants of health, defined by the World Health Organization as "the conditions in which people are born, grow, live, work, and age."[1] Social determinants include social and environmental risk and protective factors that have profound effects on health care access and health outcomes. Adolescence is a sensitive developmental period of rapid physical and brain development, in which transitions in family, peer, and educational relationships, and the development of health behaviors and coping skills, shape lifelong health and well-being.[2,3] Critical social determinants for adolescents include poverty and income inequality, access to education, safe and supportive families, safe and supportive schools, and positive and supportive peers.[3-5]

Drawing from recent multidisciplinary advances in neurosciences, developmental psychology, social sciences, and epigenetics, the American Academy of Pediatrics endorsed an ecobiodevelopmental framework for understanding the development of child and youth health and disease within the larger social and environmental contexts.[6] This framework shows how early and repeated life adversity and trauma can have lifelong, and even intergenerational, effects on physical and mental health. Persistent poverty, discrimination, neglect, or maltreatment can lead to

---

*Corresponding author
E-mail address: dvo@cw.bc.ca

"toxic stress" in childhood, which exerts effects through multiple molecular, bio-logic, endocrinologic, neurologic, and psychological pathways, to affect brain development, learning, and behavior through the life course. Acute and chronic stress in can have significant affects during adolescence on learning, social-emotional development, risk-taking behaviors, and mental health.[7]

Physicians, physician assistants, nurse practitioners, nurses, social workers, and mental health professionals (hereafter referred to as clinicians) should be aware that several populations of adolescents are socially marginalized and dispropor-tionately affected by social determinants, which place them at increased risk for a variety of physical and mental health problems. At the same time, internal and external protective factors can buffer the risk and promote resilience among youth growing up in high-risk environments.[5,8] The positive youth development and youth resilience literature proposes that clinicians working with vulnerable and marginalized youth identify and address risks while building on strengths and promoting protective factors in order to encourage healthy coping and behaviors, and foster positive development of youth into contributing members of society.[5,9]

This article draws from the North American literature and focuses on 5 vulner-able adolescent populations: (1) immigrant and refugee youth; (2) youth in care (foster or juvenile justice); (3) lesbian, gay, bisexual, transgender, and question-ing youth; (4) homeless and street-involved youth; and (5) sexually exploited youth. We explore salient health issues and specific risk and protective factors to consider for these youth when they present for acute medical and mental health concerns, particularly in the emergency department, primary care, and adoles-cent medicine specialty settings.

Providing emergency care for vulnerable youth also requires consideration of spe-cific legal and ethical issues regarding adolescent consent and confidentiality. Because of housing and family instability and concerns about confidentiality of sen-sitive issues, vulnerable youth may be more likely to present for emergency care without their parents or guardians. Youth highly value confidential interactions with their clinicians.[10] This is particularly true for youth who have experienced mistreat-ment or disrupted attachments, which can make it difficult for youth to trust adults in authority positions.[11] Although parent or guardian permission is sometimes nec-essary for medical services and procedures, often youth can consent for sensitive health services. Examples of these services include mental health care, reproductive health, sexually transmitted infections, and substance abuse treatment. Some states and provinces have mature minor legislation that allows youth to consent for certain aspects of their care. In addition, clinicians working with vulnerable youth must consider often complex legal and ethical issues related to potential child abuse or neglect, and possible referral to child protective services when necessary.

Table 1 lists general recommendations and common themes for serving diverse populations of vulnerable youth. This article discusses additional considerations for 5 specific vulnerable youth populations. The goal of this article is to help clinicians understand the context and health issues of vulnerable youth populations, address risk factors, and provide care from a strength-based, resiliency-based perspective in order to help these youth reach their optimal health potential.

IMMIGRANT AND REFUGEE YOUTH

Key Health Considerations

Immigrant and refugee youth (including first-generation or foreign-born youth, and second-generation youth whose parents are foreign-born) are a rapidly growing population. In the United States, immigrants make up one-fourth of the population younger than age 18 and are projected to make up one-third of the youth population by 2050.[12] In Canada, immigrants make up 11% of the adolescent population aged 12 to 19[13] and 9% of the population younger than 25 years,[14] with most newcomer youth from racialized "visible minority" backgrounds (defined by the Canadian government as "persons who are non-Caucasian in race or non-white in color and who do not report being Aboriginal").[15] Immigrant and refugee youth are a heterogeneous population with wide diversity with regard to race, ethnicity, socioeconomic status, country of origin, culture, religion, education, length of time in the new country, acculturation and identity development, and social support. Therefore, population-based data on "immigrant youth" or even "Latino youth," for example, should be interpreted with caution because they may obscure important differences within subpopulations of immigrant youth. This section focuses on immigrant and refugee youth who are the most vulnerable because of social determinants such as poverty, racism, immigration status, and social marginalization. In addition, refugee youth, as well as other subpopulations such as homestay youth, border children, and migrant youth, have their own special health needs, a detailed discussion of which is beyond the scope of this article.

Immigrant and refugee youth may present for emergency care for issues related to mental health, suicidality, and health risk behavior, which in turn are affected by culture- and migration-related stressors. Acculturation and social integration (the process of changes and adaptations that occur in response to living in a new environment) and ethnic identity development (developing one's sense of belonging in relationship to one's ethnic group of origin) have been found to affect health behaviors and outcomes, although many questions remain regarding the conceptualization and measurement of these constructs in the literature.[16-18] Acculturative stress (stress associated with multiple aspects of the migration and resettlement process) has been associated with a variety of mood, anxiety, and somatic symptoms.[19-21] Some research on acculturation (using a linear model of acculturation) suggest that "more acculturated" adolescents have increased health risk behaviors, such as smoking, drinking, drug use, and sexual behaviors.[18,22] Acculturation gaps, or differences between adolescents and their parents regarding cultural beliefs and acculturation styles, are a risk factor for intergenerational cultural conflict, family conflict, mental health symptoms and suicidality, substance misuse, and delinquency.[19,23-25]

Table 1
General recommendations for care of youth with social and environmental vulnerabilities

	Recommendations
Individual Clinician	• Consider and assess psychosocial issues and social determinants of health when working with vulnerable youth. Time constraints can be a challenge for psychosocial assessment in emergency settings. The commonly used "HEADSS" adolescent psychosocial interview has been modified into a screening tool called HEADS ED (home, education, activities/peers, drugs/alcohol, suicidality, emotions/behaviors, discharge resources), which is a brief validated mental health screening tool for youth designed for use in pediatric emergency departments.[a]
	• Engage and counsel vulnerable youth using a confidential, strengths-based approach that recognizes risk factors while aiming to promote protective factors and healthy behaviors.[b–f] It is advisable to explain confidentiality as well as its limitations in each encounter with an unfamiliar youth. Although these strategies are important for all adolescents, they may be particularly important when caring for marginalized youth.
	• Adopt a nonjudgmental, compassionate, trauma-informed approach to caring for vulnerable youth. Recognize the widespread effects of trauma on health and behaviors, and view traumatized youth from the perspective of "What has happened to you? instead of "What is wrong with you?"[g]
	• Youth with social and environmental vulnerabilities may not always be obvious to clinicians. Avoid stereotyping and making assumptions about a youth's health or behaviors.
	• Health risks should be assessed by behavior and epidemiology rather than through belonging to a particular group or having a particular identity.
	• It is critical that the clinician be knowledgeable about local, provincial, and state laws governing the care of adolescents.[e] When vulnerable youth present for emergency care without their parents or guardians, clinicians must quickly assess the adolescent's capacity for consent and confidentiality, weighing developmental and ethical considerations as well as jurisdiction-specific legal considerations.[h,i,j]
	• Connect youth to community-based, developmentally and culturally appropriate positive youth development activities and supports, which can include parents, positive peer supports, and non-parental adults.
	• Help youth connect to a medical home, which can serve as a central longitudinal source of care, coordination of services, and referrals. When possible, connect youth to clinicians who have expertise in serving the specific vulnerable youth population(s) in question.
	• Know your local resources and collaborate with allied health professionals and other local agencies that work with vulnerable youth to connect them with appropriate community services and follow-up.

Institutional and community advocacy	• Advocate for policies that promote financially accessible care for youth, including insurance coverage and public safety nets.[k] • Clinic, emergency, and hospital setting should adopt policies of inclusion and diversity. Waiting room materials should demonstrate a range of positive representation of diversity of race, ethnicity, culture, gender, and sexuality. • Create accessible medical homes for vulnerable youth. Locate medical, mental health, and social services in place-based community settings where diverse youth populations feel comfortable accessing services. • Advocate for community-based wraparound care models that meet youths' physical, mental, emotional, and spiritual health needs. Models should support housing; offer opportunities for meaningful community connection, particularly to a caring adult with whom youth can build a trusting relationship; provide mental health and addictions services; and offer legal support. Programs should be structured to promote attachment, safety, a lesbian, gay, bisexual, transgender, and questioning–positive environment, and timely responsiveness to the needs of youth. • Advocate for social and economic policies that reduce societal inequalities alleviate social determinants of health such as poverty, homelessness, social and educational exclusion, and discrimination.

[a]Cappelli M, Gray C, Zemek R, et al. The HEADS-ED: a rapid mental health screening tool for pediatric patients in the emergency department. *Pediatrics.* 2012;130, e321-e327.

[b]Vo DX. Reaching immigrant youth. In: Ginsburg KR, Kinsman SB, eds. *Reaching Teens: Strength-Based Communication Strategies to Build Resilience and Support Healthy Adolescent Development.* Elk Grove Village, IL: American Academy of Pediatrics; 2014:539-544.

[c]Chaffee T. Foster care youth: engaging foster care youth into care. In: Ginsburg KR, Kinsman SB, eds. *Reaching Teens: Strength-Based Communication Strategies to Build Resilience and Support Healthy Adolescent Development.* Elk Grove Village, IL: American Academy of Pediatrics; 2014:557-562.

[d]Dowshen ND, Hawkins LA, Arrington-Sanders R, et al. Sexual and gender minority youth. In: Ginsburg KR, Kinsman SB, eds. *Reaching Teens: Strength-Based Communication Strategies to Build Resilience and Support Healthy Adolescent Development.* Elk Grove Village, IL: American Academy of Pediatrics; 2014:531-538.

[e]Auerswald C. Serving homeless and unstably housed youth. In: Ginsburg KR, Kinsman SB, eds. *Reaching Teens: Strength-Based Communication Strategies to Build Resilience and Support Healthy Adolescent Development.* Elk Grove Village, IL: American Academy of Pediatrics; 2014:569-578.

[f]Diaz A. Emotional, physical, and sexual abuse. In: Ginsburg KR, Kinsman SB, eds. *Reaching Teens: Strength-Based Communication Strategies to Build Resilience and Support Healthy Adolescent Development.* Elk Grove Village, IL: American Academy of Pediatrics; 2014:489-498.

[g]Klinic Community Health Center. Trauma-informed: the trauma toolkit: a resource for service organizations and providers to deliver services that are trauma-informed, Second Edition, 2013. Available at: trauma-informed.ca. Accessed January 22, 2015.

[h]Ford CA, Sigman G. Confidential health care for adolescents: position paper of the Society for Adolescent Medicine. *J Adolesc Health.* 2004;35:160-167.

[i]Harrison C; for the Bioethics Committee, Canadian Paediatric Society. CPS position statement: treatment decisions regarding infants, children and adolescents. *Paediatr Child Health.* 2004;9:99-103.

[j]Elliott AS; for the Adolescent Health Committee, Canadian Paediatric Society. Meeting the health care needs of street-involved youth. *Paediatr Child Health.* 2013;18:317-326.

[k]English A, Park MJ, Shafer MA, Kreipe R, D'Angelo LJ; for the Society for Adolescent Medicine. Health care reform and adolescents-an agenda for the lifespan: a position paper of the Society for Adolescent Medicine. *J Adolesc Health.* 2009;45:310-315.

Researchers have reported a "healthy immigrant effect" (also called the immigrant paradox or epidemiologic paradox), in which first and second immigrants seem to fare better than later-generation immigrants and non-immigrant counterparts across a range of outcomes (social, mental health, risk behaviors, and delinquency) despite having lower socioeconomic status.[20,22,26] However, this effect may depend on specific outcomes being measured and on the time since immigration. For example, some research suggests that first-generation adolescents report more acculturative stress and internalizing symptoms compared to second-generation immigrants.[21] Other research suggests that youth who have immigrated more recently are at higher risk for psychological symptoms, particularly internalizing symptoms.[27]

Migration-related risk factors for mental health symptoms and risk behaviors include low family support and family conflict.[28-30] Some immigrant youth experience extended periods of geographic separation from their parents and families.[31,32] Some youth, particularly refugee youth, may have experienced significant migration-related trauma related to factors such as war, genocide, famine, traumatic journeys, forced family separation, and resettlement.[20,31,33-35] Rates of posttraumatic stress disorder (PTSD) among refugee youth have been estimated around 11% (with estimates ranging widely from 5%-89%).[35] After arrival, many immigrant youth and families experience multiple moves and attempts at resettlement, commonly without a community of similar cultural background and significant social isolation. Many immigrant youth experience discrimination and racism, which can have harmful effects on their mental health, academic and social adjustment, and health risk behaviors.[20,33,36,37] Some immigrant and refugee youth are vulnerable to victimization and recruitment by criminal gangs and subsequent involvement in violence and the juvenile justice system. Influences that increase this vulnerability include poverty, neighborhood disadvantage, perceived discrimination, limited English proficiency, refugee status, barriers to mental health services, and intergenerational and family conflicts.[33,38,39]

Research on suicidality among immigrant youth has yielded mixed findings, with varying rates according to ethnicity, generational status, and country of origin. Immigrant youth overall appear to have slightly lower rates of suicidality compared to native-born youth, although ethnicity-specific isolated increases in suicidality have been reported.[19,40] In the United States, suicide rates for youth of color have traditionally been lower than that of whites, but more recent population-based data suggest that Latino and Asian American/Pacific Islander youth may have slightly higher rates of suicidal ideation and attempts compared to non-Hispanic white and non-Hispanic black youth.[19] Risk factors for suicidality among immigrant youth include acculturation stress, depression, trauma, poverty, later generational status (second and higher generation vs first-generation), geographic separation from parents, and possibly loss of protective cultural factors such as family cohesion or religiosity.[19,33,40] Intergenerational cultural conflicts also seems to be an important risk factor for suicidality, especially among Asian American youth.[19]

Depending on the country of origin, immigrant and refugee children and youth may also be at risk for certain medical conditions, including regionally endemic infectious diseases (eg, tuberculosis, hepatitis A, amebiasis, parasitosis, human immunodeficiency virus [HIV]); congenital infections for which they may have not been screened; dental caries and poor dental care; hemoglobinopathies; and inadequate vaccination and vaccination records.[31,41]

Barriers and Challenges to Care

Lack of legal immigration and documentation status can be a major barrier to care for undocumented immigrants and refugees, both in the United States[22,31] and Canada.[42] Some evidence suggests that barriers related to immigration status (documented versus undocumented) and inadequate health insurance deter immigrants from seeking routine and preventive medical care both in the United States and in Canada,[22,42] thereby increasing the need for emergency care. Some evidence suggests that immigrant children and youth also face barriers to accessing mental health care[33] and emergency medical care.[43] Language barriers and inadequate translation services are significant impediments to care for immigrant adolescents and their family members with limited English proficiency.[22,31] Utilization of children and adolescents as interpreters is almost always discouraged because parents need to disclose sensitive information, disclosure may be traumatic for the child, and some immigrant adolescents may intentionally mistranslate in order to hide information from their parents.[44] Cultural barriers to care and inadequate cultural competency on the part of health care practitioners and health care systems have been well-documented.[45] For instance, some immigrant adolescents perceive that health care practitioners may make assumptions, treat them differently, or discriminate against them.[44]

Protective Factors and Strategies

Some evidence suggests that adolescents with an "integrated" acculturation style (affiliation with both their culture of origin and the new culture) seem to have optimal adaptation and functioning.[16,46] Social and academic support is protective against acculturation stress and mental health symptoms for immigrant youth.[21] Family-related factors can also influence adolescent health. For example, several studies have found that increased family efficacy (a family's confidence in its capabilities to manage different situations in order to achieve desired outcomes) is protective against risk behaviors, including tobacco use, alcohol and drug use, and sexual behaviors.[47] Increased family cohesion has been found to be protective against mental health symptoms and violence, and may buffer the harmful effects of discrimination.[28,40,48] Living in an intact family (without geographic separation between youth and parents) seems to be an important protective factor against suicidality.[29,40] Some studies suggest that the development of a positive sense of ethnic identity and bicultural self-efficacy (confidence in navigating both culture of origin and mainstream culture) may be protective against youth violence and delinquency.[39,49] Table 2 lists recommendations for serving immigrant and refugee youth.

Table 2
Recommendations for emergency care of immigrant and refugee youth

	Recommendations
Individual Clinician	• Strive to serve immigrant youth and families with cultural competence (skills to effectively serve in cross-cultural situations) and cultural humility (a strategy that emphasizes lifelong learning, self-critique, and awareness of one's own biases).[a-g] • Avoid using youth or family members as untrained language interpreters. Instead, use bilingual clinicians, professional interpreters, or remote technologies for language interpretation.[b,d,h] • Do not make cultural assumptions about health behaviors of immigrant youth. Screen and counsel immigrant youth regarding health risk behaviors the same as you would for all youth. • Be alert to potential acculturation stress, trauma, and cultural dynamics that may affect the health presentation or care plan. Assess a youth's identity and acculturation style, for example, by asking what group(s) they identify with, what language(s) and activities they prefer, and whether or not they've experienced discrimination. Ask about migration history, family conflicts and stressors, and intergenerational conflicts around culture.[e,i,j] • Support an integrated acculturation style (or bicultural identity) by encouraging youth to retain affiliation and identity with their culture(s) of origin while establishing ties with the broader mainstream society. • Help immigrant youth develop positive relationships with their families, being aware of potential intergenerational cultural conflicts and acculturation gaps. • Given barriers to routine health care for this population, consider using acute care visits as opportunities for infectious diseases screening and catch-up vaccinations as indicated, when possible. Caring for Kids New to Canada lists considerations in the medical assessment for immigrant and refugee children.[k]
Institutional and community advocacy	• Make health care accessible to all youth regardless of legal immigration or documentation status. • In administration and policy, promote the development of a more culturally effective health care, including professional training and evaluation, adequacy of linguistic services and materials, and data collection and quality improvement.[d,g] • In medical education, promote the development of a more diverse and culturally competent health care workforce.[d,g]

[a]Vo DX. Reaching immigrant youth. In: Ginsburg KR, Kinsman SB, eds. *Reaching Teens: Strength-Based Communication Strategies to Build Resilience and Support Healthy Adolescent Development*. Elk Grove Village, IL: American Academy of Pediatrics; 2014:539-544.

[b]Chilton LA, Handal GA, Paz-Soldan GJ; American Academy of Pediatrics Council on Community Pediatrics. Providing care for immigrant, migrant, and border children. *Pediatrics*. 2013;131:e2028-e2034

[c]Pumariega AJ, Rothe E. Cultural considerations in child and adolescent psychiatric emergencies and crises. *Child Adolesc Psychiatr Clin N Am*. 2003;12:723-744.

[d]Britton, CV; American Academy of Pediatrics Committee on Pediatric Workforce. Ensuring culturally effective pediatric care: implications for education and health policy. *Pediatrics*. 2004;114:1677-1685.

[e]Vo DX, Mayhew M, eds. Cultural competence for child and youth health professionals. In: *Caring for Kids New to Canada. A guide for health professionals working with immigrant and refugee children and youth* July 2014. Ottawa, ON: Canadian Paediatric Society. Available at: www.kidsnewtocanada.ca/culture/competence. Accessed January 20, 2015.

[f]Lewis VJ, Campbell K, Diaz A et al. Cultural humility. In: Ginsburg KR, Kinsman SB, eds. *Reaching Teens: Strength-Based Communication Strategies to Build Resilience and Support Healthy Adolescent Development*. Elk Grove Village, IL: American Academy of Pediatrics; 2014:145-152.

[g]Barkley L, Kodjo C, West KJ, et al; for the Society for Adolescent Health and Medicine. Promoting equity and reducing health disparities among racially/ethnically diverse adolescents: a position paper of the Society for Adolescent Health and Medicine. *J Adolesc Health*. 2013;52:804-807.

[h]Hilliard R, ed. Using interpreters in health care settings. In: *Caring for Kids New to Canada. A guide for health professionals working with immigrant and refugee children and youth*. July 2014. Ottawa, ON: Canadian Pediatric Society. Available at: www.kidsnewtocanada.ca/care/interpreters. Accessed January 20, 2015.

[i]Beiser M, Korczak D, eds. Post-traumatic stress disorder. In: *Caring for Kids New to Canada. A guide for health professionals working with immigrant and refugee children and youth*. August 2014. Ottawa, ON: Canadian Paediatric Society. Available at: www.kidsnewtocanada.ca/mental-health/ptsd. Accessed January 21, 2015.

[j]Mayhew M, ed. Adaptation and acculturation. In: *Caring for Kids New to Canada. A guide for health professionals working with immigrant and refugee children and youth*. April 2013. Ottawa, ON: Canadian Paediatric Society. Available at: www.kidsnewtocanada.ca/culture/adaptation. Accessed January 20, 2015.

[k]Hilliard R, ed. Medical assessment of immigrant and refugee children. In: *Caring for Kids New to Canada. A guide for health professionals working with immigrant and refugee children and youth*. August 2014. Ottawa, ON: Canadian Pediatric Society. www.kidsnewtocanada.ca/care/assessment. Accessed January 20, 2015.

YOUTH IN CARE

Key Health Considerations

Nearly 500,000 children and adolescents are in foster care in the United States and Canada.[50,51] They represent less than 1% of the general population of children and adolescents,[52,53] yet they are disproportionally seen in emergency care because of the increased frequency of morbidity and mortality across their lifespan. Health care disparities begin in early childhood and are multifactorial.[54] Maltreated children enter foster care with high rates of physical, emotional, and developmental risks, with estimates that every child has at least 1 physical health care diagnosis.[54] Once in care, 35% to 50% of youth have a physical health condition, and 50% to 80% have a psychiatric diagnosis.[54] Foster children are at risk for poor outcomes in adolescent and young adult years and are vastly overrepresented in at-risk youth populations.[55] Furthermore, the effects of child maltreatment are long-lasting, with longitudinal evidence linking childhood abuse and family dysfunction to chronic disease, psychiatric illness, and poor sexual health outcomes.[56-58]

Youth in care have almost twice the rates of emergency service use compared to youth with economic disadvantages.[59] Placement into a new living situation is a critical time when more children are likely to present to emergency services,[59] which reflects the destabilization that occurs with home transitions.[60] Psychiatric presentations are the most common reason for seeking emergency services.[61] Use of psychotropic medications is much more frequent in this population and is increasing, reflective of difficult-to-control behaviors and emotions without adequate therapeutic support in those with traumatic histories, disruptive attachment to parenting adults, and fragmented care.[60] Overmedication is a concern because many mental health symptoms are a reflection of challenging environmental situations rather than illness flare-ups.[62] Foster care youth also have higher rates of chronic disease, such as asthma, diabetes, hypertension, epilepsy,[63] and other chronic health conditions.[64] Sexual health issues, including early sexual initiation, adolescent pregnancy, and sexually transmitted infections, are more common.[54]

Youth involved in the juvenile justice system are a special population of youth in care. These youth have high morbidity and mortality related to both their health pre-incarceration and the stress of detainment. Health examinations at intake may identify a chronic health condition that was poorly attended to previously and thus became an urgent medical problem.[65] Suicide and injuries occur at high frequencies during detainment,[65,66] but rates may be lower with routine screening.[67] When they present to health care, this population may face significant misunderstanding and practitioner biases because of pervasive societal perceptions of young people in the juvenile justice system as being violent, dangerous, and gang-involved.[68] However, most youth in the US juvenile justice system are detained for non-violent crimes, and some may be involved in activities considered illegal only because of their age, such as truancy, curfew violations, or running away from home.[69] Gang involvement among youth presenting to the emergency department is relatively rare.[68]

Barriers and Challenges to Care

Inadequate medical histories, disruption in primary and preventive care, and inadequate uptake of community and primary care services to prevent and manage illness are challenges for those serving youth in care. Fragmented or absent medical histories stem from changes in living situations without a unified strategy to maintain continuity of medical care from one home to the next.[54] Inadequate medical services before entry into foster care is another contributing factor.[54] Although housing placements are intended to be short-term, the average foster child spends more than 2 years in care, and adolescents in foster care often experience frequent moves and subsequent disruptions.[55] Health care management is the legal responsibility of the state for youth in care yet often requires medical expertise given the complexity of the youth in care.

Similar to foster care youth, juvenile justice–involved youth have multiple interferences with continuity of health care, including numerous moves, change in custody arrangements, gaps in health insurance coverage, and disconnection from responsible adults.[65] Sentences and terms of custody vary, so youth may only have the assistance of detention staff, a case worker, probation officer, or other court-facilitated advocate for a particular duration of time, and assembling facilitated follow-up and ongoing care recommendations may be impractical.

Protective Factors and Strategies

Potential avenues to mitigate the negative effects of foster care and juvenile justice involvement on adolescent health include longitudinal mentorship, longitudinal connections to a clinician or a medical home, and case management.[54] For many youth, involvement in the foster care or juvenile justice system is their first opportunity for medical and mental health care evaluation and treatment. Nonparental adult mentors have demonstrated effectiveness in decreasing negative health outcomes.[54] State programs that have implemented medical home and case management policies demonstrate less usage of emergency care services.[70,71] Tools to assist adolescents and young adults assume responsibility for their own health care as they transition out of the pediatric system may be reasonably applied to youth in care to mitigate the disruption in health care information. On a policy level, growing evidence suggests that extended foster care support beyond age 18 leads to improved adult health, education, and employment outcomes.[54,72] Clinicians who attend to youth in care are well positioned to be advocates for the best interests of this population.[60] Table 3 lists recommendations for serving youth in care.

Table 3
Recommendations for emergency care of youth in care and juvenile justice involved youth

	Recommendations
Individual Clinician	• Presentation to the emergency department at times of crisis provides an opportunity to engage stabilizing social services but requires attention to underlying issues leading to the crisis, linkages to outpatient services, and communication with responsible and consistent adults who can adhere to follow-up plans. • Point-of-care testing, empiric treatment, and timely follow-up plans should be used for youth in care and juvenile justice–involved youth given that custody arrangements and living situations can change quickly for adolescents. • Youth should be encouraged to take charge of their own health care information and develop skills to become their own health advocates. See "MyHealth Passport" online as an example.[a]
Institutional and community advocacy	• Emergency departments and clinics should establish a protocol for identifying guardianship and living situation at triage because the health history, case management, and follow-up care plans may depend on involvement of responsible adults who have a longstanding continuous relationship with the adolescent, such as a parent, foster parent, or social worker. • Measures to prevent disruption of health insurance when entering and leaving care are critical. • Emergencies will be decreased with policies that require timely and comprehensive initial assessments that include physical, mental, dental, and developmental assessments immediately when entering care or custody. Advocate for policies that can improve outcomes for this population. Principal avenues include welfare reforms measures such as guardianship permanency, extended foster care supports beyond age 18, and health professional case management programs.

[a]Kaufman, M. The Hospital for Sick Children. Good 2 Go Transition Program—MyHealth Passport. 2007 to 2012. Available at: www.sickkids.ca/myhealthpassport. Accessed January 18, 2015.

LESBIAN, GAY BISEXUAL, TRANSGENDER, AND QUESTIONING YOUTH

Key Health Considerations

Lesbian, gay, bisexual, transgender, and questioning (LGBTQ) youth have special needs in emergency settings because of sensitivity regarding their coming out and potential experiences of discrimination, stigma, and victimization. Estimates of people that identify as LGBTQ vary from 2% to 10%,[73] but it is difficult to obtain accurate youth estimates. Identification of LGBTQ youth may not be clear to the clinician. Identification as LGBTQ does not always match behavior, and both self-identification and behaviors may shift throughout adolescence and young adulthood.[73]

Most LGBTQ youth are well adjusted,[73] although rates of depression, suicide thoughts, and suicidal attempts are more frequent among lesbian, gay, and bisexual youth.[74] Personal, family, peer, school, and community factors all influence this risk,[75] and expert opinion attributes the risk to increased discrimination, harassment, and isolation experienced by LGBTQ youth.[75] Feelings of disconnection is a common theme among LGBTQ youth.[76] Family rejection is associated with poor health outcomes during young adulthood.[77] Substance use is increased in both female and male LGBTQ youth, which is likely a reflection of negative coping behaviors.[73]

Sexual health risks are the same or increased for LGBTQ youth compared with heterosexual youth. Lesbian youth are at equal or increased risk for pregnancy and sexually transmitted infections because of heterosexual intercourse.[73] Bisexual females, compared to lesbian and heterosexual-identified youth, have higher reports of emergency contraception use, pregnancy termination, and number of lifetime male partners.[78,79] Gay-identified male youth may also impregnate a female partner and are at risk for sexually transmitted infections.[73] Inquiries should be made about sexual behaviors rather than sexual orientation, because behaviors may not be presumed by group identification. The LGBTQ youth does not want to be singled out as having increased HIV risk, yet emergency departments are important locations for identification of primary and chronic HIV among all adolescents.[80]

Higher rates of victimization of LGBTQ youth in their homes,[81] schools,[75] relationships,[82] and communities[73] have been reported and are important to assess because victimization is associated with higher rates of suicidality among all youth.[83]

Barriers and Challenges to Care

Lesbian, gay, bisexual, transgender, and questioning people face disparities and barriers in health care settings. Clinicians are poorly trained in LGBTQ issues. Three-fourths of emergency medicine programs do not provide any LGBTQ training,[84] which may explain why clinicians rarely ask adolescents about their sexuality,[85] even when they come to medical attention for mental health or sexual health reasons.[73] Only one-third of LGBTQ youth disclose their sexuality to their clinicians, mostly because the clinicians do not ask.[85]

Lesbian, gay, bisexual, transgender, and questioning youth value the same characteristics in their health care settings as do other youth. Some of the most important clinician characteristics desired are strong interpersonal skills, cleanliness, and medical expertise. The youth also appreciate clinician comfort and experience with, knowledge of, and accepting attitude toward LGBTQ youth[86,87] but do not require clinicians with the same gender or sexual orientation, nor is it necessary that clinician disclose their own sexuality.[86] Some youth require discretion about their sexuality if they have not yet come out to their family or friends.

Transgender youth require particular consideration. Little research has been done on transgender youth to guide the approach to their needs in the health care setting. Transgender individuals may delay or forgo care because of concerns about discrimination. In a survey of transgender people, of the third who used emergency care, 70% did not have their needs met, and more than half reported negative experience related to their gender identity: 32% reported hearing hurtful or insulting language; 31% reported that the practitioner did not know enough to provide care; 24% reported that the staff or practitioner thought gender marker on ID was a mistake; 24% said they were belittled or ridiculed for being transgender; and 18% reported that the practitioner refused to discuss transgender-related concerns.[88] Transgender youth may or may not be identified by clinicians, and they may be in any stage of the transition process. Most underage youth will have their biologic anatomic gender and will require the health care screening and evaluation appropriate for their biologic gender. Cross-sex hormones may contribute to health care presentation, and clinicians can reference the World Professional Association for Transgender Health guidelines for specific medication related considerations.[89]

Protective Factors and Strategies

Protective factors for LGBTQ youth include connectedness to peers, family, and a community. Family acceptance has been shown to greatly improve outcomes for LGBTQ youth.[77] Group membership as part of the coming out process is protective for many LGBT youth because it allows them to feel less singled out[76]; however, some youth may not be ready to come out. Connections among peers and family facilitate collective resistance and personal agency, which in turn contributes to improved wellness.[76] The neighborhood or region in which a person lives is also important, because mental health symptoms are associated with living in neighborhoods with higher rates of hate crimes and are less frequent when protective policies are in place.[90] With the growing public acceptance and improved legal environment for LGBTQ individuals, there is a shift in the social ecology that is likely to improve outcomes for young LGBTQ people, although the developmental differences will still persist. Table 4 lists recommendations for providing care to LGBTQ youth.

HOMELESS AND STREET-INVOLVED YOUTH

Key Health Considerations

Homeless youth are heterogeneous in terms of their pathways to homelessness, street experiences, and health needs.[91] Consistent definitions of homelessness are lacking.[92] Overlapping terms include literally homeless (youth who live out-

Table 4

Recommendations for emergency care of lesbian, gay, bisexual, transgender, and questioning youth

	Recommendations
Individual Clinician	• A non-judgmental approach and sensitivity around LGBTQ issues are essential, such as not assuming LGBTQ sexual health and human immunodeficiency virus risks.[a] Avoid assessing youth health risks according to sexual orientation; instead ask specific questions about sexual behaviors. Never assume a risk category based on someone's sexual orientation or group identification.
	• All youth need open and honest communication about sexual behaviors and mental health.
	• Clinical screening should assess isolation, runaway status, victimization, sexual safety, depression/suicide, school connection, alcohol and drug use, and family acceptance.
	• Clinicians can use acute situations to promote family, school, and community connectedness by recognizing positive acceptance among families and facilitating healthy communication and interactions. Families and youth should be connected to resources and community supports to increase acceptance and decrease rejection of the child and of the child's identity, if needed.
	• Some youth will not be ready to discuss their sexuality with their clinicians, parents, or peers. Clinicians should accept their patient's desire for confidentiality regarding these sensitive issues.
	• In cases of ongoing or significant distress, referral to an LGBTQ-sensitive mental health therapist or family therapist is important. Gender questioning and transgendered youth should be connected to a youth-friendly gender clinic or specialist for evaluation if the youth is interested.
Institutional and community advocacy	• The Society for Adolescent Health and Medicine calls for more education for clinicians around sexual development, LGBTQ youth health issues, and issues related to the coming out process.[b]
	• Health care facilities should adopt policies and practices of inclusion to decrease discrimination and health care disparities for this population. Guidelines established by national advocacy organizations can serve as a starting place.[c,d]
	• Health care facilities should avoid gender segregation, including gender-based group examination rooms and bathrooms.[e]

LGBTQ, lesbian, gay, bisexual, transgender and questioning youth.

[a]Ginsburg KR, Winn RJ, Rudy BJ, et al. How to reach sexual minority youth in the health care setting: the teens offer guidance. *J Adolesc Health*. 2002;31:407-416.

[b]Reitman DS, Austin B, Belikind U, et al; for the Society for Adolescent Health and Medicine. Recommendations for promoting the health and well-being of lesbian, gay, bisexual, and transgender adolescents: a position paper of the Society for Adolescent Health and Medicine. *J Adolesc Health*. 2013;52:506-510.

[c]Gay and Lesbian Medical Association. Guidelines for care of lesbian, gay, bisexual, and transgender patients. Available at: www.glma.org/_data/n_0001/resources/live/GLMA%20guidelines%202006%20FINAL.pdf. Accessed January 17, 2015.

[d]GLBT Health Access Project. Community standards of practice for the provision of quality health care services to lesbian, gay, bisexual, and transgender clients. Available at: www.glbthealth.org/CommunityStandardsofPractice.htm. Accessed January 17, 2015.

[e]Shaffer N. Transgender patients: implications for emergency department policy and practice. *J Emerg Nurs*. 2005;31:405-407.

doors or in abandoned buildings, or use emergency shelters or hostels); relatively homeless (youth living in unsafe, inadequate, or insecure housing, eg, staying temporarily with friends or relatives or "couch surfing"); runaways (youth who have spent more than 1 night away from home without parental permission); throwaways (youth forced to leave home by their parents); and street youth (youth living in high-risk non-traditional locations such as under bridges). An umbrella term, street-involved youth (SIY), broadly encompasses these varying degrees of housing insecurity and homelessness.[92]

Estimates of the North American population of SIY are difficult because of the hidden, variably defined, transient, and marginalized nature of the population.[93] Conservatively, on any given night 1.6 to 2 million American[94] and 150,000 Canadian youth[92] are homeless. Street-involved youth of all genders live in urban and rural areas. Reasons for street involvement and homelessness are often complex.[95] Disrupted family relationships are the most common reason young people leave home.[94] Youth exposed to violence and trauma, particularly physical or sexual abuse, are at significantly increased risk for running away.[92] Notably, the relationship between homelessness and trauma is bidirectional, with homelessness being both a consequence and a precipitator of trauma. Parental drug and alcohol abuse, poverty, residential instability, and underlying mental health issues are other key contributors.[94] Youth in care[96,97] and LGBT youth[94,96] are at especially high risk for becoming homeless.

Street-involved youth have increased mortality compared to housed peers of the same age and sex.[98] Leading causes of death are suicide, accidental injury, and substance overdose. Street-involved youth also face significant morbidity related to their physical, sexual, and mental health and social well-being.[97] Morbidity can occur both during the period of homelessness as well as afterward. Adverse health outcomes are often the result of engaging in risk behaviors to meet survival needs and cope with life on the street.[99] Levels of risk-taking are influenced not only by individual factors but also by local sociocultural environments.[100] Unsafe sexual practices, substance use, food insecurity, inadequate shelter, exposure to violence, low levels of social support, and limited access to medical care all contribute to negative health outcomes.[98,101] The longer that youth are street-involved, the more likely they are to suffer these health challenges.[95]

Clinicians should be aware of common acute physical health presentations among SIY. Generally SIY present with more advanced illness than other youth given the frequent lack of access to prevention and early intervention services.[94] Street-involved youth are particularly at risk for injuries and trauma,[101] especially that occurring secondary to substance use or violence.[92] Respiratory problems, especially asthma and tuberculosis, are more common.[100,101] Street involvement increases exposure to asthma triggers but also presents major barriers to asthma management.[101] Tuberculosis is increased because of their interactions with others at risk and their exposure to crowded shelter conditions. Street-involved youth suffer dermatologic problems, such as impetigo, infestations, acne, and atopic dermatitis; skin and soft tissue infections; and foot problems.[92,94,101] These conditions are frequently caused or exacerbated by exposure to wet and cold, inadequate footwear, and lack of access to shower facilities. Additionally, SIY often have poor dental health, especially sensitive and discolored teeth, dental caries, acute tooth pain, and broken teeth secondary to lack of oral care, poor hygiene, smoking, and alcohol use.[92,101-103] They are at high risk for hunger and malnutrition because of issues with food insecurity and comorbid drug use.[92]

Street-involved youth experience much higher rates of sexually transmitted infections, including gonorrhea, chlamydia, herpes, trichomonas, syphilis, and HIV than housed peers.[92,94,101,104] Street youth also have high rates of hepatitis B and C,[98,100] and they are vulnerable to hepatitis A acquisition because of their living conditions. As a group, SIY engage in more sexual risk behaviors than non-homeless peers,[94,104] including inconsistent condom use, multiple and concurrent sexual partners, early sexual debut, and engagement in survival sex (exchanging sex for resources such as money, food, shelter, drugs, or transportation).[105] Social and structural factors that highly contribute to negative outcomes include economic inequalities, laws, policies, criminalization, and displacement; lack of affordability of effective contraception and family planning services; higher rates of sexual abuse and exploitation; and systemic discrimination.

Runaway and homeless youth have a greater likelihood of pregnancy than non-SIY youth. Contributing factors include sexual abuse and exploitation, engaging in high-risk sexual behaviors, lack of affordability of the most effective contraception methods (ie, long-acting reversible contraceptives), and limited access to family planning services. Pregnancy represents an episode of dysequilibrium in the lives of SIY, often calling into question their desire to continue to live on the street,[106] and therefore could be viewed by youth as a hopeful or positive life event catalyzing a transition to a more stable living situation.

Street-involved youth have high levels of mental health disorders, including depression, bipolar disorder, anxiety, substance abuse, PTSD, and psychosis.[92,94] These conditions both precede homelessness and can be precipitated by the chronic stress of homelessness. Rates of psychiatric hospitalization are higher among homeless adolescents than housed peers.[101] Street-involved youth also have markedly high rates of suicidal ideation, attempts at suicide, and completed suicide.[94,107] Evidence suggests a strong and graded association between childhood trauma and subsequent attempted suicide among SIY.[107] Younger age at street life entry is associated with higher risk for depression and negative mental health outcomes.[97]

Street-involved youth commonly use substances to alter mood, cope with trauma, gain peer acceptance, and satisfy expectations of an exploiter.[95] Patterns of substance use are influenced by gender, age, length of homelessness, and sociogeographic context.[94] Youth who are totally homeless are at greatest risk for substance abuse, followed by shelter-based youth, with home-based youth at lowest risk.[101] Substance use can trigger or exacerbate mental health problems, contribute to engagement in high-risk behaviors, and lead to injuries.[94]

Barriers and Challenges to Care

Street-involved youth who present to the health setting can be challenging for clinicians because many SIY do not fit a stereotypical image of homelessness. They often appear initially healthy despite later requiring management for medical problems related to homelessness. Often SIY do not reveal they are homeless unless they are asked directly about housing or economic status. Figure 1 shows a short screening tool that can help to identify SIY.

Street-involved youth often lack money, transportation, and knowledge to access appropriate health care services. Because of their histories of trauma and disrupted attachments, SIY are often distrustful of adults and professional agencies, skeptical about psychiatric treatment, and fearful of the police and social services. The demands of finding adequate food[92,95,97,101,108] and shelter can consume significant time and energy, impairing their ability to prioritize health care. Structural factors that limit care to SIY include the need for a health card or permanent address, inaccessible health insurance, perceived need for adult con-

---

In the last 6 months, have you stayed one or more nights in any of these places because you could not stay in your home or you did not have a home?

- A shelter _____
- Outdoors _____
- A squat _____
- With a stranger or someone you did not know well _____
- A car _____
- On public transportation _____
- A single-room occupancy (SRO)/hotel _____
- Jail _____
- One or more of these places, but I don't want to say which _____

Scoring: *If participant indicates only one of these choices, ask if this was for one night or more (eg, "You said you stayed outdoors in the past 6 months. Was this for one night, or more than that?").*

If participant stayed **0 or one night total** *in any place or combination of places, participant is not to be considered unstably housed.*

If participant stayed **more than one night** *in any place or combination of places, participant is to be considered unstably housed.*

Fig 1. Unstable housing status screening tool. From Auerswald C. Serving homeless and unstably housed youth. In: Ginsburg KR, Kinsman SB, eds. *Reaching Teens: Strength-Based Communication Strategies to Build Resilience and Support Healthy Adolescent Development.* Elk Grove Village, IL: American Academy of Pediatrics; 2014:575.

sent, services that are difficult to access and poorly coordinated, clinics that are closed on evenings and weekends, long referral waitlists, services that cater to homeless adults instead of youth, and stigmatization and criminalization of SIY.[92,94,109] Given these barriers, many youth delay seeking care, which increases their risk for serious health problems and need for emergency care.[94]

Protective Factors and Strategies

Mobilization of particular personal and social resources, as well as minimizing the negative environmental influences of homelessness, have been shown to support positive health and developmental outcomes among SIY.[110-114] The relationships between protective factors, which are complex and interactive over time, remain a topic of active research.[110] The presence of natural mentors (non-parental adults to whom SIY turn for support) is associated with fewer risky sexual behaviors, higher protective sexual behaviors, and better school attendance.[111] Similarly, social support in the form of tangible aid and service is protective against depressive symptoms and subjective health status.[112] Among males and females, positive expectations for the future and decision-making skills are both correlated with healthier sexual behaviors.[113] Having self-esteem, being employed, and attending school seem to positively affect sexual health behaviors in females.[113] Finally, the importance of stable housing for homeless youth is clear; the longer they are unstably housed, the greater the erosion of mental health variables and resilience.[114] Table 5 lists recommendations for serving homeless youth and SIY.

SEXUALLY EXPLOITED YOUTH

Key Health Considerations

Sexual exploitation of adolescents is variably defined in the literature. It includes adolescents younger than 18 years engaged in commercial sex work (on the street, in brothels, through escort services, and on the Internet), sex trafficking, pornography, exotic dancing, and survival sex.[115] These situations include youth selling or trading sexual activities for resources such as money, food, shelter, drugs, or transportation.[105] Sexual exploitation of adolescents constitutes a form of coercion and violence, and it is considered to be sexual abuse and a human rights abuse by the United Nations Conventions on the Rights of the Child.[116] Although some youth may feel that they have consented to these activities and do not feel exploited, the adults who participating in sexual activities with them are exploiting them.[105,116]

The scope of sexual exploitation of youth in North America is underrecognized. The National Longitudinal Study of Adolescent Health found that 3.5% of adolescents had ever exchanged sex for drugs or money.[117] Canadian studies have found 1 in 3 SIY and 1 in 5 youth in juvenile justice custody had a history of sexual exploitation.[105] Sexually exploited youth are too often misidentified as criminals (eg, as prostitutes)

Table 5

Recommendations for emergency care of homeless and street-involved youth

	Recommendations
Individual Clinician	• Use screening strategies to identify families and youth at risk for street involvement and facilitate early connection to supportive community resources. See Figure 1 for an example of a brief screening tool that can be used to identify SIY.[a] • When street-involved youth present for acute medical concerns, screen for acute mental health and safety concerns (eg, suicidality, exploitation, drug use). • Take advantage of opportunities at acute care visits to provide point-of-care services and address immediate and routine health needs. For example, provide comprehensive sexual health assessment, treat any suspected sexually transmitted infections empirically, and offer catch-up vaccinations.[b,c] • Use harm reduction principles when counseling teens regarding health behaviors.[d] • Develop simple care plans that take into account barriers posed by street involvement. • Recognize times of dysequilibrium (eg, unplanned teen pregnancy, assault) as catalysts for potential change that could lead to exiting street involvement.[e] • Make a timely report to child protective services when there is a reasonable suspicion of maltreatment, abuse, or severe neglect (eg, being kicked out of home), in accordance with state or provincial mandated reporting laws. Reporting is not dependent on consent and may offer an opportunity for stabilization for vulnerable young persons before they become acculturated to the street.
Institutional and community advocacy	• Develop youth-specific, developmentally appropriate services for homeless and street-involved populations. • Advocate for safe, accessible, low-barrier, youth-focused shelters and transitional housing. • Develop wraparound services for street-involved youth primary care, reproductive health, mental health, housing, educational and vocational services, and assistance connecting to supportive social networks.[f]

[a]Auerswald C. Serving homeless and unstably housed youth. In: Ginsburg KR, Kinsman SB, eds. *Reaching Teens: Strength-Based Communication Strategies to Build Resilience and Support Healthy Adolescent Development.* Elk Grove Village, IL: American Academy of Pediatrics; 2014:569-578.
[b]Elliott AS; for the Adolescent Health Committee, Canadian Paediatric Society. Meeting the health care needs of street-involved youth. *Paediatr Child Health.* 2013;18:317-326.
[c]Briggs MA; American Academy of Pediatrics Council on Community Pediatrics. Providing care for children and adolescents facing homelessness and housing insecurity. *Pediatrics.* 2013;131: 1206-1210.
[d]Leslie KM; for the Adolescent Health Committee, Canadian Paediatric Society. Harm reduction: an approach to reducing risky health behaviors in adolescents. *Paediatr Child Health.* 2008;13:53-56.
[e]Auerswald CL, Eyre SL. Youth homelessness in San Francisco: a life cycle approach. *Soc Sci Med.* 2002;54:1497-1512.
[f]Smid M, Bourgois P, Auerswald CL. The challenge of pregnancy among homeless youth: reclaiming a lost opportunity. *J Health Care Poor Underserved.* 2010;21(2 Suppl):140-156.

rather than as victims.[115] Emerging data suggest that significant numbers of males are exploited, in some locales nearing equal in number to females; and most male exploiters are female.[118-120] The average age of first sexual exploitation in youth is 14 years.[105] Street-involved youth[92,101,105,121] and LGBT youth[109] in particular are over-represented in sexually exploited youth samples. A history of running away, poverty, substance use, having friends or family in prostitution, homelessness, and physical or sexual abuse are common experiences among sexually exploited youth.[117,122,123]

Predators frequently use the Internet to facilitate sexual solicitation[124] and sexual exploitation of youth, through activities such as selling or purchasing minors for prostitution, and producing, selling, and purchasing child pornography.[125] Victims in these settings are often offered or given illegal drugs or alcohol and physically assaulted as part of the crime.[125]

Sexually exploited youth are at risk for many of the same health problems as their homeless and street-involved counterparts. There is overlap in these populations (see section on Homeless and Street-Involved Youth); however, youth who have been sexually exploited include both housed and homeless individuals. Sexually exploited youth may present for emergency care of physical injuries secondary to physical and sexual violence as well as drug use.[115] They are at increased risk for reproductive health issues, including exposure to sexually transmitted infections[117,126] and increased rates of pregnancy.[127] They are also at significant risk for mental health challenges, including depression, dissociation, self-harm behaviors, substance abuse, suicidality and attempts, and PTSD.[115,128,129]

Barriers and Challenges to Care

Individual barriers to youth accessing care include their lack of viewing themselves as victims of exploitation, their belief that health issues will resolve without treatment, their fear of opening up to clinicians in authority roles, their experiences of shame and stigma, their worries about judgment and lack of confidentiality, and their past negative experiences with health care staff or services.[129,130] Structural barriers include limited wraparound youth-friendly services for this population, poor coordination of services, and poor accessibility of services, particularly evening hours and on weekends. Males who have been exploited report more forgone care, negative experiences, and reliance on emergency services compared to urban at-risk young men who have not been exploited.[131] Contributing factors include masculine ideals that shape perceptions about accessing health care and the societal stereotype that males have agency in their choices and therefore cannot be victims of exploitation.[132]

Clinicians may not be able to easily identify youth at risk for sexual exploitation. For example, despite media portrayals to the contrary, sexual exploitation is not always linked to having a pimp, perpetrators are not only men, and exploitation may occur while youth are still attending school.[120,133] Youth presenting to the emergency department with injuries or intoxications, particularly with repeat visits, should raise clinicians' level of concern for possible sexual exploitation. Given the difficulty in identifying youth with these experiences, clinicians should consider screening all adolescents for the possibility of sexual exploitation.

Screening for sexual exploitation in adolescents is challenging. A screening tool called "Spotting the Signs" is currently under evaluation, including its applicability to emergency settings.[134] Spotting the Signs focuses on key questions about education, family relationships, friendships, relationships, consent, sexual health knowledge, mood, and suicidality, with the goal of identifying evidence of coercion, overt aggression, suspicion of sexual exploitation/grooming, sexual abuse, power imbalance, and other vulnerabilities.[135]

Some experts in the field suggest that a combination of signs may indicate sexual exploitation. Some of these include attire not appropriate for climate, sudden changes in physical appearance (including expensive clothing, accessories, or electronics out of keeping with financial means), having access to cash, evidence of substance use, hunger, fatigue, homelessness or having run away, school truancy, bruising or physical trauma, evidence of PTSD (fear, anxiety, hypervigilance), tattoos of identified pimps or gangs, sexualized behavior, having an older partner, and being often seen in the proximity of a watchful older individual or situations in which the teen is not allowed privacy with a professional.[128,136]

Protective Factors and Strategies

There is a paucity of literature examining protective factors and strategies among sexually exploited youth, particularly among boys. Among sexually exploited runaway girls, family support and nurturing, involvement of caring other adults, school connectedness, health teaching, and health care are protective factors leading to better health outcomes, which include decreased self-harm and suicidality, decreased substance use, healthier sexual behaviors, better school performance, and increased hope and future planning.[137] Practitioners of emergency care for sexually exploited youth are in a position to promote connection with family, school, nurturing adults, and a medical home throughout assessment and discharge planning as well as to ensure that follow-up plans will continue to facilitate these important relationships.

Table 6 lists specific recommendations for individual clinicians working with sexually exploited adolescents as well as for institutional and community advocacy for this group.

Table 6
Recommendations for emergency care of sexually exploited youth

	Recommendations
Individual Clinician	• Recognize that sexually exploited adolescents are a heterogeneous group, involving all genders. • Be nonjudgmental and avoid imposing labels (eg, prostitute, sex worker). Not all sexually exploited youth identify as such, sometimes seeing their situation as consensual when it is exploitative, fearing discrimination or repercussions of disclosure. • Consider screening adolescents for sexual exploitation. "Spotting the Signs" is an example of a standardized approach to pick up on warning signs of sexual exploitation and can be integrated into the routine adolescent psychosocial assessment.[a] • Use acute presentations among sexually exploited youth (eg, acute physical injuries, sexual violence, intoxication, or pregnancy) as opportunities for advocacy and extrication from abusive situations. • Be familiar with regional mandatory reporting laws for sexual abuse and exploitation. Engage child protection services, law enforcement, and social work or other local agencies as indicated. To minimize potential harm to the adolescent, be aware of potential issues related to reporting sexual exploitation to authorities.[b] For further information about ethical decision-making related to reporting, refer to the Institute for Medicine report.[c] • Provide emergency medical care for acute issues such as reproductive health, sexually transmitted infections, and injuries; offer pregnancy screening, postcoital contraception, reproductive counseling, and preventive vaccinations; and plan for appropriate medical and mental health follow-up. • In cases of sexual assault, assure appropriate techniques in forensic examination are offered when youth consent. Ensure a clinician chaperone during sensitive parts of the examination. • Identify reputable referrals for youth-friendly community supports, particularly emergency shelters and substance abuse treatment centers. • Regularly ask patients about online relationships and safety and provide anticipatory guidance.[d]
Institutional and community advocacy	• Create services that offer safe and nonjudgmental services for sexually exploited youth because policies that criminalize sexually exploited youth further drive them to the margins.

[a]Rogstad K, Johnston G. Spotting the signs: a national proforma for identifying risk of child sexual exploitation in sexual health services. 2014. Available at: www.fsrh.org/pdfs/SpottingTheSigns NationalProforma.pdf. Accessed December 18, 2014.
[b]Greenbaum J, Crawford-Jakubiak JE; American Academy of Pediatrics Committee on Child Abuse and Neglect. Child sex trafficking and commercial sexual exploitation: health care needs of victims. *Pediatrics*. 2015;135:566-574.
[c]Institute of Medicine and National Research Council. *Confronting Commercial Sexual Exploitation and sex trafficking of Minors in the United States*. Washington, DC: The National Academies Press; 2013.
[d]Mitchell KJ, Finkelhor D, Wolak J. Risk factors for and impact of online sexual solicitation of youth. *JAMA*. 2001;285:3011-3014.

CONCLUSION

Emergency care clinicians should be alert to psychosocial stressors and social determinants of health that can affect the health outcomes and behaviors of the most vulnerable youth. Clinicians should strive to care for vulnerable youth from a trauma-informed, culturally effective, strength-based perspective. Health professionals should advocate for policies that promote health equity, decrease barriers to care, and address social determinants of health.

References

1. Commission on Social Determinants of Health. Closing the gap in a generation: health equity through action on the social determinants of health. Geneva, Switzerland: World Health Organization; 2008
2. Sawyer SM, Afifi R, Bearinger LH, et al. Adolescence: a foundation for future health. *Lancet.* 2012;379:1630-1640
3. World Health Organization. Health for the world's adolescents: a second chance in the second decade. Geneva, Switzerland: World Health Organization. May 2014. Available at: apps.who.int/adolescent/second-decade. Accessed January 20, 2015
4. Viner RM, Ozer EM, Denny S, et al. Adolescence and the social determinants of health. *Lancet.* 2012;379,1641-1652
5. Ginsburg KR. How a strength-based approach affects behavioral change. In: Ginsburg KR, Kinsman SB, eds. *Reaching Teens: Strength-Based Communication Strategies to Build Resilience and Support Healthy Adolescent Development.* Elk Grove Village, IL: American Academy of Pediatrics; 2014:9-18
6. Shonkoff JP, Garner AS; American Academy of Pediatrics Committee on Psychosocial Aspects of Child and Family Health. The lifelong effects of early childhood adversity and toxic stress. *Pediatrics.* 2012;129:e232-e46
7. Johnson SB, Blum RW. Stress and the brain: how experiences and exposures across the life span shape health, development, and learning in adolescence. *J Adolesc Health.* 2012;51(2 Suppl):S1-S2
8. Catalano RF, Fagan A, Gavin LE, et al. Worldwide application of prevention science in adolescent health. *Lancet.* 2012;379:1653-1664
9. Lerner RM, Lerner JV, von Eye A, Bowers EP, Lewin-Bizan S. Individual and contextual bases of thriving in adolescence: a view of the issues. *J Adolesc.* 2011;34:1107-1114
10. Ford CA, Sigman G. Confidential health care for adolescents: position paper of the Society for Adolescent Medicine. *J Adolesc Health.* 2004;35:160-167
11. Heineman TV. Relationships beget relationships: why understanding attachment theory is critical to program design for homeless youth. Sacramento, CA: California Homeless Youth Project. June 2010. Available at: cahomelessyouth.library.ca.gov/docs/pdf/HYP-Report.pdf. Accessed January 25, 2015
12. Passel JS. Demography of immigrant youth: past, present, and future. *Future Child.* 2011;21:19-41
13. Chief Public Health Officer. The Chief Public Health Officer's Report on the State of Public Health in Canada, 2011. Chapter 3: The health and well-being of Canadian youth and young adults. Ottawa, ON: Public Health Agency of Canada. 2011. Available at: www.phac-aspc.gc.ca/cphor-sphc-respcacsp/2011/cphorsphc-respcacsp-06-eng.php. Accessed January 10, 2015
14. Children and youth. In: Canada Year Book Overview 2008. Ottawa, ON: Statistics Canada. 2008. Available at: www41.statcan.gc.ca/2008/20000/ceb20000_000-eng.htm. Accessed January 10, 2015
15. Shakya Y. Determinants of mental health for newcomer youth: policy and service implications. *Canadian Issues.* 2010;Summer:98-102
16. Berry JW, Phinney JS, Lam DL, Vedder P. Immigrant youth, acculturation, identity, and adaptation. *Appl Psychol.* 2006;55:303-332

17. Li PS. Deconstructing Canada's discourse of immigrant integration. *J Int Migr Integr.* 2003; 4:315-333
18. Santelli JS, Abraido-Lanza AF, Melnikas AJ. Migration, acculturation, and sexual and reproductive health of Latino adolescents. *J Adolesc Health.* 2009;44:3-4
19. Lipsicas CB, Mäkinen IH. Immigration and suicidality in the young. *Can J Psychiatry.* 2010; 55:274-281
20. Perreira KM, Ornelas IJ. The physical and psychological well-being of immigrant children. *Future Child.* 2011;21:195-218
21. Katsiaficas D, Suárez-Orozco C, Sirin SR, Gupta T. Mediators of the relationship between acculturative stress and internalization symptoms for immigrant origin youth. *Cultur Divers Ethnic Minor Psychol.* 2013;19:27-37
22. Mendoza FS. Health disparities and children in immigrant families: a research agenda. *Pediatrics.* 2009;124(Suppl):S187-S195
23. Le TN, Stockdale G. Acculturative dissonance, ethnic identity, and youth violence. *Cultur Divers Ethnic Minor Psychol.* 2008;14:1-9
24. Fuligni AJ. Gaps, conflicts, and arguments between adolescents and their parents. *New Dir Child Adolesc Dev.* 2012;135:105-110
25. Lui PP. Intergenerational cultural conflict, mental health, and educational outcomes among Asian and Latino/Americans: qualitative and meta-analytic review. *Psychol Bull.* 2015;141:404-446
26. Kwak K, Rudmin F. Adolescent health and adaptation in Canada: examination of gender and age aspects of the healthy immigrant effect. *Int J Equity Health.* 2014;13:103-113
27. Patel SG, Kull MA. Assessing psychological symptoms in recent immigrant adolescents. *J Immigr Minor Health.* 2011;13:616-619
28. Juang LP, Alvarez AA. Discrimination and adjustment among Chinese American adolescents: family conflict and family cohesion as vulnerability and protective factors. *Am J Public Health.* 2010;100:2403-2409
29. Cho YB, Haslam N. Suicidal ideation and distress among immigrant adolescents: the role of acculturation, life stress, and social support. *J Youth Adolesc.* 2010;39:370-379
30. Bacio GA, Mays VM, Lau AS. Drinking initiation and problematic drinking among Latino adolescents: explanations of the immigrant paradox. *Psychol Addict Behav.* 2013;27:14-22
31. Chilton LA, Handal GA, Paz-Soldan GJ; for the Council on Community Pediatrics, American Academy of Pediatrics. Providing care for immigrant, migrant, and border children. *Pediatrics.* 2013;131:e2028-e2034
32. Schapiro NA, Kools SM, Weiss SJ, Brindis CD. Separation and reunification: the experiences of adolescents living in transnational families. *Curr Probl Pediatr Adolesc Health Care.* 2013;43:48-68
33. Pumariega AJ, Rothe E. Cultural considerations in child and adolescent psychiatric emergencies and crises. *Child Adolesc Psychiatr Clin N Am.* 2003;12:723-744
34. Salehi R. Intersection of health, immigration, and youth: a systematic literature review. *J Immigr Minor Health.* 2010;12:788-97
35. Beiser M, Korczak D, eds. Post-traumatic stress disorder. In: *Caring for Kids New to Canada. A guide for health professionals working with immigrant and refugee children and youth.* August 2014. Canadian Paediatric Society. Available at: www.kidsnewtocanada.ca/mental-health/ptsd. Accessed January 21, 2015
36. Basáñez T, Unger JB, Soto D, Crano W, Baezconde-Garbanati L. Perceived discrimination as a risk factor for depressive symptoms and substance use among Hispanic adolescents in Los Angeles. *Ethn Health.* 2013;18:244-261
37. Niwa EY, Way N, Hughes DL. Trajectories of ethnic-racial discrimination among ethnically diverse early adolescents: associations with psychological and social adjustment. *Child Dev.* 2014;85:2339-2354
38. Ngo H, Schleifer B. Immigrant children and youth in focus. *Canadian Issues.* 2005;29-33
39. Bersani BE, Loughran TA, Piquero AR. Comparing patterns and predictors of immigrant offending among a sample of adjudicated youth. *J Youth Adolesc.* 2014;43:1914-1933

40. Pottie K, Dahal G, Georgiades K, Premji K, Hassan G. Do first generation immigrant adolescents face higher rates of bullying, violence and suicidal behaviours than do third generation and native born? *J Immigr Minor Health*. 2015;17:1557-1566

41. Hilliard R, ed. Medical assessment of immigrant and refugee children. In: *Caring for Kids New to Canada. A guide for health professionals working with immigrant and refugee children and youth*. August 2014. Canadian Paediatric Society. Available at: www.kidsnewtocanada.ca/care/assessment. Accessed January 27, 2015

42. Caulford P, D'Andrade J. Health care for Canada's medically uninsured immigrants and refugees: whose problem is it? *Can Fam Physician*. 2012;58:725-727

43. Guagliardo MF, Teach SJ, Huang ZJ, Chamberlain JM, Joseph JG. Racial and ethnic disparities in pediatric appendicitis rupture rate. *Acad Emerg Med*. 2003;10:1218-1227

44. Vo DX, Pate OL, Zhao H, Philip SP, Ginsburg KR. Voices of Asian American youth: important characteristics of clinicians and clinical sites. *Pediatrics*. 2007;120:e1481-e1493

45. Smedley BD, Adrienne YS, Nelson AR, eds. Committee on Understanding and Eliminating Racial and Ethnic Disparities in Health Care, Board on Health Sciences Policy, Institute of Medicine. In: *Unequal Treatment: Confronting Racial and Ethnic Disparities in Health Care*. Washington, DC: National Academies Press; 2003

46. Berry JW. Acculturation: living successfully in two cultures. *Int J Intercult Relat*. 2005;29:697-712

47. Kao T-SA, Lupiya CM, Clemen-Stone S. Family efficacy as a protective factor against immigrant adolescent risky behavior: a literature review. *J Holist Nurs*. 2014;32:202-216

48. Nguyen H, Rawana JS, Flora DB. Risk and protective predictors of trajectories of depressive symptoms among adolescents from immigrant backgrounds. *J Youth Adolesc*. 2011;40:1544-1558

49. Soriano FI, Rivera LM, Williams KJ, Daley SP, Reznik VM. Navigating between cultures: the role of culture in youth violence. *J Adolesc Health*. 2004;34:169-176

50. Canadian Child Welfare Research Portal, Frequently Asked Questions. Available at: cwrp.ca/faqs#Q11. Accessed November 9, 2015

51. Child Welfare Information Gateway. Foster Care Statistics 2011. Washington, DC: U.S. Department of Health and Human Services, Children's Bureau; 2013

52. Statistics Canada. Population by sex and age group. 2012. Available at: www.statcan.gc.ca/tables-tableaux/sum-som/l01/cst01/demo10a-eng.htm. Accessed November 9, 2015

53. Childstats.gov. Child population: number of children (in millions) ages 0-17 in the United States by age 1950-2012 and projected 2013-2050. Available at: www.childstats.gov/americaschildren/tables/pop1.asp. Accessed November 9, 2015

54. Christian CW, Schwarz DF. Child maltreatment and the transition to adult-based medical and mental health care. *Pediatrics*. 2011;127;139

55. Doyle J. Child protection and child outcomes: measuring the effects of foster care. *Am Econ Rev*. 2007;97:1583-1610

56. Felitti VJ, Anda RF, Nordenberg D, et al. Relationship of childhood abuse and household dysfunction to many of the leading causes of death in adults. The Adverse Childhood Experiences (ACE) Study. *Am J Prev Med*. 1998;14:245-258

57. Edwards VJ, Holden GW, Felitti VJ, Anda RF. Relationship between multiple forms of childhood maltreatment and adult mental health in community respondents: results from the Adverse Childhood Experiences study. *Am J Psychiatry*. 2003;160:1453-1460

58. Hillis SD, Anda RF, Felitti VJ, Marchbanks PA. Adverse childhood experiences and sexual risk behaviors in women: a retrospective cohort study. *Fam Plann Perspect*. 2001;33:206-211

59. Rubin DM, Alessandrini EA, Feudtner C, Localio AR, Hadley T. Placement changes and emergency department visits in the first year of foster care. *Pediatrics*. 2004;114:e354

60. McKonnen R, Noonan K, Rubin D. Achieving better health care outcomes for children in foster care. *Pediatr Clin North Am*. 2009;56:405-415

61. Almgren G, Marenkco MO. Emergency room use among a foster care sample: the influence of placement history, chronic illness, psychiatric diagnosis and care factors. *Brief Treat Crisis Interv*. 2001;1:55-64

62. Zito JM, Safer DJ, Sai D, et al. Psychotropic medication patterns among youth in foster care. *Pediatrics*. 2008;121:e157-e163

63. Zlotnick C, Tam TW, Soman LA. Life course outcomes on mental and physical health: the impact of foster care on adulthood. *Am J Public Health*. 2012;102:534-540

64. Jee SH, Barth RP, Szilagyi MA, et al. Factors associated with chronic conditions among children in foster care. *J Health Care Poor Underserved*. 2006;17:328-341

65. Golzari M, Hunt SJ, Anoshiravani A. The health status of youth in juvenile detention facilities. *J Adolesc Health*. 2006;38:776-782

66. Joseph-DiCaprio J, Farrow J, Feinstein RA, et al; for the Ad Hoc Committee Juvenile Justice Special Interest Group, Society for Adolescent Medicine. Health care for incarcerated youth: position paper of the society for Adolescent Medicine. *J Adolec Health*. 2000;27:73-75

67. Gallagher CA, Dobrin A. The association between suicide screening practices and attempts requiring emergency care in juvenile justice facilities. *J Am Acad Child Adolesc Psychiatry*. 2005;44:485-493

68. Grewal M, McKay MP, Teitlebaum AS. Gang members in the ED: what you believe may not be true. *Am J Emerg Med*. 2011;29:834-835

69. Snyder, Howard N, Sickmund M. Juvenile Offenders and Victims: 2006 National Report. Washington, DC: US Department of Justice, Office of Justice Programs, Office of Juvenile Justice and Delinquency Prevention. Available at: http://www.ojjdp.gov/ojstatbb/nr2006/downloads/NR2006.pdf. Accessed January 28, 2015

70. Jaudes KP, Champagne V, Harden A, Masterson J, Bilaver LA. Expanded medical home model works for children in foster care. *Child Welfare*. 2012;91:9-33

71. Jaudes PK; for the Council on Foster Care, Adoption, and Kinship Care and Committee on Early Childhood, American Academy of Pediatrics. Health care of youth aging out of foster care. *Pediatrics*. 2012;130:1170-1173

72. Courtney M, Dworsky A, Lee J, Raap M. *Midwest Evaluation of the Adult Functioning of Former Foster Youth: Outcomes At Age 23 and 24*. Chicago, IL: Chapin Hall at the University of Chicago; 2009

73. Institute of Medicine. *The Health of Lesbian, Gay, Bisexual, and Transgender People: Building a Foundation for Better Understanding*. Washington, DC: The National Academies Press; 2011

74. Duncan DT, Hatzenbuehler. Lesbian, gay, bisexual, and transgender hate crimes and suicidality among a population-based sample of sexual-minority adolescents in Boston. *Am J Public Health*. 2014;104:272-278

75. Reitman DS, Austin B, Belikind U, et al; for the Society for Adolescent Health and Medicine. Recommendations for promoting the health and well-being of lesbian, gay, bisexual, and transgender adolescents: a position paper of the Society for Adolescent Health and Medicine. *J Adolesc Health*. 2013;52:506-510

76. DiFulvio, GT. Sexual minority youth, social connection and resilience: from personal struggle to collective identity. *Soc Sci Med*. 2011;72:1611-1617

77. Ryan C, Russell ST, Huebner D, Diaz R, Sanchez J. Family acceptance in adolescence and the health of LGBT young adults. *J Child Adolesc Psychiatric Nurs*. 2010;23:205-213

78. Tornello SL, Riskind RG, Patterson CH. Sexual orientation and sexual and reproductive health among adolescent young women in the United States. *J Adolesc Health*. 2014;54:160-168

79. Gangamma R, Slesnick N, Toviessi P, Serovich J. Comparison of HIV risks among gay, lesbian, bisexual and heterosexual homeless youth. *J Youth Adolesc*. 2008;37:456-464

80. Garofalo R, Guzman-Cottrill J. Adolescents, HIV, and the emergency department: opportunities and challenges. *Clin Pediatr Emerg Med*. 2003;4:47-57

81. Saewyc EM, Skay CL, Pettingell SL, et al. Hazards of stigma: the sexual and physical abuse of gay, lesbian, and bisexual adolescents in the United States and Canada. *Child Welfare League Am*. 2006;85:195-213

82. Dank M, Lachman, Zweig JM, Yahner J. Dating violence experiences of lesbian, gay, bisexual, and transgender youth. *J Youth Adolesc*. 2014;43:846-857

83. Shields JP, Whitaker K, Glassman J, Franks HM, Howard K. Impact of victimization of risk of suicide among lesbian, gay and bisexual high school students in San Francisco. *J Adolesc Health*. 2012;50:418-420

84. Moll J, Krieger P, Moreno-Walton L, et al. The prevalence of lesbian, gay, bisexual, and transgender health education and training in emergency medicine residency programs: what do we know? *Acad Emerg Med.* 2014;21:608-611

85. Meckler GD, Elliott MN, Kanouse DE, Beals KP, Schuster MA. Nondisclosure of sexual orientation to a physician among a sample of gay, lesbian, and bisexual youth. *Arch Pediatr Adolesc Med.* 2006;160:1248-1254

86. Hoffman ND, Freeman K, Swann S. Healthcare preferences of lesbian, gay, bisexual, transgender and questioning youth. *J Adolesc Health.* 2009;45:222-229

87. Ginsburg KR, Winn RJ, Rudy BJ, et al. How to reach sexual minority youth in the health care setting: the teens offer guidance. *J Adolesc Health.* 2002;31:407-416

88. Bauer GR, Scheim AI, Deutsh MB, Massarella C. Reported emergency department avoidance, use, and experiences of transgender persons in Ontario, Canada: results from a respondent-driven sampling survey. *Ann Emerg Med.* 2014;63:713-720

89. The World Professional Organization for Transgender Health. Standards of care for the health of transsexual, transgender and gender-nonconforming people, Version 7. 2012. Available at: www.wpath.org. Accessed January 23, 2015

90. Hatzenbuehler ML. Structural stigma and the health of lesbian, gay, and bisexual populations. *Cur Dir Psychol Sci.* 2014;23:127-132

91. Bantchevska D, Bartle-Haring S, Dashora P, Glebova T. Problem behaviors of homeless youth: a social capital perspective. *J Hum Ecol.* 2008;23:285-293

92. Elliott AS; for the Adolescent Health Committee, Canadian Paediatric Society. Meeting the health care needs of street-involved youth. *Paediatr Child Health.* 2013;18(6):317-326

93. Kelly K, Caputo T. Health and street/homeless youth. *J Health Psychol.* 2007;12:726-736

94. Edidin JP, Ganim Z, Hunter SJ, Karnik NS. The mental and physical health of homeless youth: a literature review. *Child Psychiatry Hum Dev.* 2012;43:354-375

95. Busen NH, Engebreston JC. Facilitating risk reduction among homeless and street-involved youth. *J Am Acad Nurse Pract.* 2008;20:567-575

96. Auerswald C. Serving homeless and unstably housed youth. In: Ginsburg KR, Kinsman SB, eds. *Reaching Teens: Strength-Based Communication Strategies to Build Resilience and Support Healthy Adolescent Development.* Elk Grove Village, IL: American Academy of Pediatrics; 2014:569-578

97. Berdahl TA, Hoyt DR, Whitbeck LB. Predictors of first mental health service utilization among homeless and runaway adolescents. *J Adolesc Health.* 2005;37:145-154

98. Boivin JF, Roy E, Haley N, Galbaud du Fort G. The health of street youth: a Canadian perspective. *Can J Public Health.* 2005;96:432-437

99. Chew Ng RA, Muth SQ, Auerswald CL. Impact of social networks on shelter use among street youth in San Francisco. *J Adolesc Health.* 2013;53:381-386

100. Auerswald CL, Eyre SL. Youth homelessness in San Francisco: a life cycle approach. *Soc Sci Med.* 2002;54:1497-1512

101. Feldmann J, Middleman AB. Homeless adolescents: common clinical concerns. *Semin Pediatr Infect Dis.* 2003;14:6-11

102. Chiu SH, DiMarco MA, Procop JL. Childhood obesity and dental caries in homeless children. *J Pediatr Health Care.* 2013;27:278-283

103. Rowan MS, Mason M, Robitaille A, Labrecque L, Tocchi CL. An innovative medical and dental hygiene clinic for street youth: results of a process evaluation. *Eval Program Plann.* 2013;40:10-16

104. Marshall BD, Kerr T, Shoveller JA, Montaner JS, Wood E. Structural factors associated with an increased risk of HIV and sexually transmitted infection transmission among street-involved youth. *BMC Public Health.* 2009;9:7

105. Saewyc EM, MacKay LJ, Anderson J, Drozda C. It's not what you think: sexually exploited youth in British Columbia. May 2008. Available at: www.nursing.ubc.ca/PDFs/ItsNotWhatYouThink.pdf. Accessed December 6 2014

106. Smid M, Bourgois P, Auerswald CL. The challenge of pregnancy among homeless youth: reclaiming a lost opportunity. *J Health Care Poor Underserved.* 2010;21(2 Suppl):140-156

107. Hadland SE, Marshall BDL, Kerr T, et al. Suicide and history of childhood trauma among street youth. *J Affect Disord*. 2012;136:377-380

108. McCay E, Langley J, Beanlands H, et al. Mental health challenges and strengths of street-involved youth: the need for a multi-determined approach. *Can J Nurs Res*. 2010;42:30-49

109. Marshall BD, Shannon K, Kerr T, Zhang R, Wood E. Survival sex work and increased HIV risk among sexual minority street-involved youth. *J Acquir Immune Defic Syndr*. 2010;53:661-664

110. Resnick MD. Protective factors, resiliency, and healthy youth development. *Adolesc Med*. 2000;11:157-165

111. Dang MT, Conger KJ, Breslau J, Miller E. Exploring protective factors among homeless youth: the role of natural mentors. *J Health Care Poor Underserved*. 2014;25:1121-1138

112. Unger JB, Kipke MD, Simon TR, et al. Stress, coping and social support among homeless youth. *J Adolesc Res*. 1998;13:134-157

113. Tevendale HD, Lightfoot M, Slocum S. Individual and environmental protective factors for risky sexual behavior among homeless youth: a exploration of gender differences. *AIDS Behav*. 2009;13:154-164

114. Cleverley K, Kidd SA. Resilience and suicidality among homeless youth. *J Adolesc*. 2011;34:1049-1054

115. Greenbaum J, Crawford-Jakubiak JE; American Academy of Pediatrics Committee on Child Abuse and Neglect. Child sex trafficking and commercial sexual exploitation: health care needs of victims. *Pediatrics*. 2015;135:566-574

116. United Nations General Assembly, Convention on the Rights of the Child. November 20, 1989. United Nations, Treaty Series, Volume 1577, p. 3. Available at: www.refworld.org/docid/3ae6b38f0.html. Accessed January 23, 2015

117. Edwards JM, Iritani BJ, Hallfors DD. Prevalence and correlates of exchanging sex for drugs or money among adolescents in the United States. *Sex Transm Infect*. 2006;82:354-358

118. Cockbain E, Brayley H, Ashby M; Department of Security and Crime Science. Not just a girl thing: a large-scale comparison of male and female users of child sexual exploitation services in the UK. August 2014. Available at: www.barnardos.org.uk/16136_not_just_a_girl_thing_v6.pdf. Accessed December 15 2014

119. Curtis R, Terry K, Dank M, Dombrowski K, Khan B. Commercial sexual exploitation of children in New York City, volume one: the CSEC population in New York City: size, characteristics, and needs. September 2008. Available at: www.ncjrs.gov/pdffiles1/nij/grants/225083.pdf. Accessed December 14, 2014

120. Saewyc EM, Miller BB, Rivers R, et al. Competing discourses about youth sexual exploitation in Canadian news media. *Can J Hum Sex*. 2013;22:95-105

121. Halcón LL, Lifson AR. Prevalence and predictors of sexual risks among homeless youth. *J Youth Adolesc*. 2004;33:71-80

122. Klatt D, Cavner D, Egan V. Rationalising predictors of child sexual exploitation and sex-trading. *Child Abuse Negl*. 2014;38:252-260

123. Lalor K, McElvaney R. Child sexual abuse, links to later sexual exploitation/high-risk sexual behavior, and prevention/treatment programs. *Trauma Violence Abuse*. 2010;11:159-177

124. Mitchell KJ, Finkelhor D, Wolak J. Risk factors for and impact of online sexual solicitation of youth. *JAMA*. 2001;285:3011-3014

125. Mitchell KJ, Finkelhor D, Jones LM, Wolak J. Internet-facilitated commercial sexual exploitation of children: findings from a nationally representative sample of law enforcement agencies in the United States. *Sex Abuse*. 2011;23:43-71

126. Greenbaum VJ. Commercial sexual exploitation and sex trafficking of children in the United States. *Curr Probl Pediatr Adolesc Health Care*. 2014;44:245-269

127. Saewyc EM, Magee LL, Pettingell SE. Teenage pregnancy and associated risk behaviors among sexually abused adolescents. *Perspect Sex Reprod Health*. 2004;36:98-105

128. Grace LG, Starck M, Potenza J, Kenney PA, Sheetz AH. Commercial sexual exploitation of children and the school nurse. *J Sch Nurs*. 2012;28:410-417

129. MacKay L, Saewyc E, Hirakata P, Roelefson D, Oliffe J. The unmet health needs of young men who trade sex for money or goods. *J Adolesc Health*. 2011;48:S101

130. Justice Institute of British Columbia. *Commercial Sexual Exploitation: Innovative Ideas for Working with Children and Youth*. New Westminster, BC: Justice Institute of British Columbia; 2002

131. Rivers R, Saewyc EM, MacKay L, et al. Masculinities and marginalized young men's patterns of accessing health care services. *J Adolesc Health*. 2013;52:S21

132. Dennis JP. Women are victims, men make choices: the invisibility of men and boys in the global sex trade. *Gender Issues*. 2008;25:11-25

133. Harpin SB, Edinburgh LD, Pape-Blabolil J, Saewyc EM. Beyond the stereotypes: variation in sexual exploitation experiences of youth evaluated at a hospital-based child advocacy centre. *J Adolesc Health*. 2014;54:S25-S26

134. Rogstad K, Ashby J, Wilkinson D. New tool to aid detection of child sexual exploitation. *BMJ*. 2014;349:g6454

135. Rogstad K, Johnston G. Spotting the signs: a national proforma for identifying risk of child sexual exploitation in sexual health services. 2014. Available at: www.fsrh.org/pdfs/SpottingTheSignsNationalProforma.pdf. Accessed December 18, 2014

136. Chaffee TC. Hidden Among us: sexually exploited and trafficked youth (handout). In: Ginsburg KR, Kinsman SB, eds. *Reaching Teens: Strength-Based Communication Strategies to Build Resilience and Support Healthy Adolescent Development*. Elk Grove Village, IL: American Academy of Pediatrics; 2014:578

137. Saewyc EM, Edinburgh LD. Restoring healthy developmental trajectories for sexually exploited young runaway girls: fostering protective factors and reducing risk behaviors. *J Adolesc Health*. 2010;46:180-188

Adolesc Med 026 (2015) 619–646

Human Immunodeficiency Virus: Adolescent Emergencies

Caroline Salas-Humara, MD[a]*;
Sarah M. Wood, MD[b];
Lawrence J. D'Angelo, MD, MPH[c];
Nadia Dowshen, MD[d]

[a]*Adolescent Medicine Fellow, Craig-Dalsimer Division of Adolescent Medicine, Children's Hospital of Philadelphia, Philadelphia, Pennsylvania; [b]Adolescent Medicine Fellow, Craig-Dalsimer Division of Adolescent Medicine, Children's Hospital of Philadelphia, Philadelphia, Pennsylvania; [c]Chief, Division of Adolescent and Young Adult Medicine, Children's National Medical Center, Washington, DC; [d]Assistant Professor of Pediatrics and Director of Adolescent HIV Services, Craig-Dalsimer Division of Adolescent Medicine, Children's Hospital of Philadelphia, Philadelphia, Pennsylvania

INTRODUCTION

Adolescents are at high risk for human immunodeficiency virus (HIV) infection, and often the emergency department (ED) setting is where at-risk and HIV-infected adolescents are seen as their sole source of care. It is important to have a high index of suspicion for acute HIV infection and to consider HIV screening during these evaluations. Physicians must make every effort to adhere to state policies on HIV testing and to uphold the adolescent's right for confidential care. If a diagnosis of HIV infection is made, immediate referral and linkage to care with a physician specializing in comprehensive HIV care for adolescents and young adults should be made. Management of the patient infected with HIV should include evaluation for potential opportunistic infections, immune reconstitution inflammatory syndrome, and medication side effects, as well as potential drug interactions in those receiving antiretroviral therapy. Human immunodeficiency virus postexposure prophylaxis may substantially reduce the risk of HIV infection and should be recommended if there is concern for a recent sexual or needlestick exposure. Physicians who see adolescents in acute care settings are well positioned to have an effect on the well-being of adolescents both by preventing new infections and by improving health outcomes for youth living with HIV.

---

*Corresponding author
E-mail address: salashumarac@email.chop.edu

HUMAN IMMUNODEFICIENCY VIRUS IN ADOLESCENTS

More than 1.1 million people in the United States are living with human immunodeficiency virus (HIV) infection.[1] Over the past decade, the number of people living with HIV has increased, although the overall annual number of new infections has remained static.[2] However, the pace of new infection is high among certain groups, notably adolescents and young adults, among whom there was a 21% increase in HIV incidence in those aged 13 to 29 years.[3] This age group accounted for almost 40% of new HIV infections in the United States in 2009 despite comprising less than 25% of the population.[4] An increase in the number of adolescents and young adults living with HIV who are behaviorally infected is paralleled by the large number of perinatally infected youth who are now living into adulthood. Although this longevity was not expected at the outset of the epidemic, these perinatally infected teenagers now comprise 22% of the adolescents living with HIV or acquired immunodeficiency syndrome (AIDS).[4]

Most new infections in adolescents are occurring among young men who have sex with men (MSM). Although MSM accounted for only 4% of the male population in the United States in 2010,[5] MSM accounted for 78% of new infections among males and 68% of new infections overall.[6] Specifically, young black/black and Hispanic/Latino MSM are disproportionately affected and have high rates of new infection.[4] In 2010, the largest number of new HIV infections among MSM occurred in young black/black MSM aged 13 to 24 years. In fact, young black MSM accounted for 45% of new infections among black MSM overall.[1] Male-to-female transgender youth or young transgender women also have high incidences of new infection. A review of studies estimated that HIV prevalence for transgender women was nearly 50 times as high as for other adults of reproductive age.[7]

Many of these youth are unaware of their infection. Despite having a higher incidence of new infection compared to adults, adolescents and young adults are far behind in serostatus knowledge. Approximately 80% of HIV-infected adults are aware of their status[8] compared to only 40% of adolescents and young adults.[9] Similarly, estimates from the Centers for Disease Control and Prevention (CDC) demonstrate that not only are testing rates low among youth (12.9% among high school students), but more than half of those youth (59.5%) infected were unaware of their infection.[10] Serostatus knowledge has important implications for preventing onward transmission as well as improving individual health outcomes for those who are infected.

SCREENING FOR HIV IN ADOLESCENTS

The overall benefits of screening for HIV in adolescents are substantial. Early diagnosis of adolescents can lead to improved health outcomes and has potential beneficial public health consequences.[11] A recent study demonstrated that the prevalence of high-risk sexual behavior is reduced significantly after HIV-infected individuals become aware of their infection.[12] In addition, after the initiation of antiretroviral therapy (ART), a reduced viral load may reduce transmission of HIV to other persons.[13] A large multinational randomized controlled trial demonstrated that early initiation of ART can lead to a decrease in HIV transmission.[14] Early testing and diagnosis of HIV not only may lead to earlier initiation of ART and decreased transmission but also allows for initiation of ART at higher baseline CD4 lymphocyte counts, thus affording patients the best opportunity for immune function preservation.[9]

Conversely, later diagnosis is associated with an increased risk for HIV-associated morbidity and mortality. Patients diagnosed later are more likely to present with an AIDS-defining illness and require hospitalization.[15] In addition, there is a substantial increase in health care costs for those diagnosed later in the course of their disease. One study found that total annual expenditures for patients with CD4 cell counts less than 50 cells/μL were 2.6 times greater than for patients with counts of 350 cells/μL or more because of additional costs for medication and hospitalization.[16]

Because of these major public and individual health benefits, the CDC, the US Preventive Services Task Force (USPSTF) and the American Academy of Pediatrics (AAP) all recommend routine universal screening rather than a targeted approach to HIV testing. In 2006, the CDC put forth revised recommendations indicating that all individuals aged 13 to 64 years should be offered opt-out HIV screening in all health care settings regardless of risk.[17] Specifically, they recommend screening patients after notifying them that the test will be performed. Assent is inferred unless the patient declines testing.[17] Furthermore, they recommend at least yearly screening (every 3-6 months) for persons at high risk for HIV infection, such as injection-drug users and their sex partners, persons who exchange sex for money or drugs, sex partners of HIV-infected persons, and MSM or heterosexual persons who themselves or whose sex partners have had more than 1 sex partner since their most recent HIV test.[17] Similarly, in response to the growing incidence of HIV infection in adolescents, in 2011 the AAP recommended universal routine screening for all adolescents at least once by the time they reach 16 to 18 years of age.[18] Finally, in 2013 the USPSTF reviewed new evidence on the effectiveness of treatments in HIV-infected persons and concluded that it was beneficial to recommend screening all adolescents and adults aged 15 to 65 years for HIV infection (grade A recommendation).[19] However, despite these recommendations, nationwide only 12.9% of youth report being screened for HIV.[10]

Early diagnosis of HIV infection may have particularly important public health benefits. Patients with acute infection are typically highly infectious because of a high viral load burden in blood and genital secretions and therefore are more likely to transmit the virus to others during this stage of infection.[20] Identifying acute HIV infection (AHI) is extremely important given this risk of increased infectivity and potential transmission through unprotected sex.[21-23] Despite this potential benefit and the fact that most patients are symptomatic, the diagnosis of AHI is frequently missed in medical evaluations.[24] In 1 case series, the diagnosis of HIV infection was only considered in 26% of patients presenting with symptoms consistent with acute infection.[25] The diagnosis of AHI is likely often missed, in part, because the symptoms overlap those of other viral syndromes, including Epstein-Barr virus (EBV), and are non-specific and so mild that those experiencing the symptoms do not seek medical attention. This is particularly important for ED physicians because some of the most common reasons for youth presenting to the ED are non-specific viral complaints.[26]

HUMAN IMMUNODEFICIENCY VIRUS TESTING IN THE ED SETTING

Despite recommendations for routine screening, testing rates remain low. The ED and the acute care setting, in addition to the primary care setting, are important venues for HIV screening of adolescents. The ED often serves as the primary source of care for adolescents because of their lack of access to health services, so the ED can be the setting to provide sexual health screening.[27] Adolescents who use the ED are more likely to have higher levels of sexual risk behaviors, which emphasizes the importance of HIV screening in this setting.[27] In addition, the emergency setting is often where adolescents present with signs and symptoms of AHI or opportunistic infections (OIs); thus, the ED is an important place for diagnosis of infection. As a result, acute care physicians are in a unique position to prevent, diagnose, and ensure appropriate treatment of adolescents living with, or who are at high risk for, HIV infection.

Overview of Diagnostic Tests

The sequence of different laboratory markers detected after infection can be helpful in determining the most appropriate diagnostic test to use in a given clinical encounter (see Figure 1). Immediately after HIV-1 infection, low levels of HIV-1 ribonucleic acid (RNA) may not yet be detectable in the blood. Approximately 7 to 10 days after infection, HIV-1 RNA becomes detectable by the nucleic acid amplification test (NAAT), and levels rise quickly.[28-32] Next, HIV-1 p24 antigen is expressed, and its level becomes high enough to be detected by the fourth-generation antigen/antibody tests approximately 10 to 14 days after infection. Next, immunoglobulin M antibodies are expressed, which can be detected by third- and fourth-generation immunoassays approximately 20 to 30 days after infection. Finally, immunoglobulin G antibodies are expressed and remain positive throughout chronic infection. First- and second-generation immunoassays vary as to how soon they can detect immunoglobulin G antibodies, with time to positivity ranging from 25 to 45 days after initial infection.[33-36]

Acute infection is defined as the interval between detectable HIV-1 RNA and the appearance of antibodies.

In 2014, the CDC released updated recommendations for laboratory testing for the diagnosis of HIV infection.[37] They no longer recommend the use of enzyme immunoassay antibody testing with a confirmatory western blot (third-generation immunoassay). Instead, they recommend initial testing with a US Food and Drug Administration (FDA)-approved antigen/antibody combination (fourth-generation) immunoassay that detects both HIV-1 and HIV-2 antibodies as well as HIV-1 p24 antigen to screen for both HIV-1 or HIV-2 chronic

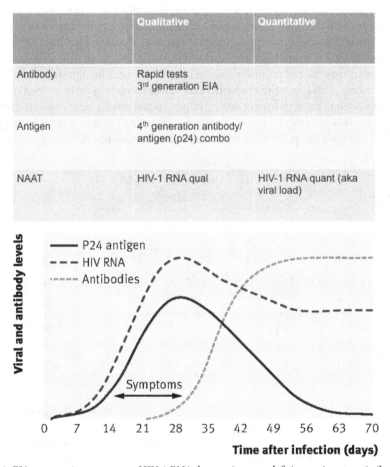

	Qualitative	Quantitative
Antibody	Rapid tests 3rd generation EIA	
Antigen	4th generation antibody/ antigen (p24) combo	
NAAT	HIV-1 RNA qual	HIV-1 RNA quant (aka viral load)

Fig 1. EIA, enzyme immunoassay; HIV-1 RNA, human immunodeficiency virus type 1 ribonucleic acid; NAAT, nucleic acid amplification test. From Centers for Disease Control and Prevention and Association of Public Health Laboratories. Laboratory Testing for the Diagnosis of HIV Infection: Updated Recommendations. Available at: stacks.cdc.gov/view/cdc/23447. Published June 27, 2014. Accessed October 13, 2014

infection and acute HIV-1 infection. The rationale for this change is that the fourth-generation test will often detect p24 antigen during acute infection when antibodies are not yet detectable. A positive fourth-generation test should then be followed by an HIV-1/2 antibody differentiation immunoassay (multispot) for confirmation. If results are discordant, then a NAAT should be used to distinguish acute infection from a false-positive result. An additional benefit of this new algorithm is that the time to confirmation of a diagnosis can be a matter of a few hours as opposed to more than 1 week for western blot results (Figure 2).

Advantages and Disadvantages of Rapid Tests

Rapid antibody tests can be performed in the laboratory, in community-based settings, or at home. They have the advantage of offering preliminary results in the same patient encounter, with the results usually available in less than 20 minutes. Additionally, the rapid tests are most often performed as an oral swab or finger stick, and they do not require venipuncture, which may be a deterrent for many adolescents. This type of test is particularly advantageous in certain situations, for example, when patients cannot wait or return for test results, or in resource-limited settings. This test may be preferable in the ED setting because it does not require follow-up with the patient for results, a barrier commonly cited by practitioners

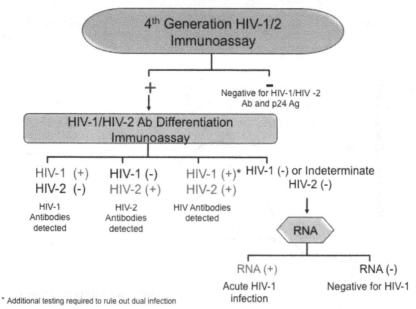

* Additional testing required to rule out dual infection

Fig 2. Newly proposed Centers for Disease Control and Prevention/Association of Public Health Laboratories (CDC/APHL) testing algorithm for human immunodeficiency virus (HIV) diagnosis. Ab, antibody; Ag, antigen; RNA, ribonucleic acid. From Centers for Disease Control and Prevention and Association of Public Health Laboratories. Laboratory Testing for the Diagnosis of HIV Infection: Updated Recommendations. Available at: stacks.cdc.gov/view/cdc/23447. Published June 27, 2014. Accessed October 13, 2014

for universal HIV screening in the ED.[38,39] In fact, studies demonstrate that adolescents prefer rapid HIV testing,[40] specifically in the ED.[41] At this time, most rapid tests are third-generation tests and only detect the presence of the antibody and not the p24 antigen. Therefore, when this test is used, the result is non-reactive, and if AHI is suspected in a patient, a separate NAAT to identify HIV-1 RNA or a fourth-generation test that detects p24 antigen must be performed to rule out acute infection. This is especially important to keep in mind when choosing a test in the setting of a patient presenting with signs or symptoms potentially consistent with AHI in the emergency setting because using the western blot can produce a false-negative test during seroconversion.[42,43] In fact, the previous testing algorithm, using third-generation antibody testing, failed to identify acute infection in 4% to 32% of all new infections in some populations, particularly MSM.[42,44-46] Currently an FDA-approved single-use rapid fourth-generation combination antigen/antibody immunoassay test is available for rapid testing. However, the test is not widely available, and as of April 2014 the CDC has not officially recommended it as an initial assay in the testing algorithm because of insufficient data available, although this may change in the future.[37] Refer to Figure 1 for the different types of HIV tests and the CDC (www.cdc.gov/hiv/pdf/testing_Advantages&Disadvantages.pdf) for advantages and disadvantages of different tests.

Confidentiality and Consent Laws for Testing

In general, separate written consent for HIV is not required; rather, general consent for medical care should be sufficient to include HIV testing.[17] Adolescents older than 18 years may consent to their own medical care. Similarly, individuals younger than 18 years who are self-supporting or are married, parents, or members of the armed services may consent to their own health care without the need for parental involvement.[47] In addition, legal statutes allow for confidential medical evaluation and treatment of minors for sexually transmitted infections (STIs) without the knowledge or consent of the parent or guardian. However, only 31 states explicitly include HIV testing and treatment as part of this STI package to which minors may consent on their own.[47,48] Information regarding state policies can be found at the Guttmacher Institute (www.guttmacher.org/statecenter/spibs/spib_MASS.pdf). Physicians should be aware of the laws of the state in which they practice and aim to uphold the adolescent's request for privacy. The Compendium of State HIV Testing Laws from the National HIV/AIDS Physicians' Consultation Center (www.nccc.ucsf.edu) can also help physicians clarify how their state laws and the CDC recommendations apply in practice.[18]

Human Immunodeficiency Virus Test Counseling, Delivery of Results, and Linkage to Care

Counseling associated with HIV testing is not a straightforward topic. According to the new CDC guidelines, prevention counseling is not required as part of a patient screening; however, in the United States, state laws vary as to what is required.[49] At the minimum, patients should be informed that they are being tested. The International Antiviral Panel similarly stated in its most recent recommendations (2014) that pretest counseling should only be sufficient to meet the individual's needs and to comply with local regulations.[50] Prevention counseling is recommended for patients at high risk for HIV and other STIs.[17] Reviewing negative results with a patient can be an opportunity for further HIV and STI prevention counseling. A positive test result should be discussed with a patient in person and not over the telephone.[18] For the patient who is HIV positive, every attempt should be made to make an immediate referral and linkage to care with a physician who specializes in comprehensive HIV care for adolescents and young adults.[51]

ACUTE HIV INFECTION IN THE EMERGENCY SETTING

There are a number of different ways to define AHI based on virologic markers and clinical symptoms. Here we will use the term AHI to refer to symptomatic early infection and the time during which a patient is viremic but has not yet produced antibodies to the infection. The prevalence of acute infection of patients presenting to care varies depending on the patient population examined; however, the literature suggests that it is likely more prevalent than most physicians suspect.[52,53] One study found that 1% of patients presenting to an urban urgent care setting with viral symptoms were diagnosed with AHI.[52] The diagnosis is often missed in clinical settings; as many as 83% of infections may be missed at the first medical encounter.[54] A diagnosis may prove elusive for several reasons: the syndrome often is non-specific and mimics other viral illnesses, the physician makes an insufficient assessment of patient risk factors for HIV, the physician fails to consider AHI as a potential diagnosis, and the physician has insufficient knowledge regarding diagnostic testing. It is essential that physicians in acute care settings have a high index of suspicion for AHI so that these youth can be identified quickly. Identifying those with recent infection will lead to health benefits on both the public health and individual levels. Specifically, this subset of patients is highly infectious and is responsible for a disproportionate number of new infections, so identifying and treating those with early infection may help to improve their clinical outcomes.[23,55]

The clinical syndrome can range from asymptomatic to severe disease. The exact proportion of those who develop symptoms is difficult to estimate given that those who are detected generally have symptoms and those without symptoms do not seek medical care and therefore go undetected; those who develop symptoms range from 50% to 89%.[22,56] The usual time from HIV exposure to the development of symptoms is 1 to 4 weeks after transmission. The symptoms usually self-resolve after 2 to 4 weeks, although the incubation period and severity vary among patients.[57,58] Symptoms typically include fever, fatigue/malaise, headache, rash, myalgias or arthralgias, vomiting or diarrhea, anorexia or weight loss, pharyngitis, lymphadenopathy, and mucocutaneous ulcers.[22] The original descriptions characterized the illness as "mononucleosis-like" or "influenza-like".[59] Fever, fatigue, and myalgias are the most common symptoms reported by patients with AHI.[56,60] Non-tender adenopathy is typically seen in the second week of illness and involves the axillary, cervical, and occipital nodes. None of these symptoms are specific for AHI; however, the rash and mucocutaneous ulcers are more distinctive manifestations. The rash is typically non-pruritic and maculopapular, presenting on the upper thorax and collar region, with lesions frequently on the face and scalp. Lesions may also appear on the extremities, particularly the palms and soles.[61] Mucocutaneous ulcers are painful and may occur on the oral mucosa, esophagus, anus, or penis. They are typically round, shallow white ulcers surrounded by a thin area of erythema.[61] It is important to exclude other potential causes of ulcers because they may indicate acute infection or a concomitant infection with syphilis, herpes simplex virus (HSV), or chancroid. The gastrointestinal tract can be involved, given that it is a primary target of infection. Patients can suffer from weight loss, nausea, diarrhea, or anorexia. Headache is commonly seen, but other rare, more serious neurologic manifestations occur, including aseptic meningitis.[56] Laboratory findings, including transaminitis, thrombocytopenia, and atypical lymphocytosis, can be seen in those with acute infection.[58,62]

The constellation of symptoms typically seen is non-specific and therefore can easily be mistaken for other viral syndromes. When a patient presents with these symptoms in an acute care setting, it is important to include AHI in the differential diagnosis, in addition to EBV, non-EBV mononucleosis syndromes (eg, cytomegalovirus [CMV]), syphilis, streptococcal infection, influenza, and viral hepatitis. New-onset autoimmune disorders can also resemble AHI. Importantly, a positive heterophile antibody test does not exclude the diagnosis of HIV because it can be positive during AHI.[63] Whether this represents a false-positive result or reactivation of EBV is not clear.[64]

Acute HIV infection should be strongly considered in patients with a recent high-risk exposure or in patients with a recent diagnosis of another STI regardless of symptoms. It should also be considered in patients presenting with the clinical symptoms described, regardless of high-risk behavior, because adolescents may not be forthcoming in disclosing their sexual behavior or may not perceive their behavior as high risk.

Diagnosis, Delivery of Results, and Linkage to Care

Once a diagnosis of HIV infection is made in the acute care setting, you will need to keep in mind several issues when delivering results to the patient. At this point it would be appropriate to reach out to your local adolescent and HIV specialist colleagues for support. Ensuring timely linkage to the care team with appropriate expertise is essential. Table 1 lists tips for delivering HIV test results.

Table 1
Tips for delivering HIV test results

When preparing to give a positive result, be in touch and keep your own emotions in check before meeting with the patient. Keep in mind that although this is difficult news, it may not be the most difficult thing going on in this young person's life, and you do not want to present the diagnosis as more of catastrophe than the adolescent would have otherwise perceived it to be.	It may be helpful to provide support in the form of appropriate touch: putting your hand on the adolescent's shoulder can be comforting and remind youth that they are worthy of respect and love.
Sit on the same level as the youth and make sure you are not physically blocking exit from room.	Allow time for the patient to react and ask questions. Explain that she may initially want to disclose her diagnosis to 1 or 2 people whom she feels will be supportive and trust to keep her information private.
Be calm but matter of fact when you speak and allow pause for the youth to react.	Remember that listening may be more important than talking. The patient will guide you about his needs.
It is important to convey a message of hope while also not diminishing the pain and sadness that accompany this diagnosis. As with patients with other chronic diseases such as diabetes, HIV-positive people can lead long, productive, healthy lives.	Finally, assess for safety, establish a plan for close follow-up, and connect the patient to an appropriate HIV care provider in her community as soon as possible.

HIV, human immunodeficiency virus.

CARE OF THE HIV-INFECTED ADOLESCENT

Despite the advent of combination ART, HIV-infected adults and adolescents continue to access the ED at higher rates than their uninfected peers.[2] Among patients on ART, many have well-controlled HIV with minimal immune suppression and low risk for OI. In these patients, the cause of illness is less likely related to HIV or an OI.[2,65] However, despite the wide availability of ART and the recommendation for early initiation of treatment, many adolescent patients may not achieve immunologic recovery and virologic suppression. Although it is estimated that 20% to 28% of the total HIV-infected population is virologically suppressed, this proportion is estimated to be substantially lower in adolescents.[8,9] Thus, OIs and HIV-related complications remain important considerations in evaluating acutely ill, HIV-infected adolescents.

A detailed history is essential to best tailor differential diagnosis and management. It is important to remember that care should be patient-centered and confidential. Do not assume that parents, friends, or other people accompanying the patient are aware of the HIV diagnosis. Patients should be interviewed alone, and they should be asked about who knows about their status and with whom they are comfortable discussing their HIV diagnosis and care. Practitioners should be familiar with state laws governing confidentiality of HIV care and treatment of adolescents. As of 2014, 31 states allow minors to consent to HIV testing and treatment. Eighteen states allow physicians to inform a minor's parent if the child is seeking or receiving HIV treatment, but only Iowa requires parental notification of a positive HIV test.[48]

The history of present illness should include the presence and duration of systemic symptoms such as weight loss, fever, and new or worsening lymphadenopathy, as well as a detailed review of systems. A detailed HIV-specific history should include the date of HIV diagnosis, any OI or co-infections including hepatitis B, hepatitis C, and tuberculosis, and the most recent CD4 counts and viral load. A CD4 count less than 200 suggests severe immune suppression and should heighten the physician's concern for OI. Table 2 lists OI presentation, treatment, and prophylaxis. The medication history should focus on whether the patient is on ART or OI prophylaxis, what medications they are taking, the duration of therapy, and an assessment of adherence. A rough estimate of adherence can be obtained by asking the patient about the number of doses missed in the last 3 and 7 days, as well as the last month. The patient's immunization status should be assessed, with special attention to pneumococcal, meningococcal, influenza, and varicella vaccinations.

The physical examination should help the physician narrow the differential diagnosis. Fever, hemodynamic instability, or respiratory compromise should be noted on vital signs. Weight should be assessed with attention to recent loss. A careful head, eyes, ears, nose, and throat examination should include funduscopy and inspection of the oral mucosa for thrush or oral lesions. Many HIV-infected patients, particularly those not on ART, may have lymphadenopathy at baseline, but any new or significantly increased lymphadenopathy or signs of lymphadenitis should be noted. On respiratory examination, observation of tachypnea, increased work of breathing, rales, and other adventitious breath sound can be helpful in diagnosing pneumonia. On cardiovascular examination, physicians should observe for any new murmur, friction rub, or extra heart sound. Abdominal examination should note any new or worsening hepatosplenomegaly, or mass. Every patient with related complaints should undergo a careful genitourinary examination, with close attention to the presence of lesions or urethral discharge suggestive of STI. The skin examination should note any rashes, with particular attention to distribution and mucous membrane involvement. Finally, a complete neurologic examination is essential and should include evaluation of the cranial nerves, strength and sensory testing, and assessment of mental status.

As previously noted, the differential diagnosis of the acutely ill HIV-infected adolescent is quite broad, and history and physical examination should be used to tailor the management approach. In addition to opportunistic pathogens, many of the common bacterial and viral illnesses that typically affect adolescents, such as bacterial pneumonia and skin and soft tissue infections, may present with more severe disease in HIV-infected patients. The following discussion will focus on presentations of HIV-specific illness and complications, as well as the diagnostic workup.

Table 2
Prophylaxis and treatment of opportunistic infections in HIV-infected adolescents

Opportunistic infection[a]	Prophylaxis[b]	Treatment	Clinical clues to diagnosis
Pneumocystis jirovecii pneumonia (PCP)	Trimethoprim-sulfamethoxazole (TMP-SMX) 1 double-strength (DS) tablet daily[c] or 1 single-strength (SS) tablet daily Alternative: Dapsone 100 mg PO daily or 50 mg BID or atovaquone 1500 mg PO daily[d]	Mild-to-Moderate PCP: TMP-SMX: (TMP 15-20 mg and SMX 75-100 mg)/kg/day, given PO in 3 divided doses or TMP-SMX: (160 mg/800 mg or DS) 2 tablets PO TID Moderate-to-Severe PCP: TMP-SMX: (TMP 15-20 mg and SMX 75-100 mg)/kg/day IV given q6h or q8h, may switch to PO after clinical improvement Duration of therapy: 21 days[e]	Subacute onset of progressive dyspnea, fever, nonproductive cough, chest discomfort that worsens within days to weeks
Toxoplasma gondii encephalitis	TMP-SMX 1 DS tablet daily Alternative: Dapsone 50 mg PO daily + (pyrimethamine 50 mg + leucovorin 25 mg) PO weekly	Acute Infection: Pyrimethamine 200 mg PO 1 time, followed by weight-based therapy: If ≤60 kg: Pyrimethamine 50 mg PO once daily + sulfadiazine 1000 mg PO q6h + leucovorin 10-25 mg PO once daily If ≥60 kg: Pyrimethamine 75 mg PO once daily + sulfadiazine 1500 mg PO q6h + leucovorin 10-25 mg PO once daily Duration of acute therapy: at least 6 weeks; longer duration if clinical or radiologic disease is extensive or response is incomplete at 6 weeks	Focal encephalitis with headache, confusion, motor weakness, fever
Disseminated Mycobacterium avium complex (MAC) disease	Azithromycin 1200 mg PO once weekly Or Clarithromycin 500 mg PO BID Alternative: Rifabutin (dose adjusted based on concomitant ART)	At least 2 drugs as initial therapy: Clarithromycin 500 mg PO BID + ethambutol 15 mg/kg PO daily ± rifabutin[f] Duration of therapy: at least 12 months	Early symptoms: fever, night sweats, weight loss, fatigue, diarrhea, abdominal pain
Mycobacterium tuberculosis infection (TB)	Latent Tuberculosis Infection (LTBI) Treatment: Isoniazid (INH) 300 mg PO + pyridoxine 25 mg PO daily × 9 months Alternative: Rifampin 600 mg PO daily × 4 months	Active Pulmonary Disease[g]: Initial phase: INH + rifampin (RIF) or rifabutin (RFB) + pyrazinamide (PZA) + ethambutol (EMB) daily administered for 2 months, followed by INH and RIF (or RFB) for 4 additional months[h]	Latent: asymptomatic Active: fever, sweats, weight loss, productive cough, fatigue Extrapulmonary disease more common in HIV-infected persons

Histoplasma capsulatum infection	Itraconazole 200 mg PO daily	Less severe disseminated histoplasmosis: *Initial therapy:* Itraconazole 200 mg PO TID for 3 days, followed by 200 mg BID for at least 12 months Moderately severe to severe disseminated histoplasmosis: *Induction therapy:* Liposomal amphotericin B 3 mg/kg IV daily for ≥2 weeks (or until improved clinically), followed by itraconazole 200 mg PO TID for 3 days and then 200 mg BID[i]	Fever, fatigue, weight loss, hepatosplenomegaly, lymphadenopathy Cough, chest pain, dyspnea occur in approximately 50% of patients
Candidiasis	Routine prophylaxis not recommended	Oropharyngeal candidiasis: *Oral therapy:* Fluconazole 100 mg PO daily *Topical therapy:* Clotrimazole troches 10 mg PO 5 times daily Duration of therapy: 7-14 days Esophageal candidiasis: Fluconazole 100 mg (up to 400 mg) PO or IV daily or itraconazole oral solution 200 mg PO daily Duration of therapy:14-21 days Vulvovaginal candidiasis: *Uncomplicated:* Oral fluconazole 150 mg for 1 dose or topical azoles (clotrimazole, butoconazole, miconazole, tioconazole, or terconazole) Duration of therapy: 3-7 days *Recurrent or severe:* Fluconazole 100-200 mg PO daily for ≥7 days, or topical antifungal for ≥7 days	Oropharyngeal candidiasis: painless, creamy white, plaquelike lesions of buccal or oropharyngeal mucosa or tongue surface Esophageal candidiasis: retrosternal burning pain or discomfort, odynophagia Vulvovaginitis: white vaginal discharge associated with mucosal burning and itching
Cryptococcus neoformans	Routine antifungal prophylaxis not recommended	Meningitis: *Induction therapy (for at least 2 weeks, followed by consolidation therapy):* Liposomal amphotericin B 3-4 mg/kg IV daily + flucytosine[j] 25 mg/kg PO QID *Consolidation therapy (for at least 8 weeks, followed by maintenance therapy):* Fluconazole 400 mg PO (or IV) daily *Maintenance therapy:* Fluconazole 200 mg PO daily for at least 12 months	Meningoencephalitis with fever, malaise, headache
Cryptosporidium	Data insufficient to recommend prophylaxis	ART with immune restoration	Acute or subacute onset of profuse, nonbloody, watery diarrhea
Coccidioides immitis	Fluconazole 400 mg PO daily[k]	Mild infection (eg, focal pneumonia): Fluconazole 400 mg PO daily or itraconazole 200 mg PO BID Severely ill (non-meningeal infection) or diffuse pulmonary disease: Amphotericin B deoxycholate 0.7-1.0 mg/kg IV daily Duration of therapy: until clinical improvement, then switch to azole Meningeal infection: Fluconazole 400-800 mg IV or PO daily[l]	Syndromes: focal pneumonia, diffuse pneumonia (presenting as apparent PCP), cutaneous involvement, meningitis, liver or lymph node involvement

(continued)

Table 2
Prophylaxis and treatment of opportunistic infections in HIV-infected adolescents (*continued*)

Opportunistic infection[a]	Prophylaxis[b]	Treatment	Clinical clues to diagnosis
JC virus (progressive multifocal leukoencephalopathy infection)	Routine prophylaxis not recommended	No specific established therapy exists; main approach is ART to reverse immunosuppression	*Progressive multifocal leukoencephalopathy:* neurologic syndrome characterized by cognitive dysfunction, dementia, seizures, ataxia and cranial nerve deficits; evolves over weeks to months
Bacterial enteric infections (most common: *Salmonella, Shigella, Campylobacter*)	For travelers, antimicrobial prophylaxis can be considered, depending on the level of immunosuppression and the region and duration of travel Consider fluoroquinolones or rifaximin	Empiric treatment[m]: Ciprofloxacin 500-750 mg PO (or 400 mg IV) q12h *Salmonella*[n]: Ciprofloxacin 500-750 mg PO (or 400 mg IV) q12h, if susceptible Duration of therapy: *For gastroenteritis without bacteremia:* If CD4 count ≥200 cells/μL: 7-14 days If CD4 count <200 cells/μL: 2-6 weeks *For gastroenteritis with bacteremia:* If CD4 count ≥200/μL: 14 days If CD4 count <200 cells/μL: 2-6 weeks *Shigella:* Ciprofloxacin 500-750 mg PO (or 400 mg IV) q12h Duration of therapy: *Gastroenteritis:* 7-10 days *Bacteremia:* ≥14 days *Recurrent infections:* 2-6 weeks *Campylobacter:* *Mild disease and if CD4 count >200 cells/μL:* Withhold therapy unless symptoms persist for more than several days *Mild-to-moderate disease (if susceptible):* Ciprofloxacin 500-750 mg PO (or 400 mg IV) q12h or azithromycin 500 mg PO daily *Campylobacter bacteremia:* Ciprofloxacin 500-750 mg PO (or 400 mg IV) q12h + an aminoglycoside	Fever, bloody diarrhea, weight loss, possible bacteremia (bloody diarrhea more common with *Shigella* but can occur with *Salmonella* and *Campylobacter*)

| Bacterial respiratory disease (pneumonia) | *For those who never received any pneumococcal vaccine:* Single dose of PCV13 regardless of CD4 count (PCV13 0.5 mL IM ×1) *For those with CD4 count ≥200 cells/µL:* PPV23 0.5 mL IM or SQ at least 8 weeks after PCV13 vaccine *For those with CD4 count <200 cells/µL:* Offer PPV23 at least 8 weeks after receiving PCV13 or can wait until CD4 count increased to ≥200 cells/µL. *For individuals who previously received PPV23:* One dose of PCV13 should be given at least 1 year after the last receipt of PPV23 | Empiric outpatient: PO beta-lactam + PO macrolide (preferred beta-lactams: high-dose amoxicillin and amoxicillin-clavulanate), (preferred macrolides: azithromycin and clarithromycin) *For penicillin-allergic patients:* Levofloxacin 750 mg PO once daily or moxifloxacin 400 mg PO once daily Duration of therapy: 7-10 days. Should be afebrile for 48-72 hours and clinically stable before discontinuing Empiric non-ICU inpatient: IV beta-lactam + macrolide (preferred beta-lactams are ceftriaxone, cefotaxime, or ampicillin-sulbactam) (preferred macrolides: azithromycin and clarithromycin) *For penicillin-allergic patients:* Levofloxacin, 750 mg IV once daily or moxifloxacin 400 mg IV once daily Empiric treatment of ICU patients: IV beta-lactam + IV azithromycin or IV beta-lactam + (levofloxacin 750 mg IV once daily or moxifloxacin 400 mg IV once daily) Empiric therapy for patients at risk for methicillin-resistant *Staphylococcus aureus* Pneumonia: Add vancomycin IV or linezolid (IV or PO) to the antibiotic regimen Empiric therapy for patients at risk for pseudomonas pneumonia: IV antipneumococcal, antipseudomonal beta-lactam + (ciprofloxacin 400 mg IV q8-12h or levofloxacin 750 mg IV once daily) (Preferred beta-lactams: piperacillin-tazobactam, cefepime, imipenem, or meropenem) | Acute onset (3-5 days) of symptoms, including fevers, chills, rigors, chest pain, cough productive of purulent sputum, dyspnea |

(continued)

Table 2
Prophylaxis and treatment of opportunistic infections in HIV-infected adolescents (continued)

Influenza	Inactivated influenza vaccine annually (per recommendation for the season) Live-attenuated influenza vaccine is contraindicated in HIV-infected patients	Fever, headache, fatigue, myalgia

ART, antiretroviral therapy; BID, twice daily; HIV, human immunodeficiency virus; ICU, intensive care unit; IM, intramuscular; IV, intravenous; PO, by mouth; QID, four times daily; SQ, subcutaneous; TID, three times daily.

[a]Table adapted from: Panel on Opportunistic Infections In HIV-Infected Adults and Adolescents. Guidelines for the prevention and treatment of opportunistic infections in HIV-infected adults and adolescents: recommendations from the Centers for Disease Control and Prevention, the National Institutes of Health, and the HIV Medicine Association of the Infectious Diseases Society of America. Available at http://aidsinfo.nih.gov/contentfiles/lvguidelines/adult_oi.pdf. Accessed October 13, 2015.

[b]The doses recommended above are intended for patients with normal renal function; the doses of some of these agents must be adjusted in patients with renal insufficiency.

[c]TMP-SMX dose preferred for prevention of PCP when toxoplasmosis prophylaxis also indicated.

[d]Examples of alternatives; there are others that exist.

[e]Patients with documented or suspected PCP and moderate-to-severe disease (defined by room air pO_2 <70 mm Hg or arterial-alveolar O_2 gradient >35 mm Hg) should receive adjunctive corticosteroids as early as possible, and certainly within 72 hours after starting specific PCP therapy.

[f]Initial treatment of MAC disease should consist of 2 or more anti-mycobacterial drugs to prevent or delay the emergence of resistance. Consider adding third drug (rifabutin) for patients with advanced immunosuppression (CD4 counts <50 cells/μL), high mycobacterial loads (>2 log CFU/mL of blood), or in the absence of effective ART.

[g]Should collect specimen for culture and molecular diagnostic tests before beginning empiric TB treatment in individuals with clinical and radiographic presentation suggestive of TB.

[h]RIF is not recommended for patients receiving HIV PI because of its induction of PI metabolism.

[i]For persons with confirmed meningitis, liposomal amphotericin B should be administered as initial therapy for 4-6 weeks at a dosage of 5 mg/kg daily. This should be followed by maintenance therapy with itraconazole at a dose of 200 mg 2 or 3 times daily for a total of ≥1 year and until resolution of abnormal CSF findings.

[j]Patients receiving flucytosine should have either blood levels monitored or close monitoring of blood counts for development of cytopenia. Dosage should be adjusted in patients with renal insufficiency.

[k]Within an area where the disease is endemic, a positive IgM or IgG serologic test indicates an increased risk for the development of active infection and treatment is recommended if the CD4 count is <250 cells/μL.

[l]Therapy should be lifelong in patients with meningeal infections because relapse occurs in 80% of HIV-infected patients after discontinuation of azole therapy.

[m]Empiric antibiotic therapy is indicated for patients with advanced HIV (CD4 count <200 cells/μL or concomitant AIDS-defining illnesses), with clinically severe diarrhea (≥6 stools per day or bloody stool) and/or accompanying fever or chills. Fecal specimens should be obtained before initiation of empiric antibiotic therapy.

[n]All HIV-infected patients with salmonellosis should receive antimicrobial treatment because of an increase of bacteremia and mortality (by up to 7-fold) compared to HIV-negative individuals.

Complications of ART

Immediate and long-term complications of ART should be considered in the acutely ill HIV patient. Almost all of the antiretroviral medications have extensive toxicity profiles (Table 3).[66] In particular, the protease inhibitors are associated with gastrointestinal intolerance, including nausea, vomiting, and diarrhea, which may be particularly severe at the time of initiation. Adverse effects may range from nausea and vomiting with the protease inhibitors, to lactic acidosis with the nucleoside reverse transcriptase inhibitors, to hepatic failure and Stevens-Johnson syndrome with the non-nucleoside reverse transcriptase inhibitors. Long-term use of ART may lead to hyperlipidemia, metabolic disorder, and type 2 diabetes, all of which increase the risk for a myocardial event.[66] Finally, for patients who have recently initiated ART, the immune reconstitution inflammatory syndrome (IRIS) may present with symptoms ranging from fever and lymphadenopathy to altered mental status based on the underlying pathogen. Reactivation of the previously suppressed immune system results in an exaggerated response to either an unknown pathogen or disease process (unmasking IRIS) or to worsening presentation of a known OI (paradoxical IRIS), most commonly tuberculosis (TB), *Cryptococcus*, or CMV. Patients with CD4 counts less than 50 at ART initiation are at highest risk for these complications.[67]

Fever/Lymphadenopathy

Evaluation of the febrile HIV-infected patient includes a search for typical bacterial and viral causes, malignancy, and OIs (see Table 2). *Mycobacterium tuberculosis* typically presents as fever, sweats, weight loss, productive cough, and fatigue. However, in patients with advanced immune suppression, TB is more likely to present with extrapulmonary disease such as lymphadenitis, pleuritis, pericarditis, or meningitis. *Mycobacterium avium* complex (MAC) may present with fever, weight loss, nausea, vomiting, hepatosplenomegaly, and lymphadenopathy, typically in patients with CD4 counts less than 50. It may also cause localized syndromes such as lymphadenitis, osteomyelitis, soft tissue abscesses, pneumonitis, or central nervous system (CNS) infection. Infections by *Bartonella* species are another common cause of fever in patients with CD4 counts less than 100.[68]

Pulmonary Disease

Bacterial pneumonia, most often caused by *Streptococcus pneumoniae*, occurs with high frequency in HIV-infected patients. It presents with fever, cough, tachypnea, and respiratory distress. Conversely, PCP usually has a more subacute presentation of progressive dyspnea, chest tightness, cough, and fever, which evolves over days to weeks. Pulmonary cryptococcosis and CMV pneumonitis are rare causes of pulmonary disease in patients with advanced immunosuppression.[68]

Table 3
Characteristics of antiretroviral agents

Antiretroviral class	Medications*	Common adverse effects
Nucleoside reverse transcriptase inhibitors (NRTIs)	Abacavir/ABC (Ziagen) Didanosine/DDI (Videx) Emtricitabine/FTC (Emtriva) Lamivudine/3TC (Epivir) Stavudine/D4T (Zerit) Tenofovir/TDF (Viread) Zidovudine/ZDV (Retrovir)	Hypersensitivity (Abacavir) Gastrointestinal intolerance Lactic acidosis PR prolongation QT prolongation Nephrolithiasis Pancreatitis Hyperlipidemia, hyperglycemia Renal insufficiency (Tenofovir) Rash (including Stevens-Johnson syndrome) Anemia/neutropenia (Zidovudine)
Non-nucleoside reverse transcriptase inhibitors (NNRTIs)	Efavirenz/EFV (Sustiva) Etravirine/ETR (Intelence) Nevirapine/NVP (Viramune) Rilpivirine/RPV (Edurant)	Hepatoxicity Gastrointestinal intolerance Neuropsychiatric symptoms (Efavirenz) Rash (including Stevens-Johnson syndrome) Gastrointestinal intolerance Neuropsychiatric symptoms (Efavirenz) Rash (including Stevens-Johnson syndrome)
Protease inhibitors (PIs)	Atazanavir/ATV (Reyataz) Darunavir/DRV (Prezista) Fosamprenavir/FPV (Lexiva) Indinavir/IDV (Crixivan) Lopinavir/ritonavir LPV/r (Kaletra) Nelfinavir/NFV (Viracept) Saquinavir/SQV (Invirase)	Hypersensitivity reaction (Abacavir) Gastrointestinal intolerance PR prolongation QT prolongation Nephrolithiasis Rash (including Stevens-Johnson syndrome)
Integrase strand transfer inhibitors (INSTIs)	Dolutegravir/DTG (Tivicay) Elvitegravir/ELV (in Stribild) Raltegravir/RAL (Isentress)	Gastrointestinal intolerance Hypersensitivity reaction Rhabdomyolysis (Raltegravir) Headache
CCR5 antagonist	Marviroc/MVC (Selzentry)	Gastrointestinal intolerance Rash Dizziness/orthostatic hypotension Pyrexia Hepatotoxicity
Fusion inhibitors	Enfurvitide (Fuseon)	Injection site reactions Hypersensitivity

*Combination formulations include: ABC+3TC (Epzicom), ABC+3TC+DTV (Triumeq), TDF+FTC (Truvada), TDF+FTC+EFV (Sustiva), TDF+FTC+EFV+cobicistat (Stribild), TDF+FTC+RPV (Complera), ZDV+3TC (Combivir), ZDV+3TC+ABC (Trizivir).

Oral and Gastrointestinal Disease

Candida albicans causes most cases of oropharyngeal candidiasis (thrush) and esophageal candidiasis. Thrush is characterized by creamy white plaques on the oral mucous membranes. Esophagitis typically presents with chest pain, retrosternal burning, or odynophagia. In the United States, there are high rates of coinfection with HIV and hepatitis B (estimated ~10%) and hepatitis C (estimated 20%-30%) in the adult population. Patients with jaundice, fatigue, and evidence of hepatitis should be tested for hepatitis A, B, and C. Diarrhea is a common cause of morbidity in HIV-infected patients. Severe diarrhea in the HIV patient may be caused by common bacterial pathogens such as *Salmonella, Shigella*, and *Clostridium difficile*, which is the leading cause of bacterial diarrhea in patients with HIV infection. Enteric viruses are found frequently, as are atypical agents such as *Cryptosporidium parvum, Giardia lamblia, Isospora belli*, and microsporidia. Notably, CMV can cause both esophagitis and colitis in patients with CD4 counts less than 50.[68]

Neurologic Disease

In addition to the typical causes of bacterial meningitis and viral encephalitis, it is important to consider OI in patients with low CD4 counts presenting with altered mental status. Toxoplasmosis presents with altered mental status, headache, or weakness and fever. Cryptococcal meningitis usually has a subacute presentation with headache, fever, and malaise, occasionally associated with encephalopathy. Syphilis, caused by the spirochete *Treponema pallidum*, can present with neurologic involvement at any stage of disease. Cytomegalovirus, herpes simplex virus (HSV), and varicella zoster virus (VZV) can cause encephalitis in the HIV-infected patient. In patients with advanced HIV/AIDS, JC virus can cause progressive multifocal leukoencephalopathy, a neurologic syndrome characterized by cognitive dysfunction, dementia, seizures, ataxia, and cranial nerve deficits that evolve over weeks to months.[68,69]

Genitourinary Disease

Herpes simplex virus typically causes ulcerative disease of the oral or genital mucosal lesions. Primary infection may also cause systemic symptoms, including fever, myalgias, and encephalitis. Adolescents with advanced HIV infection are at risk for both more frequent recurrences and more severe ulcerative disease. Primary syphilis manifests as solitary painless anal or genital ulcer, or chancre. However, patients with HIV may present with multiple chancres. Secondary syphilis is characterized by a diffuse maculopapular rash involving the palms and soles. Condyloma lata (broad, moist-appearing papules typically occur in the anogenital region and axilla) are another hallmark of secondary syphilis. The presence of urethral or vaginal discharge should prompt evaluation for gonorrhea and chlamydia in all patients and trichomoniasis in females. It is important to remember that dysuria or discharge in the adolescent or young adult male represents an STI and should be treated empirically as such until proven otherwise. The presence of a single STI should prompt evaluation for others. Prompt diagnosis and treatment of STIs are of key importance because the presence of STIs substantially increases the risk or HIV transmission.[70,71]

Dermatologic Disease

Numerous infectious pathogens can cause rash in the HIV-infected adolescent. Varicella zoster virus typically causes a vesicular eruption in both primary varicella and herpes zoster reactivation disease. Herpes zoster may occur at any CD4 count and presents as a painful, vesicular eruption that follows a dermatomal distribution. Patients with severe immunosuppression may also present with disseminated zoster, characterized by multidermatomal or diffuse rash and CNS or ocular involvement. Cryptococcosis may present with disseminated skin lesions that can be vesicular or papular and often mimic molluscum. Other common dermatologic manifestations of HIV infection include papular pruritic eruption, bacillary angiomatosis, seborrheic dermatitis, dermatophyte fungal infections, folliculitis, and prurigo nodularis. Physicians should also consider drug hypersensitivity reactions that may present as maculopapular or morbilliform eruptions.[68]

Ophthalmologic Disease

Patients infected with HIV who have visual complaints should be seen urgently by an ophthalmologist. A number of OIs can present with ocular complaints and rapidly lead to vision loss. Cytomegalovirus retinitis often presents with scotoma, "floaters" in the visual field, visual field defects, and decreased visual acuity. Funduscopic examination reveals intraretinal hemorrhage and retinal infiltrates. HSV and VZV both are causes of acute retinal necrosis.[68]

Hematologic and Oncologic Disease

Anemia, neutropenia, and thrombocytopenia all can occur as a consequence of untreated HIV infection. Drug-induced marrow suppression may occur from treatment with zidovudine, ganciclovir, or foscarnet. Infections such as MAC or parvovirus may also cause myelosuppression. It is important to consider lymphoma in patients with cytopenia, particularly in those who also present with fever, weight loss, or lymphadenopathy. Individuals infected with HIV are at much higher risk for non-Hodgkin lymphoma than the general population, and absence of ART and low CD4 count further increase this risk. Other HIV-associated malignancies, such as Burkitt or Hodgkin lymphoma, also occur frequently, even in patients with high CD4 counts. Kaposi sarcoma, a malignancy associated with human herpes virus-8 (HHV-8), presents with purple or brown, non-tender, firm skin lesions. Oral and visceral dissemination may occur as well.[68]

DIAGNOSTIC EVALUATION

The diagnostic workup should be determined by the patient's presentation and degree of immune suppression. For a well-appearing patient with minimal immune suppression (CD4 count >500), an extensive diagnostic workup is rarely necessary. However, for the ill-appearing or immunosuppressed patient, the laboratory workup should be directed at both identifying the cause as well as assessing the patient's state of health.

For ill-appearing patients, it is prudent to obtain complete blood count (CBC) with differential, comprehensive metabolic panel with liver and kidney function, and blood culture. In patients with severe immune suppression or those with concern for mycobacterial disease, blood should also be sent for acid-fast bacilli (AFB) smear and culture, interferon gamma release assay to identify *M tuberculosis*, and cryptococcal rapid antigen. If there is concern for malignancy, uric acid and lactate dehydrogenase (also typically elevated in PCP) are important to assess for tumor lysis. There is a high incidence of *Salmonella* bacteremia in HIV patients, so all patients with fever and diarrhea should undergo tests for blood culture in addition to stool studies. For patients with moderate to severe diarrhea, stool studies should include bacterial culture for salmonella and shigella, ova and parasites, cryptosporidium and Giardia, and *C difficile*.[68]

Obtaining CD4 counts and a quantitative HIV RNA assay (viral load) is not recommended in the acute care setting. Acute illness transiently lowers the CD4 count and may elevate the viral load.[66] Values in the ED may not reflect the patient's current immune status outside of the acute illness, and results are typically not available in a time frame that would influence clinical decision-making. The absolute lymphocyte count, derived by the CBC, can be used as a surrogate marker for CD4 when no recent value is available. Markers of inflammation, such as C-reactive protein and erythrocyte sedimentation rate, are often unreliable in HIV infection because they may be chronically elevated. However, they may be useful in monitoring response to long courses of antibiotic therapy for illnesses such as osteomyelitis.

Chest radiography is important to assess for pneumonia, PCP, TB, or mediastinal lymphadenopathy in patients with suspected lymphoma. PCP usually appears as bilateral, symmetric ground glass infiltrates. In patients with minimal immune suppression, TB will typically appear as upper lobe and cavitary disease. However, for patients with severe immune suppression, cavitation is rare, and there may be middle and lower lobe involvement or miliary infiltrate. Sputum smear and culture should be obtained if TB is suspected. For patients with severe respiratory distress or those with suspected PCP, arterial blood gas measurement should be obtained with calculation of the alveolar-arterial O_2 gradient to characterize the severity of hypoxemia and need for corticosteroid treatment in PCP.[68]

For patients with altered mental status, computerized tomography of the brain with intravenous contrast should be obtained before lumbar puncture to assess for increased intracranial pressure and identify CNS mass lesions. *Toxoplasma* and CNS lymphoma both typically present as ring-enhancing lesions. The lesions of toxoplasmosis are typically located in the basal ganglia or cortical gray matter with pronounced edema, whereas CNS lymphoma often involves the corpus callosum or periventricular areas.[69] It is important to obtain opening pressure by manometry with lumbar puncture because increased pressure is associated with significant morbidity and mortality in cryptococcal meningitis. In addition to cell counts, protein, glucose, and bacterial culture, additional cerebrospinal fluid should be obtained for cryptococcal rapid antigen, VDRL, fungal, and AFB cultures. In addition, cerebrospinal fluid can be evaluated by polymerase chain reaction for EBV (which will be elevated in primary CNS lymphoma), *Toxoplasma*, HSV, CMV, VZV, or JC virus (elevated in progressive multifocal leukoencephalopathy).[68,69]

Treatment should be directed based on clinical and laboratory findings. For up-to-date treatment recommendations for OIs, physicians should consult "Guidelines for the Prevention and Treatment of Opportunistic Infections in HIV-infected Adults and Adolescents" available at www.aidsinfo.nih.gov/guidelines.[68] It is important to note when starting new medications, many antiretroviral (ARV) drugs have significant drug-drug interactions that may either impair the effectiveness of ART or other drugs prescribed. Physicians should consult the DHHS "Guidelines for the Use of Antiretroviral Agents in Adolescents and Adults" available at www.aidsinfo.nih.gov/guidelines to assure that any new medications will not interact with the patient's existing ARV regimen.[66] For patients on ARVs, altering or changing ART without guidance from an HIV specialist is not recommended. For patients who meet criteria for OI prophylaxis by CD4 count or clinical history (see Care of the HIV Infected Adolescent section) it is important to assure they are on the appropriate prophylaxis regimen at discharge (Table 2).

HUMAN IMMUNODEFICIENCY VIRUS POSTEXPOSURE PROPHYLAXIS

Physicians have an important role to play in the management of patients with HIV exposures. Sexual and needlestick exposures are common occurrences, and the first site of presentation is typically the primary care office or ED. HIV postexposure prophylaxis (PEP) may substantially reduce the risk of HIV infection when implemented promptly, that is, as close to the exposure time as possible and not beyond 72 hours.[72,73] A clear history of the timing and nature of exposure is essential in the physician's assessment of whether PEP is warranted. Key elements of the history include the timing of exposure, the type of exposure with attention to the body fluid involved and site of inoculation, the HIV status of the source, and the medical comorbidities of the exposed patient. The risk of HIV transmission per contact varies depending on the type of sexual exposure, and an understanding of this risk should help inform the decision to initiate PEP. The estimated risks are 1% to 30% with receptive anal intercourse, 0.1% to 10% with insertive anal intercourse or receptive vaginal intercourse, and 0.1% to 1% with insertive vaginal intercourse.[74]

In general, PEP should be recommended in cases of unprotected receptive and insertive vaginal or anal intercourse, needle sharing, or exposure to blood or potentially infected fluid for which the source is HIV infected or of unknown HIV status. Postexposure prophylaxis should be considered on a case-by-case basis for lower-risk exposures, including oral-vaginal, oral-penile, and oral-anal contact. In all cases, it is important to consider the source's HIV status, viral load, presence of HIV on non-intact mucosa (eg, mucosal lesions or gingivitis), and presence of genital ulcer disease or other STI that may increase the risk of HIV transmission.[75] Additionally, PEP is recommended for sexual assault victims, especially because genital trauma can increase the likelihood of HIV transmission. Consultation with an infectious diseases or HIV specialist is recommended in situations in which the indication for PEP or the choice of regimen is unclear. In addition, physicians can contact the 24-hour National Physicians' Consultation Center PEPline at 1-888-448-4911 for guidance on providing PEP.

Before starting PEP, baseline laboratory testing for all patients should include HIV testing (preferably by fourth generation antibody/antigen combination assay), comprehensive metabolic panel with creatinine and liver function tests, and hepatitis B and C serology. The patient should be vaccinated for hepatitis B if there is no evidence of immunity and offered immunoglobulin B if the patient was exposed to a source with hepatitis B infection. For sexual exposures, the patient should be tested for other STIs, including gonorrhea, chlamydia, and syphilis, and empiric treatment should be considered. Women should be tested for pregnancy and offered emergency contraception. A CBC should be performed if starting a zidovudine-based regimen because of the risks of anemia and neutropenia. Postexposure prophylaxis should not be delayed while waiting for the results of these tests.

When the HIV status of the exposure source is unknown, every attempt should be made to test the source. However, starting PEP should not be delayed while the source's status is being determined. If the source is available and consents for testing, an FDA-approved rapid test or laboratory-based immunoassay should be performed. If the source or patient has an HIV exposure in the previous 6 weeks, a plasma HIV RNA assay should also be obtained to rule out acute infection in the window period. In all cases, PEP should be continued for a full 28 days or until the source is found to be definitively HIV negative.

Guidelines for the provision of PEP changed in 2013 to recommend a 3-drug regimen given for 28 days, irrespective of exposure type.[76] The preferred PEP regimen for patients 13 years or older and Tanner III or greater is a tenofovir/ emtricitabine (Truvada) 300/200 mg tablet once daily and Raltegravir (Isentress) 400 mg twice daily.[75,76] Use of tenofovir/emtricitabine is not recommended for patients with renal disease, those younger than 13 years, or those less than Tanner stage III. Preferred and alternate regimens for PEP are listed in Table 4. Whenever possible, patients should be sent home with a 5-day supply of medications in hand and a prescription for the remainder of the 28-day course. Patients should be counseled regarding possible drug toxicities and drug-drug interactions. The importance of adherence to the PEP regimen should be stressed. For patients who feel unable to adhere to twice-daily dosing, alternate once-daily regimens can be recommended (Table 4). Patients should be counseled regarding HIV risk reduction, both for long-term health maintenance and for prevention of secondary HIV transmission until the patient is confirmed to be HIV negative. For patients with a history of high-risk sexual behavior or repeated HIV exposures, counseling regarding HIV preexposure prophylaxis should be incorporated into patient education.

Ensuring timely follow-up of patients with a physician knowledgeable in the management of PEP is essential. Patients should be seen within 72 hours of initial presentation to assess side effects and tolerability, determine whether the PEP prescription has been filled and covered by insurance, and provide additional counseling and adherence support. Patients should be followed again 2 weeks after starting PEP for ongoing monitoring of PEP toxicity, with renal and hepatic function tests at this time, as well as a CBC if using a zidovudine-based

Table 4
Preferred and alternate PEP regimens after HIV exposure

Preferred Regimen	
Age >13 years who are Tanner III or higher	• Raltegravir: One 400-mg tablet BID **PLUS** • Tenofovir/emtricitabine (Truvada) 300/200 mg tablet once daily[a]
Alternate Regimens	
Once-daily dosing Age >13 years who are Tanner III or higher	• Tenofovir/emtricitabine (Truvada)[a] 300/200 mg tablet once daily **PLUS** • Darunavir 800 mg PO daily *OR* atazanavir 300 mg PO daily **AND** • Ritonavir 100 mg PO daily
Age 6-12 years who are >30 kg and *can* swallow whole tablets/caplets OR Age >13 years who are less than Tanner III	• Raltegravir: 400 mg BID **PLUS** lamivudine/ zidovudine (Combivir)[b] 150/300 mg BID

BID, twice daily; HIV, human immunodeficiency virus; PO, by mouth.
[a]If patient has history of renal disease, replace tenofovir/emtricitabine with lamivudine/zidovudine (Combivir) 150/300 mg BID unless severe anemia
[b]Unless severe anemia

regimen. Finally, follow-up HIV testing should be performed at 4 to 6 weeks and 12 weeks after the initial exposure if a fourth-generation antigen/antibody combination assay is used. If a third-generation is used, the final HIV test should occur 6 months after exposure.

SUMMARY

Many adolescents are at high risk for HIV infection, and those who are infected or at-risk commonly present to the ED, often as their only or frequent source of care. It is important to consider routine screening and to have a high index of suspicion for AHI in this setting. If a diagnosis of HIV infection is made, immediate linkage to care with a specialist in adolescent and young adult HIV infection should be prioritized. For the known HIV-infected patient, management must consider unique possibilities of OIs, IRIS, and medication side effects. For any patient on ART, drug-drug interactions must be noted as part of any treatment plan. If a young person presents with a recent sexual or needlestick exposure of concern, every effort to prescribe and ensure follow-up for PEP should be made. It is essential for physicians to understand and comply with local regulations regarding HIV testing and adolescents' rights for associated confidential care. Finally, physicians who see adolescents in acute care settings have a tremendous opportunity to make a difference in ensuring improved health outcomes for youth living with HIV and to prevent new infections.

References

1. Centers for Disease Control and Prevention. Monitoring selected national HIV prevention and care objectives by using HIV surveillance data—United States and 6 U.S. dependent areas—2011. *HIV Surveillance Supplemental Report* 2013;18(No. 5). Available at: www.cdc.gov/hiv/library/reports/surveillance/. Published October 2013. Accessed October 13, 2015
2. Mohareb AM, Rothman RE, Hsieh YH. Emergency department (ED) utilization by HIV-infected ED patients in the United States in 2009 and 2010—a national estimation. *HIV Med.* 2013;14:605-613
3. Prejean J, Song R, Hernandez A, et al. Estimated HIV incidence in the United States, 2006-2009. *PloS One.* 2011;6:e17502
4. Centers for Disease Control and Prevention. HIV Among Youth 2011. Available at: www.cdc.gov/hiv/pdf/library_factsheet_HIV_amongYouth.pdf. Accessed October 13, 2015
5. Purcell DW, Johnson CH, Lansky A, et al. Estimating the population size of men who have sex with men in the United States to obtain HIV and syphilis rates. *Open AIDS J.* 2012;6:98-107
6. Centers for Disease Control and Prevention. Estimated HIV incidence in the United States, 2007–2010. HIV Surveillance Supplemental Report 2012. December 2012;17(4). Available at: www.cdc.gov/hiv/pdf/statistics_hssr_vol_17_no_4.pdf. Accessed October 13, 2015
7. Centers for Disease Control and Prevention. HIV Among Transgender People in the United States. November 2013. Available at: www.cdc.gov/hiv/pdf/risk_transgender.pdf. Accessed October 13, 2015
8. Gardner EM, McLees MP, Steiner JF, Del Rio C, Burman WJ. The spectrum of engagement in HIV care and its relevance to test-and-treat strategies for prevention of HIV infection. *Clin Infect Dis.* 2011;52:793-800
9. Zanoni BC, Mayer KH. The adolescent and young adult HIV cascade of care in the United States: exaggerated health disparities. *AIDS Patient Care STDS.* 2014;28:128-135
10. Kann L, Kinchen S, Shanklin SL, et al. Youth risk behavior surveillance—United States, 2013. *MMWR Surveill Summ.* 2014;63(Suppl 4):1-168

644   C. Salas-Humara et al / Adolesc Med 026 (2015) 619–646

11. US Preventive Services Task Force. Screening for HIV: recommendation statement. *Ann Intern Med.* 2005;143:32-37
12. Marks G, Crepaz N, Senterfitt JW, Janssen RS. Meta-analysis of high-risk sexual behavior in persons aware and unaware they are infected with HIV in the United States: implications for HIV prevention programs. *J Acquir Immune Defic Syndr.* 2005;39(4):446-453
13. Sanders GD, Bayoumi AM, Sundaram V, et al. Cost-effectiveness of screening for HIV in the era of highly active antiretroviral therapy. *N Engl J Med.* 2005;352:570-585
14. Cohen MS, Chen YQ, McCauley M, et al. Prevention of HIV-1 infection with early antiretroviral therapy. *N Engl J Med.* 2011;365:493-505
15. Sabin CA, Smith CJ, Gumley H, et al. Late presenters in the era of highly active antiretroviral therapy: uptake of and responses to antiretroviral therapy. *AIDS.* 2004;18:2145-2151
16. Chen RY, Accortt NA, Westfall AO, et al. Distribution of health care expenditures for HIV-infected patients. *Clin Infect Dis.* 2006;42:1003-1010
17. Branson BM, Handsfield HH, Lampe MA, et al. Revised recommendations for HIV testing of adults, adolescents, and pregnant women in health-care settings. *MMWR Recomm Rep.* 2006;55(RR-14):1-17
18. American Academy of Pediatrics Committee on Pediatric AIDS; Emmanuel PJ, Martinez J. Adolescents and HIV infection: the pediatrician's role in promoting routine testing. *Pediatrics.* 2011;1281023-1029
19. Moyer VA; U.S. Preventive Services Task Force. Screening for HIV: U.S. Preventive Services Task Force Recommendation Statement. *Ann Intern Med.* 2013;159:51-60
20. Daar ES, Little S, Pitt J, et al. Diagnosis of primary HIV-1 infection. Los Angeles County Primary HIV Infection Recruitment Network. *Ann Intern Med.* 2001;134:25-29
21. Brenner BG, Roger M, Routy JP, et al. High rates of forward transmission events after acute/early HIV-1 infection. *J Infect Dis.* 2007;195:951-959
22. Kahn JO, Walker BD. Acute human immunodeficiency virus type 1 infection. *N Engl J Med.* 1998;339:33-39
23. Wawer MJ, Gray RH, Sewankambo NK, et al. Rates of HIV-1 transmission per coital act, by stage of HIV-1 infection, in Rakai, Uganda. *J Infect Dis.* 2005;191:1403-1409
24. Tindall B, Barker S, Donovan B, et al. Characterization of the acute clinical illness associated with human immunodeficiency virus infection. *Arch Intern Med.* 1988;148:945-949
25. Schacker T, Collier AC, Hughes J, Shea T, Corey L. Clinical and epidemiologic features of primary HIV infection. *Ann Intern Med.* 1996;125:257-264
26. Massin MM, Montesanti J, Gerard P, Lepage P. Spectrum and frequency of illness presenting to a pediatric emergency department. *Acta Clin Belg.* 2006;61:161-165
27. Wilson KM, Klein JD. Adolescents who use the emergency department as their usual source of care. *Arch Pediatr Adolesc Med.* 2000;154:361-365
28. Keele BF, Giorgi EE, Salazar-Gonzalez JF, et al. Identification and characterization of transmitted and early founder virus envelopes in primary HIV-1 infection. *Proc Natl Acad Sci U S A.* 2008;105:7552-7557
29. Lee HY, Giorgi EE, Keele BF, et al. Modeling sequence evolution in acute HIV-1 infection. *J Theor Biol.* 2009;261:341-360
30. Lindback S, Karlsson AC, Mittler J, et al. Viral dynamics in primary HIV-1 infection. Karolinska Institutet Primary HIV Infection Study Group. *AIDS.* 2000;14:2283-2291
31. Lindback S, Thorstensson R, Karlsson AC, et al. Diagnosis of primary HIV-1 infection and duration of follow-up after HIV exposure. Karolinska Institute Primary HIV Infection Study Group. *AIDS.* 2000;14:2333-2339
32. Vermeulen M, Coleman C, Mitchel J, et al. Comparison of human immunodeficiency virus assays in window phase and elite controller samples: viral load distribution and implications for transmission risk. *Transfusion.* 2013;53(10 Pt 2):2384-2398
33. Masciotra S, McDougal JS, Feldman J, et al. Evaluation of an alternative HIV diagnostic algorithm using specimens from seroconversion panels and persons with established HIV infections. *J Clin Virol.* 2011;52(Suppl 1):S17-S22

34. Fiebig EW, Wright DJ, Rawal BD, et al. Dynamics of HIV viremia and antibody seroconversion in plasma donors: implications for diagnosis and staging of primary HIV infection. *AIDS.* 2003;17:1871-1879

35. Owen SM, Yang C, Spira T, et al. Alternative algorithms for human immunodeficiency virus infection diagnosis using tests that are licensed in the United States. *J Clin Microbiol.* 2008;46:1588-1595

36. Tomaras GD, Yates NL, Liu P, et al. Initial B-cell responses to transmitted human immunodeficiency virus type 1: virion-binding immunoglobulin M (IgM) and IgG antibodies followed by plasma anti-gp41 antibodies with ineffective control of initial viremia. *J Virol.* 2008;82:12449-12463

37. Centers for Disease Control and Prevention. National HIV Testing Day and new testing recommendations. *MMWR Morb Mortal Wkly Rep.* 2014;63(25):537

38. Arbelaez C, Wright EA, Losina E, et al. Emergency provider attitudes and barriers to universal HIV testing in the emergency department. *J Emerg Med.* 2012;42:7-14

39. Fincher-Mergi M, Cartone KJ, et al. Assessment of emergency department health care professionals' behaviors regarding HIV testing and referral for patients with STDs. *AIDS Patient Care STDS.* 2002;16:549-553

40. Kowalczyk Mullins TL, Braverman PK, et al. Adolescent preferences for human immunodeficiency virus testing methods and impact of rapid tests on receipt of results. *J Adolesc Health.* 2010;46:162-168

41. Haines CJ, Uwazuoke K, Zussman B, et al. Pediatric emergency department-based rapid HIV testing: adolescent attitudes and preferences. *Pediatr Emerg Care.* 2011;27:13-16

42. Centers for Disease Control and Prevention. Detection of acute HIV infection in two evaluations of a new HIV diagnostic testing algorithm—United States, 2011-2013. *MMWR Morb Mortal Wkly Rep.* 2013;62:489-494

43. Styer LM, Sullivan TJ, Parker MM. Evaluation of an alternative supplemental testing strategy for HIV diagnosis by retrospective analysis of clinical HIV testing data. *J Clin Virol.* 2011;52 (Suppl 1):S35-S40

44. Stekler JD, Swenson PD, Coombs RW, et al. HIV testing in a high-incidence population: is antibody testing alone good enough? *Clin Infect Dis.* 2009;49:444-453

45. Pilcher CD, Fiscus SA, Nguyen TQ, et al. Detection of acute infections during HIV testing in North Carolina. *N Engl J Med.* 2005;352:1873-1883

46. Patel P, Klausner JD, Bacon OM, et al. Detection of acute HIV infections in high-risk patients in California. *J Acquir Immune Defic Syndr.* 2006;42:75-79

47. American Academy of Pediatrics Committee on Pediatric AIDS, Committee on Adolescence. Adolescents and human immunodeficiency virus infection: the role of the pediatrician in prevention and intervention. *Pediatrics.* 2001;107:188-190

48. Guttmacher Institute: State Policies in Brief. Minors' access to STI services. Available at: http://www.guttmacher.org/statecenter/spibs/spib_MASS.pdf. Accessed August 10, 2014

49. Centers for Disease Control and Prevention. State HIV Laws. Available at: www.cdc.gov/hiv/policies/law/states/index.html. Accessed August 11, 2014

50. Marrazzo JM, del Rio C, Holtgrave DR, et al. HIV prevention in clinical care settings: 2014 recommendations of the International Antiviral Society-USA Panel. *JAMA.* 2014;312:390-409

51. D'Angelo LJ, Samples C, Rogers AS, Peralta L, Friedman L. HIV infection and AIDS in adolescents: an update of the position of the Society for Adolescent Medicine. *J Adolesc Health.* 2006;38:88-91

52. Pincus JM, Crosby SS, Losina E, et al. Acute human immunodeficiency virus infection in patients presenting to an urban urgent care center. *Clin Infect Dis.* 2003;37:1699-1704

53. Rosenberg ES, Caliendo AM, Walker BD. Acute HIV infection among patients tested for mononucleosis. *N Engl J Med.* 1999;340:969

54. Weintrob AC, Giner J, Menezes P, et al. Infrequent diagnosis of primary human immunodeficiency virus infection: missed opportunities in acute care settings. *Arch Intern Med.* 2003;163:2097-2100

55. Zaunders JJ, Munier ML, Kaufmann DE, et al. Early proliferation of CCR5(+) CD38(+++) antigen-specific CD4(+) Th1 effector cells during primary HIV-1 infection. *Blood.* 2005;106: 1660-1667

56. McKellar MS, Cope AB, Gay CL, et al. Acute HIV-1 infection in the Southeastern United States: a cohort study. *AIDS Res Hum Retroviruses*. 2013;29:121-128

57. Ridzon R, Gallagher K, Ciesielski C, et al. Simultaneous transmission of human immunodeficiency virus and hepatitis C virus from a needle-stick injury. *N Engl J Med*. 1997;336:919-922

58. Chu C, Selwyn PA. Diagnosis and initial management of acute HIV infection. *Am Fam Physician*. 2010;81:1239-1244

59. Cooper DA, Gold J, Maclean P, et al. Acute AIDS retrovirus infection. Definition of a clinical illness associated with seroconversion. *Lancet*. 1985;1:537-540

60. Daar ES, Pilcher CD, Hecht FM. Clinical presentation and diagnosis of primary HIV-1 infection. *Curr Opin HIV AIDS*. 2008;3:10-15

61. Lapins J, Gaines H, Lindback S, Lidbrink P, Emtestam L. Skin and mucosal characteristics of symptomatic primary HIV-1 infection. *AIDS Patient Care STDS*. 1997;11:67-70

62. Zetola NM, Pilcher CD. Diagnosis and management of acute HIV infection. *Infect Dis Clin North Am*. 2007;21(1):19-48, vii

63. de Jong MD, Hulsebosch HJ, Lange JM. Clinical, virological and immunological features of primary HIV-1 infection. *Genitourin Med*. 1991;67:367-373

64. van Essen GG, Lieverse AG, Sprenger HG, Schirm J, Weits J. False-positive Paul-Bunnell test in HIV seroconversion. *Lancet*. 1988;2:747-748

65. Josephs JS, Fleishman JA, Korthuis PT, Moore RD, Gebo KA. Emergency department utilization among HIV-infected patients in a multisite multistate study. *HIV Med*. 2010;11:74-84

66. US Department of Health and Human Services. Panel on Antiretroviral Guidelines for Adults and Adolescents. Guidelines for the use of antiretroviral agents in HIV-1-infected adults and adolescents. Available at: www.aidsinfo.nih.gov/ContentFiles/AdultandAdolescentGL.pdf. Accessed October 13, 2014

67. Muller M, Wandel S, Colebunders R, et al. Immune reconstitution inflammatory syndrome in patients starting antiretroviral therapy for HIV infection: a systematic review and meta-analysis. *Lancet Infect Dis*. 2010;10:251-261

68. Panel on Opportunistic Infections in HIV-Infected Adults and Adolescents. Guidelines for the prevention and treatment of opportunistic infections in HIV-infected adults and adolescents: recommendations from the Centers for Disease Control and Prevention, the National Institutes of Health, and the HIV Medicine Association of the Infectious Diseases Society of America. Available at: aidsinfo.nih.gov/contentfiles/lvguidelines/adult_oi.pdf. Accessed October 2014.

69. Ho EL, Jay CA. Altered mental status in HIV-infected patients. *Emerg Med Clin North Am*. 2010;28:311-323

70. Ward H, Ronn M. Contribution of sexually transmitted infections to the sexual transmission of HIV. *Curr Opin HIV AIDS*. 2010;5:305-310

71. Workowski KA, Berman S. Sexually transmitted diseases treatment guidelines, 2010. *MMWR Recomm Rep*. 2010;59(RR-12):1-110

72. Cardo DM, Culver DH, Ciesielski CA, et al. A case-control study of HIV seroconversion in health care workers after percutaneous exposure. Centers for Disease Control and Prevention Needlestick Surveillance Group. *N Engl J Med*. 1997;337:1485-1490

73. Schechter M, do Lago RF, Mendelsohn AB, et al. Behavioral impact, acceptability, and HIV incidence among homosexual men with access to postexposure chemoprophylaxis for HIV. *J Acquir Immune Defic Syndr*. 2004;35:519-525

74 Smith DK, Grohskopf LA, Black RJ, et al. Antiretroviral postexposure prophylaxis after sexual, injection-drug use, or other nonoccupational exposure to HIV in the United States: recommendations from the U.S. Department of Health and Human Services. *MMWR Recomm Rep*. 2005;54 (RR-2):1-20

75. New York State Department of Public Health. HIV prophylaxis after non-occupational exposure 2013. Available at: www.hivguidelines.org/clinical-guidelines/post-exposure-prophylaxis/hiv-prophylaxis-following-non-occupational-exposure/. Accessed October 13, 2014

76. Kuhar DT, Henderson DK, Struble KA, et al. Updated US Public Health Service guidelines for the management of occupational exposures to human immunodeficiency virus and recommendations for postexposure prophylaxis. *Infect Contr Hosp Epidemiol*. 2013;34:875-892

Adolesc Med 026 (2015) 647–657

Evaluation and Treatment of the Adolescent Sexual Assault Patient

Cynthia J. Mollen, MD, MSCE[a]*; Monika Goyal, MD, MSCE[b]; Jane Lavelle, MD[a]; Philip Scribano, DO, MSCE[a]

[a]Children's Hospital of Philadelphia, University of Pennsylvania, Perelman School of Medicine, Philadelphia, Pennsylvania; [b]Children's National Medical Center, The George Washington University, Washington, DC

Emergency medicine (EM) physicians are often the first practitioners to care for survivors of sexual assault. Although estimates of the prevalence of sexual assault vary, adolescents and young adults have the highest rates of sexual assault of any age group nationally, and the statistics likely underestimate the true rates because of underreporting.[1] According to the 2013 Youth Risk Behavior Surveillance Survey, 10.5% of female high school students and 4.2% of male high school students reported being forced to have sexual intercourse. Among the 74% who had dated within the prior 12 months, 10.4% of male and female (combined) adolescents had been kissed, touched, or physically forced to have sexual intercourse against their wishes by someone they were dating. More than 14% of females and more than 6% of males reported sexual violence.[2] A recent study found that almost 11% of adolescent girls aged 14 to 17 years experienced sexual assault.[3] Saltzman et al[4] analyzed data from the National Electronic Injury Surveillance System and found that preadolescents and adolescents (aged 10-19 years) were more frequently evaluated after a sexual assault in the ED than people of other ages. Of note, rates of visits for males were highest in the 0- to 9-year age group, compared to females, for whom the highest rate was in the 10- to 19-year age group; this may reflect, in part, an underreporting bias for adolescent males.[4] Additionally, adolescents reported a significant prevalence of dating physical violence with their intimate partner, with an annual estimate of 1.5 million high school students experiencing this form of violence.[5] Up to 30% of adolescents report some form of dating violence, with higher odds of violence among sexual minority youth compared to their heterosexual counterparts.[6] Given the preva-

*Corresponding author
E-mail address: mollenc@email.chop.edu

lence of sexual assault, it is critical that EM physicians familiarize themselves with how to care for survivors of acute sexual assault and remain aware of institutional and local protocols for medical care, reporting to child protective services and/or law enforcement agencies, and providing access to support services.

Several authors have found that the emergency department (ED) care of pediatric survivors of sexual assault is less than ideal. For example, Merchant et al[7] reviewed the medical records of adolescent patients seeking care for sexual assault in 11 Rhode Island EDs and found that many patients did not receive the American Academy of Pediatrics recommended tests and prophylaxis. In addition, they noted that boys received fewer tests than girls and that testing and prophylaxis varied by the type of ED. More specifically, of the adolescent female sexual assault patients evaluated in the ED within 72 hours, only 12.3% were offered the full set of tests and prophylaxis, and none of the boys received all of the possible applicable tests and prophylaxis. Of note, adolescent females were more likely to be offered testing for pregnancy, *Neisseria gonorrhea* (GC), and *Chlamydia trachomatis* (CT), and were less likely to receive syphilis testing, emergency contraception, and prophylaxis for GC and chlamydia. Additionally, more tests and prophylaxis were offered to adolescents at the women's health care specialty hospital and the children's hospital compared with the 9 general hospitals included in the study.[7]

Similarly, Rovi and Shimoni[8] analyzed data from the National Hospital Ambulatory Medical Care Survey (NHAMCS) for 1994 to 1999 and found that none of the identified cases of sexual assault were provided the full regimen of antibiotics for sexually transmitted infection (STI) recommended by the Centers for Disease Control and Prevention (CDC). Similarly, through analysis of 2003 NHAMCS data, Straight and Heaton[9] found that only 7% of ED visits for a sexual offense resulted in appropriate antibiotic prophylaxis.

Given the complexities of caring for pediatric sexual assault survivors, one option that may provide consistency in quality and improve the examination and management of these patients is a sexual assault response team. These teams usually include specially trained nurse examiners as well as specific protocols, and their existence has been demonstrated to shorten time to evaluation, increase consistency of STI and pregnancy testing and prophylaxis, and increase the rate of forensic evidence collection.[10-12] In a qualitative study of 2 sexual assault nurse examiner programs, adolescents reported that the nurses were sensitive to both their physical and emotional needs and that the nurses were compassionate and caring.[13]

However, because the development and maintenance of these programs are labor-intensive and because such programs continue to be rare, especially in pediatric EDs, it is imperative for physicians who will be caring for these patients to have the necessary skills to provide comprehensive, consistent, high-quality care. In locations where a dedicated program does not exist, a standardized order set may assist with adherence to recommended treatment. Britton et al[14] found that adherence with CDC guidelines increased from 4.4% to 82.4% after implementation of an order set specific for survivors of sexual assault.

TRIAGE AND PRESENTATION

Many patients who have experienced a sexual assault present with a clear chief complaint outlining the event. However, the EM physician should consider the potential for sexual assault in patients with injuries that do not match the provided history; physical injuries resulting from peer (and possible dating) violence; psychiatric emergencies that may have been triggered by such a trauma event; and intoxicated patients for whom there is no clear history of preceding events.

Patients with a history concerning for sexual assault should be triaged according to the Emergency Severity Index (ESI) as a level 2. In patients who have been acutely sexually assaulted, it is crucial to identify injuries and to collect forensic evidence as soon as possible after the event; therefore, these patients should be prioritized and cared for immediately. Patients should be triaged as an ESI level 2 if they report any of the following: acute assault (within 72 hours); evidence of trauma; or complaints of abdominal pain, vaginal bleeding, dysuria, or rectal pain. Patients with altered mental status or evidence of significant injury with concerning vital signs should be triaged as ESI level 1. Acute psychiatric disturbances may also be present and should prompt rapid evaluation. Such patients should be placed in a treatment room as soon as possible and instructed to remain clothed and not to eat, drink, or urinate, if possible.

EMERGENCY DEPARTMENT EVALUATION

Whenever possible, a team approach should be used for the assessment and treatment of these patients, which will limit the number of times a history is given and the number of times a patient is examined. Patients who are clinically unstable or have significant injuries should be treated as all other trauma patients, but an attempt to preserve clothing and other potential evidence is imperative. For patients who are stable, the evaluation can begin with history taking, ideally with all relevant team members (physician, nurse, sexual assault examiner [if available], social worker [if available]) present.

HISTORY

A comprehensive, detailed history is not be needed for most patients. The goals of the history are to determine the minimal facts around the sexual contact to guide evaluation and treatment decisions and to assist with interpreting physical examination findings. Optimally, an interview by a trained forensic interviewer, a police detective, or child protective services caseworker will follow the initial medical evaluation. Information regarding the timing of the assault; the circumstances of the assault (ie, known perpetrator, age of perpetrator, and whether assault was in the context of a dating relationship vs. unknown assailant); type of sexual contact; location of the incident; whether there is reason for concern for drug-facilitated sexual assault; and symptoms of traumatic injury are considered "minimal facts" to gather in the history. For sexually active teens, it is important to determine the last consensual sexual contact if forensic evidence will be collected; otherwise, an unsuspecting consenting partner's DNA identification may cause difficulties in the investigation. Therefore, it is often unnecessary to obtain additional, specific details about the event in the ED setting. Because forensic interviewing requires specific training and is beyond the scope of skills of most professionals, avoiding in-depth interviewing can minimize the potential for inconsistent or confusing information.

The adolescent patient should be interviewed alone, unless the patient objects to the parent leaving the room. In the context of a perpetrator who may have been romantically involved with the patient, assessment of other intimate partner violence (physical, emotional, and prior sexual) experiences is important to determine timing of follow-up care.

Key features to the adolescent interview include using open-ended questions, developmentally appropriate language, and the patient's own words for genital anatomy. When making a determination about forensic evidence collection, the physician should remember that the details of the event can become more specific over time. For this reason, selective forensic evidence collection is not recommended; if forensic evidence collection is indicated, the entire evidence kit should be completed (see Forensic Evidence Collection section).

Documentation of the history should include a thorough description of the event as told by the patient, including specific questions asked and verbatim answers from the patient's disclosure. The physician should document who was present for the interview in the medical record.

PHYSICAL EXAMINATION

The adolescent patient should provide consent for both the physical examination and the collection of evidence. The primary goal of the physical examination is to document injuries that may have been sustained during the assault. The physician should be careful to ensure that the physical examination is performed in a manner that does not increase the patient's psychological trauma. This can include allowing the presence of support people for the patient and providing pain control or possibly sedation or anxiolysis. Regardless of the gender of the patient or physician, all examinations should be performed in the presence of a chaperone, who is a trained member of the medical staff, who can assist in examination procedures, and serves as an unbiased witness to the examination.[15] The genital examination occurs as part of a full general physical examination looking for other physical findings of trauma. The examination should include careful inspection of the penis and scrotum in males, the labia, introitus, and hymen in females, and the anus in all patients. Rarely is a speculum or bimanual examination required in adolescent patients, unless the patient has symptoms concerning for pelvic inflammatory disease, foreign body, or significant vaginal bleeding. Use of a Bluemaxx light source may assist in identifying areas of potential semen staining, which can aid in forensic evidence collection. In addition, a complete head-to-toe examination should be completed, with photo-documentation of all injuries. It may be useful to photo-document a normal genital examination as well. A colposcope or other photo-documentation system, if available, should be used to provide optimal visualization with magnification capabilities and best-quality photo-documentation. Documentation should include detailed written examination descriptions and diagrams, if appropriate.

Of note, urgent physical examination is not required for a patient more than 72 hours after sexual assault, unless the patient has ongoing symptoms such as genital pain, bleeding, or discharge, or the family is in crisis, as an examination may provide immediate therapeutic benefit under this circumstance. Otherwise, it may be preferable to refer the patient for a timely outpatient examination with a specialist in child abuse or sexual assault; optimal timing should include consideration that the patient could be pregnant.

Importantly for the EM practitioner, adolescents who have been sexually assaulted may have a normal genital examination, in part because of rapid healing of the mucosa, elasticity of the estrogenized hymen, and the fact that many assaults do not involve enough force to cause visible injury. A normal physical examination does not rule out sexual assault, and this information should be communicated to the patient and the family. However, the EM practitioner should be prepared to find evidence of injury. For example, a recent study noted that 30% of patients had an abnormal ano-genital examination[12]; 20% had injuries consistent with acute assault, but another 10% had an ano-genital examination that was concerning for acute assault but was not diagnostic per the criteria of Adams et al.[16] For the patient who has been injured, specific findings are indicative of penetrating trauma from sexual assault. For example, acute injuries, such as lacerations of the inferior aspect of the hymen or posterior fourchette, ecchymosis of the hymen, or perianal lacerations, are consistent with recent blunt force penetrating trauma to those tissues. In addition, some acute genital injuries are concerning but not diagnostic of sexual assault, such as bruising or lacerations of the vulva, penis, scrotum, perineum, or perianal area. These injuries can be caused by accidental mechanisms, but this history is usually clear and plausible at the time of presentation for medical care.

Although extensive injury is infrequent, medical or surgical treatment of associated injuries, if required, should follow standard procedure with immediate consultation by urology, gynecology, general surgery, or other consulting specialty services as indicated to manage significant trauma or uncontrolled hemorrhage. Determining the extent of trauma and the need for additional surgical intervention may require the use of sedation or completion of the examination under anesthesia for optimal outcomes. During initial medical evaluation and stabilization, all reasonable attempts should be made to preserve potential evidence (see Emergency Department Evaluation section). If possible, avoid cutting through holes found in clothing, collect clothing and other material in paper bags and leave them with the patient until chain of custody can be confirmed. Avoid cleansing particular areas of the body (ie, genital, anal) prior to obtaining important trace and/or DNA evidence for analysis. It is important to remember, however, that the management of serious coexisting injuries or other acute medical conditions takes precedence over preservation of forensic evidence. If needed, a forensic examination can be completed in the operating room while other serious injuries are being managed.

FORENSIC EVIDENCE COLLECTION

Once the decision to collect forensic evidence has been made, the evidence should be collected as soon as possible. Although the time frame in which forensic evidence can be collected varies by jurisdiction, for adolescent patients presenting within 72 hours of assault, the collection of forensic evidence has significantly high yield with a 20% to 34% range of positive evidence collection kits in pubertal survivors of acute sexual assault.[17,18] These outcomes are particularly significant, in light of current forensic laboratory procedures with DNA analyses. Before any forensic examination, patients who experienced a sexual assault should be advised to not change their clothes, bathe or shower, or eat or drink, if possible. If the patient needs to urinate before being examined, he should be handed a urine specimen cup that can be saved for possible evidence collection. The patient's clothes should be stored in a paper bag. A significant amount of trace forensic evidence can been retrieved from objects such as linens and clothing.

Alcohol or other drugs play an important role in many sexual assaults, whether they were voluntarily ingested by the person who was assaulted, were surreptitiously given by the assailant, or were ingested under force or coercion. Adolescents often report using alcohol or drugs immediately before a sexual assault. Increasing rates of drug-facilitated sexual assault have been associated with the availability of alcohol and benzodiazepines. Although "date rape" drugs (ie, flunitrazepam [Rohypnol], Y-hydroxybutyrate [GHB], ketamine) have received much attention, they are rarely identified as the offending agent. In fact, the most common substance associated with sexual assault is alcohol. If there is any suspicion of drug-facilitated assault, drug testing should be considered. Drug testing should be performed if a patient demonstrates clinical signs of intoxication, reports drug-facilitated assault, or cannot recall details of the assault. Patients should be reminded that even if drug use was voluntary, it is important to provide a history of intoxication preceding assault. Discussion with the toxicology laboratory at each institution is recommended because date rape drugs and many other drugs of abuse are not included in standard drug screening panels.

DIAGNOSTIC TESTING

Pregnancy testing should be performed in all pubertal females. Most experts recommend that pubertal survivors of sexual assault undergo STI testing because of the high prevalence of preexisting asymptomatic infection in this group. Therefore, although identification of an STI may represent an infection acquired before the assault, "shield" laws in all 50 states strictly limit the evidentiary use of a survivor's previous sexual history, including evidence of previously acquired STIs, as part of an effort to undermine the credibility of the survivor's testimony. Additionally, STI tests have been found to be positive as a result of an assault when obtained within 72 hours of the assault. Testing for STIs should occur before beginning any treatment that could interfere with the diagnosis. Furthermore, if a patient is thought to have a specific STI, she should also be tested for other common STIs. Because of the legal and psychosocial consequences of a false-positive diagnosis, only tests with high specificities should be used.

For adolescent patients, determination of which sites to sample should be based on areas of possible contact with the assailant's bodily fluids and can include vaginal, urethral, ano-rectal, throat, and blood. Because the history of the assault provided or recalled may change with time, the physician should consider testing for STIs from multiple sources. If possible, STI testing before prophylactic treatment (described below) is recommended. Nucleic acid amplification tests (NAATs) for GC and CT are the preferred diagnostic tests for adolescent survivors of sexual assault, regardless of the sites evaluated (genital and extragenital). Testing for *Trichomonas vaginalis* (TV) should be performed by rapid antigen testing or NAAT (preferred) or by culture or wet mount of a vaginal swab specimen. The wet mount can also be used to evaluate for bacterial vaginosis and candidiasis if vaginal discharge, malodor, or itching is evident; however, these infections are not generally the result of the acute assault. Syphilis testing should be performed using the rapid plasma reagin (RPR) test, and hepatitis B testing should be performed if the patient has not been fully immunized against this infection. Testing for HIV should be performed after the patient is appropriately counseled and is informed that the test result will only provide evidence of infection acquired 6 months before testing, although the new fourth-generation HIV immunoassays can detect more acute HIV-1 infection with a window of 3 months.

THERAPEUTIC INTERVENTIONS

All pubertal patients should be offered STI prophylaxis because of the poor follow-up rates in this patient population. Empiric antibiotics should be provided for treatment of GC, CT, and TV. Patients who have not been previously vaccinated against hepatitis B should receive the hepatitis B vaccination. If the alleged perpetrator is known to be positive for hepatitis B, then hepatitis B immunoglobulin should be added.[19]

HUMAN IMMUNODEFICIENCY VIRUS PROPHYLAXIS

Human immunodeficiency virus prophylaxis is not universally recommended because the frequency of HIV seroconversion in people whose only risk factor is sexual assault probably is low. Several factors affect the medical recommendation for HIV postexposure prophylaxis (PEP). These include the likelihood of the assailant having HIV; any exposure characteristics that might increase the risk for HIV transmission based on type of sexual contact (ie, single episode vs. multiple/chronic episodes); the time elapsed after the event; and the potential benefits and risks associated with PEP. Often, an assailant's HIV status at the time of the assault examination is unknown. Therefore, it is important to consider any known HIV risk behaviors of the perpetrator, local epidemiology of HIV/AIDS, and exposure characteristics of the assault. With regard to exposure characteristics, it is important to determine whether vaginal or anal penetration occurred, whether ejaculation occurred on mucous membranes, whether multiple assailants were involved, and whether mucosal lesions are present in the assailant or patient.

The rationale for HIV PEP is the window during which the viral load can be controlled by the immune system. The addition of antiretroviral medications during this window may end viral replication. Although a definitive statement of benefit cannot be made regarding PEP after sexual assault, the possibility of HIV exposure from the assault should be assessed at the time of the post-assault examination. If PEP is offered to a patient, it is important to discuss the relative risks and benefits of antiretroviral medications, the importance of close follow-up, and the need for strict adherence to the recommended dosing so that the patient and caregiver can make an informed decision about whether to start prophylaxis. Postexposure prophylaxis is most effective the sooner after exposure it is initiated, up to 72 hours after the assault. Physicians should emphasize that PEP is usually well tolerated, and serious adverse effects are rare. If initiating PEP, specialist consultation is recommended regarding treatment. No large studies examining different treatment regimens in survivors of sexual assault have been performed, but based on current occupational exposure guidelines, 2 nucleoside reverse transcriptase inhibitors and 1 of either a nonnucleoside reverse transcriptase inhibitor or a protease inhibitor for 28 days are typically recommended. Because these medications may not be readily available at some pharmacies, patients in whom PEP is initiated should be offered a 3- to 5-day supply of PEP, and a follow-up should be initiated (telephone or office visit) for several days after the initial visit to allow for additional counseling, to assess tolerance of medications, and to ensure that the patient has filled the prescription. Additionally, if PEP is started, depending upon the medications prescribed, a complete blood cell count and serum chemistry (including liver transaminases) should be performed for baseline levels as well as an HIV antibody test. Follow-up monitoring of these tests should be performed at approximately the midpoint (2 weeks) of therapy, at the peak of potential side effects.

PREGNANCY PROPHYLAXIS

Pregnancy prevention and emergency contraception should be addressed with every pubertal female patient and should include risks of prophylaxis failure and options for pregnancy management. Pubertal females should be offered emergency contraception within 120 hours of assault if they have been vaginally penetrated or had genital contact with ejaculate. Progestin-only emergency contraceptive pills are most favorable in terms of safety, adverse effects, and efficacy. A total of 1.5 mg of levonorgestrel can be taken at once, with or without ondansetron, to mitigate nausea and or vomiting as a possible side effect. Emergency contraception has been cited to be up to 90% effective in pregnancy prevention, with greater efficacy the sooner after unprotected sexual intercourse it is taken. No studies to date show untoward effects on a fetus should pregnancy occur despite emergency contraception, as emergency contraception has been found to be non-teratogenic and will not disrupt an already implanted pregnancy. Repeat pregnancy testing is recommended at 2 weeks, given the possibility of an initial, rare false-negative test.

REPORTING

Physicians and other health care professionals are mandated reporters under US law and, therefore, are required to report suspected as well as known cases of child abuse to the child protective services agency. Most adolescent sexual assaults are perpetrated by an acquaintance or relative of the adolescent. Depending on the patient's age, the identity of the alleged perpetrator, and state law, the assault may have to be reported. Statutory rape, defined as consensual sexual intercourse between an older person and a person younger than the state-mandated age of consent, continues to be a controversial issue. In these cases, the assault may have to be reported to the child protective services agency or law enforcement agency, even if the adolescent does not want it to be reported. Lastly, if injuries occur because of co-occurring intimate partner violence, physicians must be sensitive to this association and appropriate safety planning is warranted.

DISCHARGE AND FOLLOW-UP

In most cases, the sexual assault survivor may be discharged from the ED in the care of relatives. On occasion, hospitalization is necessary for significant injuries requiring urgent management or continued observation; exacerbation of preexisting or new medical conditions; or suicidal, homicidal, or psychotic reactions. If the patient is deemed medically stable for discharge and has a safe place to go once leaving the ED, follow-up care should be arranged before final discharge with appropriate referrals provided in written form.

Survivors of sexual assault should be discharged from the ED with a specific plan of care that includes adequate follow-up with their primary care physician, child abuse specialist, child advocacy center, and psychological/mental health services. Patients should be counseled to follow up with their primary care physician or child abuse specialist within 2 weeks to assess injury healing and/or as a follow-up for HIV PEP surveillance, and sooner if symptoms occur. Survivors of sexual assault are at risk for short- and long-term psychological disturbances, such as post-traumatic stress disorder, depression, and suicidality. Law enforcement contact information should be provided so that the patient can determine the status of a report or make an initial report if previously declined by the patient.

Because infectious agents acquired through assault may not produce sufficient concentrations of organisms to be detected during initial testing, evaluation for STIs can be repeated within 1 to 2 weeks of the assault, unless prophylaxis antibiotic treatment was provided. Serologic tests for syphilis can be repeated 6 weeks, 3 months, and 6 months after the assault if initial test results were negative and infection in the assailant cannot be ruled out. Completion of the hepatitis B vaccine series can also be conducted at follow-up 1 to 2 months and 4 to 6 months after the first dose, if the patient was not previously vaccinated and had received the first dose during the initial evaluation. If initial HIV testing was negative and a third-generation test was performed, repeat testing should occur at 6 weeks, 3 months, and 6 months. If a fourth-generation test was performed, repeat testing should occur at 4 weeks and 12 weeks. Finally, if HIV PEP was initiated, follow-up to monitor side effects and adherence to regimen is recommended, as described in the section Human Immunodeficiency Virus Prophylaxis.

CONCLUSION

Care of adolescent sexual assault survivors is a complex process that requires a competent, knowledgeable multidisciplinary team that is able to interface effectively with law enforcement, child protective services, and other community resources. Successful emergency department management of the acute sexual assault patient requires effective protocols and electronic order sets in place to assist the evaluating physicians. Additionally, educational programs are necessary to ensure physician competence with these rare events. A continuous quality improvement program should be put in place so that data can inform the team on further improving care provided to these adolescents.

References

1. Rand MR. Criminal victimization, 2007. Washington, DC: Bureau of Justice Statistics Bulletin; 2008. Available at: bjs.ojp.usdoj.gov/content/pub/pdf/cv07.pdf. Accessed November 10, 2015
2. Centers for Disease Control and Prevention. Youth Risk Behavior Surveillance–United States, 2009. *MMWR Surveill Summ*. 2010;59(No. SS-5):6-7
3. Finkelhor D, Shattuck A, Turner HA, Hamby SL. The lifetime prevalence of child sexual abuse and sexual assault assessed in late adolescence. *J Adolesc Health*. 2014;55:329-333
4. Saltzman LE, Basile KC, Mahnedra RR, et al. National estimates of sexual violence treated in emergency departments. *Ann Emerg Med*. 2007;49:210-217
5. Centers for Disease Control and Prevention. Physical dating violence among high school students–United States, 2003. *MMWR*. 2006;55:532-535
6. Luo F, Stone DM, Tharp AT. Physical dating violence victimization among sexual minority youth. *Am J Public Health*. 2014;104:e66–e73
7. Merchant RC, Kelly ET, Mayer KH, et al. Compliance in Rhode Island emergency departments with American Academy of Pediatrics recommendations for adolescent sexual assaults. *Pediatrics*. 2008;121:e1660-e1667
8. Rovi S, Shimoni N. Prophylaxis provided to sexual assault victims seen at US emergency departments. *J Am Med Womens Assoc*. 2002;57:204-207
9. Straight JD, Heaton PC. Emergency department care for victims of sexual offense. *Am J Health Syst Pharm*. 2007;64:1845-1850
10. Bechtel K. Ryan E, Gallagher D. Impact of sexual assault nurse examiners on the evaluation of sexual assault in a pediatric emergency department. *Pediatr Emerg Care*. 2008;24:442-447
11. Sampel K, Szobota L, Joyce D, et al. The impact of a sexual assault/domestic violence program on ED care. *J Emerg Nurs*. 2009;35:282-289
12. Goyal MK, Mollen CJ, Hayes KL, et al. Enhancing the emergency department approach to pediatric sexual assault care: implementation of a pediatric sexual assault response team program. *Pediatr Emerg Care*. 2013;29:969-973
13. Campbell R, Greeson MR, Fehler-Cabral G. With care and compassion: adolescent sexual assault victims; experiences in sexual assault nurse examiner programs. *J Forensic Nurs*. 2013;9:68-75
14. Britton DJ, Bloch RB, Strout TD, et al. Impact of a computerized order set on adherence to Centers for Disease Control guidelines for the treatment of victims of sexual assault. *J Emerg Med*. 2013;44:528-535
15. American Academy of Pediatrics Committee on Practice and Ambulatory Medicine. Use of chaperones during the physical examination of the pediatric patient. *Pediatrics*. 2011;127:991-993
16. Adams JA, Kaplan RA, Starling SP, et al. Guidelines for medical care of children who may have been sexually abused. *J Pediatr Adolesc Gynecol*. 2007;20:163-172
17. Thackeray JD, Hornor G, Benzinger EA, et al. Forensic evidence collection and DNA identification in acute child sexual assault. *Pediatrics*. 2011;128:227-232
18. Girardet R, Bolton K, Lahoti S, et al. Collection of forensic evidence from pediatric victims of sexual assault. *Pediatrics*. 2011;128:233-238
19. American Academy of Pediatrics. Hepatitis B. In: Kimberlin DW, Brady MT, Jackson MA, Long SS, eds. *Red Book: 2015 Report of the Committee on Infectious Diseases*. 30th ed. Elk Grove Village, IL: American Academy of Pediatrics;2015:413

Adolesc Med 026 (2015) 658–674

Update on Meningitis in Adolescents and Young Adults

Stephen Thacker MD, FAAP[a];
Caroline Cruce, PharmD Candidate[b];
John D. Rowlett, MD, FAAP, FACP[c]*

[a]*Assistant Professor of Pediatrics, Mercer School of Medicine, Children's Hospital at Memorial Health University Medical Center, Savannah, Georgia;* [b]*2016 Doctoral Candidate, University of Georgia College of Pharmacy, Athens, Georgia;* [c]*Director, Pediatric Emergency Medicine, Georgia Emergency Associates, Savannah, Georgia; Professor of Pediatrics, Medical College of Georgia at Georgia Regents University, Augusta, Georgia*

If, in a fever, the neck be turned awry on a sudden, so that the sick can hardly swallow, and yet no tumour appear, it is mortal (fatal).
Aphorisms of Hippocrates ~400 BC

More than 350 years have passed since the English neuroanatomist Thomas Willis described patients with "inflammation of the meninges with a continual fever" (1661) during what is now recognized as an outbreak of meningitis. In the early 1800s, Eliza North first detailed an epidemic of meningococcal meningitis in Massachusetts, the fatal course of which had been recognized nearly 2.5 millennia earlier by Hippocrates. Premorbid cerebrospinal fluid (CSF) analysis was made possible by Quincke's introduction of the lumbar puncture in 1891. Despite improved diagnostics and evolving understanding of the epidemic nature of the disease, no significant change in the management of bacterial meningitis occurred until the introduction of serum therapy for meningococcal meningitis by the German physician Joachmann and the American medical icon Simon Flexner. Vaccines and antimicrobial therapy in the form of sulfonamides (Francois Schwentker) and penicillin (Chester Keefer) began in the 20th century.[1-3] A century later, vaccines remain the mainstay of prevention and antibiotics the cornerstone of therapy.

Discussion of the diagnosis and clinical management of bacterial meningitis is beyond the scope of this review. The details of diagnosing meningitis (bacterial

---

*Corresponding author
E-mail address: drrowlett@gmail.com

and viral), including performing and interpreting the lumbar puncture, have been extensively reviewed by Straus et al[4] and Attia et al.[5] Clinical management of bacterial meningitis is a dynamic and fluid process, and practitioners should consult the most recent resources for current recommendations, including empiric drug coverage and other potentially beneficial therapies.[6-9] This review will discuss the effect of vaccinations on bacterial meningitis, new vaccine recommendations, and an overview of aseptic (viral) meningitis.

Antibiotics and the evolution of critical care medicine have served to greatly lower case mortality for bacterial meningitis compared to earlier years; however, recent data suggest that although the incidence of meningitis is decreasing, the "modern era" mortality has not substantially changed. In a recent 10-year period (1998-2007), there was a 31% decrease in the incidence of bacterial meningitis, but the case fatality rate was essentially the same (15.7% in 1998, 14.3% in 2007).[10] Future advances in treatment may further decrease the mortality and morbidity, but it is clear that the major instrument for decreasing the burden of bacterial meningitis is the continued development and implantation of effective vaccines.

Before the introduction of the vaccine in 1986, *Haemophilus influenza B* (HIB) was the leading cause of bacterial meningitis in children. The initial HIB vaccine was given to children aged 2 years and older, but because it used a traditional polysaccharide antigen, it was ineffective in infants and younger children. The original vaccine was subsequently replaced by the conjugated HIB vaccine (polysaccharide antigen conjugated to a protein moiety), which allowed for immunization of infants beginning at age 2 months. The conjugated HIB vaccine has been one of the true successes in preventive medicine. Before the introduction and widespread use of the conjugate HIB vaccine, the incidence of bacterial meningitis secondary to HIB in the United States was 54 cases per 100,000 children (age birth to 5 years). In less than a decade, the case rate (1995) had dropped to less than 1 case per 100,000 population.[11] All forms of invasive HIB disease (meningitis, pneumonia, osteomyelitis, and epiglottitis) have all but been eliminated in fully immunized children.[12] In 1986, the median age for meningitis in the United States was 15 months; by 1995 the median age had increased to 25 years of age. Consequently, although physicians fear the diagnosis of bacterial meningitis in infants and children, the disease is most likely diagnosed in the adolescent and adult populations.

Streptococcus pneumoniae remains the leading cause of bacterial meningitis in the United States.[13] Similar to the success with HIB, there has been a marked reduction in the incidence of invasive pneumococcal disease (including meningitis) since the introduction of the heptavalent protein-polysaccharide pneumococcal conjugate vaccine (PCV7) in 2000. The PCV7 vaccine contained the serotypes most associated with invasive pneumococcal disease in 2000 (4, 6B, 9V, 14, 18C, 19F, and 23F). Invasive pneumococcal disease declined 75% in children younger than 5 years, including a 99% reduction in PCV7 serotypes. Furthermore, in adults

65 years and older, there was a 92% reduction in PCV7 serotypes, and invasive disease from all serotypes decreased by 37%.[14-16] Between 2001 and 2004, PCV7 is estimated to have prevented an estimated 3330 cases (and nearly 400 deaths) of pneumococcal meningitis.[17] Unfortunately, children and adults who get pneumococcal meningitis, regardless of serotype, do poorly; 1 in 7 die, and two-thirds of the survivors are left with significant neurologic deficits.[18] Since the widespread use of PCV7, there has been a shift in serotypes causing invasive disease. Serotype 19A has emerged as the most common cause of invasive pneumococcal disease in persons previously immunized with PCV7. In 2010, the United States licensed the 13-valent pneumococcal vaccine (PCV13), which includes the addition of serotype 19A as well as 1, 3, 5, 6A, and 7F to the serotypes in PCV7.[19] Although to date there are insufficient data to report on the effect on these new serotypes in the US population, when the PCV13 vaccine was introduced in France, the number of cases of pneumococcal meningitis decreased by 27% (2009-2013), including a 66% reduction in cases caused by the additional 6 serotypes contained in PCV13.[20] Currently there is no routine recommendation for the administration of PCV13 or PCV23 to otherwise healthy unimmunized adolescents. However, routine immunization is recommended for adolescents with high-risk conditions (Table 1).[21] Despite this longstanding recommendation, recent data (2015) suggest that adherence with providing pneumococcal immunization in some populations is highly inadequate.[22]

Neisseria meningitidis is the second leading cause of bacterial meningitis in adolescents and young adults and is associated with significant mortality (10%) and morbidity. A discussion of the clinical presentation, treatment, and management of invasive meningococcal disease is beyond the scope of this review, but several points are worth mentioning. First, meningococcal disease may be very difficult to diagnose in the early stages because the presenting symptoms are frequently nonspecific (fever, decreased appetite, irritability), resembling a common viral illness.

Table 1
High-risk conditions in infants, children, and adolescents for which routine pneumococcal immunization is recommended

Cerebrospinal leaks	Cochlear implants
Sickle cell anemia and other hemoglobinopathies	Functional or anatomic asplenia
Congenital or acquired immune deficiencies	Human immunodeficiency virus/acquired immune deficiency syndrome
Chronic renal failure	Nephrotic syndrome
Malignant neoplasms	Leukemias
Hodgkin disease	Lymphomas
Solid organ transplants	Multiple myeloma
Chronic heart disease (especially cyanotic)	Chronic lung disease
Diabetes mellitus	Chronic liver failure
Other diseases treated with immune suppressive drugs (eg, lupus)	Chronic steroid use

Second, disease progression can be very rapid, with death occurring within 24 hours of the onset of the often vague symptoms. In a study of more than 400 children who were 16 years or younger with meningococcal disease, most had non-specific symptoms in the first 8 hours, but many were near death within 24 hours. Median time for hospitalization was 19 hours after symptom onset; more classic symptoms including hemorrhagic rash and meningismus occurred between 13 and 22 hours after symptom onset. In this group, the fatality rate was nearly 25% (103/448 cases).[23,24] Persons 15 to 24 years of age account for more than 1 in 5 of all deaths from meningococcal disease and experienced substantially more deaths than individuals of any other decade of age. Five serotypes (A, B, C, Y, and W135) are responsible for invasive meningococcal disease (Table 2.).[25,26]

Opportunities for improving the early diagnosis and more effective clinical treatment are limited, so it is incumbent on practitioners to maximize prevention of invasive meningococcal disease through immunization. Epidemic meningococcal disease has been recognized in military recruits living in barracks and in college communities. In addition to crowded living conditions (dorms, barracks), other identified risk factors for meningococcal disease include alcohol use, respiratory infections, and smoking. Targeted immunization campaigns have reduced the overall number of cases of meningitis; nearly 70% of new college students have received at least 1 meningococcal immunization.[27] Although the number of total invasive meningococcal disease cases has decreased, the incidence of group B meningococcal disease has increased. Between 1997 and 1999, there were 780 cases of meningococcal disease among 11- to 24-year-olds. Group B meningococcal disease was the cause of 18% of those cases. However, although there were only 106 cases between 2010 and 2012, the percentage of cases attributed to group B increased to 27%.[28] Disease caused by covered serogroups decreased somewhat, but it is not as simple as was seen with the implementation of the PCV7 vaccine. Other factors are thought to be involved in the continued changing epidemiology of epidemic meningococcal disease.[29]

Table 2
Clinically significant *Neisseria meningitidis* serogroups

Serogroup	Clinical manifestations/epidemiology
A	Rare in the United States; common in sub-Saharan Africa but thought to be able to easily migrate to other areas
B	Predominant cause of invasive *Neisseria meningitidis* disease in infants in United States and recent college outbreaks; new vaccine licensed in 2014
C	Major cause of endemic (non-epidemic) disease in the United States; incidence of disease caused by group C decreased in Europe after widespread use of vaccine
Y	Affects all age groups; more common in persons 65 years of age or older; more likely to cause pneumonia
W135	Rare in the United States but has been associated with outbreaks

Three types of meningococcal vaccinations are available in the United States: meningococcal conjugate, meningococcal polysaccharide, and serogroup B meningococcal vaccines. The conjugate and polysaccharide vaccinations protect against serotypes A, C, W, and Y (with the exception of MenHibrix, which protects against serotypes C and Y and HIB). The serogroup B meningococcal (MenB) vaccines (Trumenba and Bexsero) are the most recently licensed vaccinations against meningococcal infections and are highly effective in the short- and near-term prevention of serogroup B disease. Presently the MenB vaccines are only licensed for persons aged 10 to 25 years. Recommendations for the use of meningococcal vaccines have been extensively debated and continue to evolve. Currently, there is no consensus recommendation for the immunization of healthy children younger than 10 years with any of the available meningococcal vaccines. However, children 2 months and older with high-risk conditions should receive 1 of the available conjugate vaccines (Table 3).[30] *Routine use of the quadrivalent meningococcal vaccine is recommended for all adolescents. The initial dose should be given between 11 and 12 years of age, with a booster dose given at age 16 years.* Adolescents who receive their initial dose at or after age 16 years do not require a booster dose.[31] At the time of the release of these recommendations from the American Academy of Pediatrics, no vaccines licensed in the United States included serogroup B. However, now, in addition to the quadrivalent meningococcal vaccinations, in February 2015 the Advisory Committee on Immunization Practices (ACIP) recommended use of MenB vaccines in persons aged 10 years or older at increased risk for serogroup B meningococcal disease (Table 3), *excluding persons traveling to endemic areas* (usually not serogroup B). Interim recommendations from the Centers for Disease Control and Prevention (CDC) suggest consideration of vaccination during outbreaks in which 2 or more cases of serogroup B *Neisseria meningitidis* are reported within a 6-month period in organizations of fewer than 5000 persons.[32] Furthermore, the current recommendations do not include children younger than 10 years, first-year college students living in dorms, military recruits, or the general adolescent population. In part, these groups have been initially excluded

Table 3
Persons at increased risk for meningococcal disease

Factors	Modifier
Persistent compliment deficiencies, including C3, C5-C9, properdin, factor D, and factor H	Military recruits in barracks
Anatomic or functional asplenia	Travel to or residence in an area with hyperendemic or epidemic disease
Medical researchers working closely with the *Neisseria meningitidis* bacterium	Unvaccinated or previously vaccinated first-year college students through age 21 years living in residence halls who received their last dose before their 16th birthday
Residence in a community with a meningococcal outbreak	Patients on certain immunosuppressant regimens, including eculizumab (Soliris)

because the vaccines were fast-tracked for use in epidemics. Further study for approval for widespread use is ongoing.[33] It is widely expected that much broader recommendations for the use of MenB vaccines will be shortly forthcoming. Given the dynamic nature of these recommendations, practitioners are referred to recognized authorities (CDC, ACIP, American Academy of Pediatrics *Red Book)* for current guidelines.[34]

Invasive meningococcal disease is highly contagious. Household and close contacts are 500 to 800 times more likely to become infected than the general population (Table 4). *Therefore, postexposure chemoprophylaxis should be initiated within 24 hours of identification of the index patient. Prophylaxis initiated more than 2 weeks after exposure is ineffective.* Multiple drugs, including rifampin, ceftriaxone, ciprofloxacin, and azithromycin are effective. Patients with invasive disease treated with drugs other than third-generation cephalosporins (ceftriaxone, cefotaxime) require chemoprophylaxis to eradicate carriage despite treatment with other systemic antibiotics (penicillin). In addition to traditional antimicrobial chemoprophylaxis, the development of the MenB vaccines led to emergency use of these vaccinations during meningococcal outbreaks at college campuses. In 2013, the US Food and Drug Administration (FDA) approved the emergency use of Bexsero (Novartis Vaccines and Diagnostics, Siena, Italy) for use during an epidemic of invasive meningococcal disease at a New Jersey University. Bexsero had previously been licensed and used in Europe and Australia and therefore was chosen over Trumenba. Use of the vaccine in students on the college campus was considered successful. There were no serogroup B meningococcal disease cases in any person who received 1 or more doses of the MenB vaccine. The authors concluded that the vaccine might have protected vaccinated individuals from the disease, but they did note that because 1 case occurred in an unvaccinated close contact of students at the university, herd immunity might not be attained through these vaccinations.[35] Trumenba was shown to be efficacious in a similar outbreak in Rhode Island in 2015. The combination of chemoprophylaxis and vaccination (Trumenba) effectively eliminated nasopharyngeal carriage of the outbreak strain.[36]

Table 4
Persons requiring postexposure chemoprophylaxis for documented invasive *Neisseria meningitidis* disease

Exposure to oral secretions through close social contact (kissing, sharing of eating utensils, toothbrushes)
Childcare and daycare contacts within previous 7 days
Housemates who slept in the same dwelling in the previous 7 days
Airline passengers seated directly proximate to patient for flight of 8 hours or longer
Health care workers *only if* intimate direct exposure to secretions, such as through unprotected resuscitation, intubation, or suctioning *before* or less than 24 hours after initiation of appropriate antibiotics

Table 5
Major viral causes of aseptic meningitis

Most Common	Rare
• Enteroviruses	• Influenza virus
○ Coxsackieviruses	• Parainfluenza virus
○ Echoviruses	• Adenovirus
○ Other enteroviruses	• Lymphocytic choriomeningitis virus
• Arboviruses	• Herpes simplex virus type 1
○ West Nile Virus	• Human herpesvirus 6
○ St. Louis encephalitis virus	• Epstein-Barr virus
○ La Crosse encephalitis virus	• Cytomegalovirus
○ Western equine encephalitis virus	• Varicella zoster virus
○ Colorado tick fever	
Less Common	
• Herpes simplex virus type 2	
• Mumps virus	
• Human immunodeficiency virus	

ASEPTIC AND VIRAL MENINGITIS

Aseptic meningitis is a syndrome first described by Walden in 1925, with refinement in definition in 1951 that has since persisted.[37] Aseptic meningitis has been defined as meningeal inflammation and CSF pleocytosis with a bacteriologically sterile specimen. Use of the term has expanded to include numerous infectious and non-infectious conditions (Table 5).

VIRAL MENINGITIS VERSUS ENCEPHALITIS

Viral meningitis describes a central nervous system (CNS) infection defined by meningeal irritation without brain parenchymal disease, making it distinctly different from viral encephalitis, a disease marked by parenchymal infection and dysfunction. This review will discuss the most common causes of viral meningitis presenting in the adolescent. Because of the passive nature of CDC reporting and the typical self-resolution of many acute events of viral meningitis, epidemiologic data are limited for many of the diseases discussed.

Picornaviridae

The most clinically important members of the Picornaviridae family of viruses are Enteroviruses and Parechoviruses.[38] Enteroviruses cause most of the cases of Picornaviridae meningitis. It has been estimated that at least 75,000 cases of enteroviral meningitis occur annually in the United States among all age groups, but the true incidence in children is not known.[39] Most reported case series demonstrate the highest incidence in children younger than 4 years.[40,41] Some recent studies suggest that the incidence of human parechovirus may be rising in comparison to enterovirus, especially in infants.[42-44]

The *Enterovirus* family includes several species and serotypes. Enteroviruses have a global distribution with seasonality dependent on the climate of the geographic region. In the United States, incidences peak in the summer and fall.[2] When an etiology of aseptic meningitis is identified in children, it is estimated that greater than 70% of cases are caused by enteroviruses.[38,45]

Parechovirus, a genus originally believed to be an enterovirus, also is known to cause viral meningitis in children and adolescents.[46,47] Neuroinvasive infection with *Parechovirus* shares a seasonality with enteroviruses, with peaks in the summer and fall in the United States. The most common type of parechovirus that causes viral meningitis is human parechovirus type 3. Although true disease incidence is likely higher because of underreporting, up to 7% of enterovirus-negative CSF specimens have been attributed to *Parechovirus* in the setting of aseptic meningitis.[48]

Enterovirus Meningitis Diagnosis and Treatment

The diagnosis of enteroviral meningitis is often confirmed in the setting of epidemiologic suspicion. Studies of CSF typically demonstrate a broad range of CSF pleocytosis, with a median of 100 white blood cells per microliter and a lymphocyte predominant.[49] Testing for enterovirus is commercially available for reverse transcriptase polymerase chain reaction and has become the gold standard for detection, with newer assays demonstrating almost 100% sensitivity and specificity with use of CSF.[50-52]

Treatment of enteroviral and parechovirus meningitis continues to remain largely supportive. Although no FDA-approved treatments exist for enteroviral disease, there are reports of clinical success in treatment of severe neonatal enteroviral disease with intravenous immune globulin or immune serum globulin, although definitive clinical trials have not been completed.[53] The novel anti-picornaviral drug Pleconaril was found to be beneficial in accelerating resolution of headache in the setting of enteroviral meningitis but ultimately did not achieve FDA licensure.[54,55]

Arboviruses

A large number of viruses and viral families comprise the arboviruses, whose hallmark is their transmission by an arthropod vector (eg, flies, ticks, mosquitoes). There are more than 500 viruses in this group, but fewer than 10 cause neuroinvasive disease, such as meningitis, in North America. Of these, most are caused by West Nile virus (WNV) and La Crosse virus (LCV) (Table 6). Human-to-human transmission is rare and, when confirmed, is caused by transmission of infected blood products in most cases. Mosquitoes are the vectors for most clinically significant arboviruses in North America.[56] Exceptions include Colorado tick fever and Powassan viruses (transmitted by ticks).[57-60] Arbovirus disease follows the seasonality of their respective vectors, which in North America leads to increased incidences in the summer and fall.

Currently, WNV is the most common cause of arboviral infection in the United States.[61] West Nile virus was originally described in 1937 in the West Nile province in Uganda; however, it was not recognized as a significant pathogen in North America until a 1999 encephalitis epidemic in New York City.[62,63] Nearly 80% of WNV infections are believed to be asymptomatic. Less than 1% of total infections in adults and children result in CNS disease, with most of the CNS disease presentations affecting adults. In the United States, when children do have CNS infection with WNV, meningitis is the most common presentation. Pediatric cases largely present in the United States from the months of July to September. The median annual incidence is 0.07 cases per 100,000 children. The highest number of cases have occurred in the Midwest, but cases have been reported in 47 states and the District of Columbia.[64] The CDC has a dynamic map on its Web site displaying real-time incidence of West Nile Virus Neuroinvasive disease by state (www.cdc.gov/westnile/statsmaps/preliminary-mapsdata/incidencestatedate.html; accessed October 15, 2015). More recently, questions and concerns have been raised about the persistence of WNV and its role in renal disease. Murray et al[65] described finding RNA in the urine of 5 of 25 patients who had been infected by WNV 1 to 6 years earlier. However, a sec-

Table 6
Characteristics of neuroinvasive arboviral disease in US children

Virus	Geographic distribution	Arthropod vector	Annual incidence per million <18 years*
West Nile	United States, Canada, Mexico	Mosquito	0.68
La Crosse	North Central and Northeast United States	Mosquito	0.90
Eastern equine encephalitis	Upper New York, Michigan, Atlantic and Gulf Coast states, eastern Canada	Mosquito	0.04
Powassan	North Central and Northeast United States	Tick	0.01
St. Louis encephalitis	United States, Canada, Mexico	Mosquito	0.01
Colorado tick fever virus	Rocky Mountain range states, Canada	Tick	<0.01

*From Gaensbauer JT, Lindsey NP, Messacar K, Staples J E, Fischer M. Neuroinvasive arboviral disease in the United States: 2003 to 2012. *Pediatrics.* 2014;134:e642-e650.

ond study found no evidence of WNV RNA in urine samples obtained 6 years after acute WNV infection.[66] Further study of WNV persistence is required to fully understand the health effect this may have on adolescents and adults.

La Crosse Virus

La Crosse virus (LCV) is the most common cause of neuroinvasive arboviral disease of childhood reported in North America, causing 55% of cases in those younger than 18 years.[67] Over the period from 2003 to 2012, 88% of LCV cases reported to ArboNET, the national arboviral surveillance system, occurred in those younger than 18 years.

Although 21 states reported LCV neuroinvasive disease during this same period, 4 (Ohio, West Virginia, North Carolina, and Tennessee, in decreasing order of incidence) accounted for 81% of the reported cases. The estimated average annual incidence is 91.65 cases per million children. Similar to other arboviral infections, LCV demonstrates a seasonal trend, with most cases occurring from July to September.[67,68] Although most (78%) of the reported neuroinvasive LCV infections presented as encephalitis, 20% of presentations were described as meningitis alone.

Arboviral Meningitis Diagnosis and Treatment

The diagnosis of neuroinvasive arboviral disease is most often confirmed by the presence of immunoglobulin M (IgM) antibody production in the CSF or serum. Detection of CSF IgM is the preferred diagnostic method because some arboviruses, such as WNV, can have long-lasting serum IgM response ranging from months to years in the serum.[69] Production of WNV IgM can be detected within 3 to 5 days of illness, whereas detection of Colorado tick fever encephalitis virus by serology often does not occur until after 10 days of illness.[70] A nucleic acid amplification test (NAAT) is commercially available for WNV; NAATs for other arboviruses have been developed for research purposes but may not be readily available.[71]

Although most arboviral meningitis cases will be admitted to exclude bacterial etiologies, the treatment of arboviral meningitis is largely supportive, focusing on intravenous fluid therapy, antipyretics, and analgesics. No FDA-licensed specific therapies for neuroinvasive arboviral disease are available at this time.

Paramyxoviruses

Clinically relevant members of the Paramyxoviridae family that can cause CNS infection include mumps, measles, and the parainfluenza viruses. In the prevaccination era, mumps was a major cause of aseptic meningitis in the United States, causing up to 15% of all aseptic meningitis cases.[72,73] Although cases of mumps meningitis have declined in the postvaccination era, the most recent US outbreaks included cases of meningitis.[74-76]

Parainfluenza viruses can cause aseptic meningitis.[77] The dominant serotype identified has been parainfluenza type 3. Although measles is known to cause encephalitis, measles infection can be also be associated with CSF pleocytosis, usually without signs or symptoms of meningitis.[78]

Diagnosis and Treatment

Diagnosis for these paramyxoviruses can be confirmed through CSF viral culture, CSF serology, or more commonly NAAT.[79-81] As with many causes of aseptic meningitis, treatment is largely supportive. For mumps and measles, the risk of disease can be greatly reduced with routine vaccinations.

Herpesviruses

Nearly every member of the human herpesviruses family, including Epstein-Barr virus, *Cytomegalovirus*, and human herpesviruses 6 and 7, have been associated with aseptic meningitis in children.[82-85] However, the most clinically recognized and frequently seen herpes viruses that cause aseptic meningitis are varicella zoster virus (VZV) and herpes simplex virus type 2 (HSV-2). Varicella zoster virus meningitis has been reported in immune-competent children and young adults with and without skin lesions.[86-92] Herpes simplex virus type 2 and less often HSV-1 have been detected in the CSF individuals of all ages presenting with aseptic meningitis.[93-97]

Diagnosis and Treatment

Unlike the case for HSV encephalitis, the efficacy of acyclovir in the treatment of HSV meningitis has not been proven, although numerous reports and case series describe accelerated resolution of symptoms.[97] Treatment of children aged 3 months to 11 years often ranges from 30 to 45 mg/kg/day divided every 8 hours for 21 days. For adolescents 12 years or older, the dose is 30 mg/kg/day divided every 8 hours for 21 days.

Mollaret Meningitis

Mollaret[98,99] first described recurrent aseptic meningitis in 1944, providing a description of 3 patients he cared for over a period of 15 years. The disease is characterized by symptomatic periods of several days with interval asymptomatic periods ranging from weeks to months. Individuals suffering from Mollaret meningitis complain of fever, headache, and vomiting during symptomatic periods. Sampling of the CSF during symptomatic periods reveals pleocytosis with lymphocyte predominance and "fantomes cellulaires" or ghost cells, which are large monocyte/macrophage lineage cells, called Mollaret cells.[100] Invariably, symptomatic periods spontaneously resolve without specific directed therapy.

Most published cases of Mollaret meningitis reported the detection of HSV-2 or HSV-1, either by culture or nucleic acid amplification.[94,101-107] Less commonly reported pathogens causing Mollaret presentations include toxoplasmosis and human herpesvirus 6, and less common non-infectious etiologies include lupus, abnormal CNS anatomy, and extramedullary spinal teratoma.[108-112]

Arenaviruses

The most clinically relevant arenavirus causing aseptic meningitis is lymphocytic choriomeningitis virus (LCMV). Originally described in the 1930s as a pathogen of aseptic meningitis, reported cases have been on the decline for unclear reasons. The disease is acquired from rodents, pets, and animals in the wild. Lymphocytic choriomeningitis virus is considered endemic in wild mice. One study estimated that 9% of wild mice captured in Baltimore, Maryland, were infected with LCMV.[113] Congenital LCMV infection has been well described in mothers who acquire infection in pregnancy, although the true incidence is not known. Postnatal acquisition can occur at any age, including adolescence, and the seasonality of infection, with increased incidences in late autumn and early winter, is dictated by the seasonal movement of mice into houses during cold periods.[114-116]

Pathogenesis and Clinical Manifestations
Acquired LCMV infection typically begins with inhalation of aerosolized virus particles with deposition in the lung, leading to viral replication and pneumonia. After establishment of pulmonary infection, the virus spreads to reach the CNS and meninges, further replicating and resulting in inflammation and the clinical findings of meningitis. Although many infections lead to a mild febrile illness from which the patient self recovers, LCMV can cause a biphasic illness course that begins with malaise, fever, headache, and vomiting. The CNS disease often follows an interval period of perceived recovery, presenting with increased headache, fever, photophobia, and vomiting. Examination findings are consistent with meningeal inflammation.

Diagnosis and Treatment
The CSF findings are similar to those from other causes of aseptic meningitis, with a lymphocytic predominant CSF pleocytosis, which can be associated with hypoglycorrhachia and elevated CSF protein. The most common approach to diagnosis has been the detection of IgG or IgM antibodies from the blood or, more specifically, the CSF.[117] Polymerase chain reaction studies have been used in diagnosis but are not widely commercially available.[118]

Targeted antiviral therapy against LCMV and other arenaviruses currently is not commercially available, leaving supportive care the gold standard of therapy. Off-label use of ribavirin has been reported for treatment of severe cases of arenavirus infection.[119] Novel agents, such as favipiravir, an antiviral with potent activity against arenaviruses, hold promise for future therapies but have yet to be clinically tested.[120]

References

1. Tyler KL. A history of bacterial meningitis. *Handb Clin Neurology.* 2010;95:417-433
2. Quincke HI. *Die Technik der Lumbalpunktion.* Berlin & Vienna; 1902
3. Schwentker FF, Gelman S, Long PH. Landmark article April 24, 1937. The treatment of meningococcic meningitis with sulfanilamide. Preliminary report. *JAMA.* 1984;251:788-790
4. Straus SE, Thorpe KE, Holroyd-Leduc J. How do I perform a lumbar puncture and analyze the results to diagnose bacterial meningitis? *JAMA.* 2006;296:2012-2022
5. Attia J, Hata R, Cook DJ, et al. Does this adult patient have acute meningitis? *JAMA.* 1999; 282:175-181
6. Strange GR, Ahrens WR. Meningitis: Evidence to guide an evolving standard of care. *Pediatr Emerg Pract.* 2005;2:1-24
7. Sosa RG, Epstein L. Approach to central nervous system infections in the emergency department. *Clin Pediatr Emerg Med.* 2015;16:11-19
8. Sadoun T, Singh A. Adult acute bacterial meningitis in the United States: 2009 update. *Emerg Med Pract.* 2009;11:1-28
9. Tunkel AR, Hartman BJ, Kaplan SL, et al. Practice guidelines for the management of bacterial meningitis. *Clin Infect Dis.* 2004;39:1267-1284
10. Thigpen MC, Whitney CG, Messonnier NE, et al. Bacterial meningitis in the United States, 1998-2007. *N Engl J Med.* 2011;364:2016-2025
11. Petola H. Worldwide *Haemophilus influenza* type b disease at the beginning of the 21st century: global analysis of the disease burden 25 years after the use of the polysaccharide vaccine and a decade after the advent of the conjugates. *Clin Microbiol Rev.* 2000;13:302-317
12. American Academy of Pediatrics. Meningococcal infections. In: Kimberlin DW, Brady MT, Jackson MA, Long SS, eds. *Red Book: 2015 Report of the Committee on Infectious Diseases.* 30th ed. Elk Grove Village, IL: American Academy of Pediatrics; 2015:547-558
13. Castelblanco RL, Lee M, Hasbun R. Epidemiology of bacterial meningitis in the USA from 1997 to 2010: a population-based observational study. *Lancet Infect Dis.* 20014;14:813-819
14. Whitney CG, Farley MM, Hadler J, et al. Decline in invasive pneumococcal disease after the introduction of protein-polysaccharide conjugate vaccine. *N Engl J Med.* 348;2003:1737-1746
15. Direct and indirect effects of routine vaccination of children with 7-valent pneumococcal vaccine on incidence of invasive pneumococcal disease—United States, 1998-2003. *MMWR.* 2005;54:893-897
16. Haddy RI, Perry K, Chacko CE, et al. Comparison of incidence of invasive *Streptococcus pneumoniae* disease among children before and after the introduction of conjugated pneumococcal vaccine. *Pediatr Infect Dis J.* 2005;24:320-323
17. Tsai CJ, Griffin MR, Nuoriti JP, et al. Changing epidemiology of pneumococcal meningitis after the introduction of pneumococcal conjugate vaccine in the United States. *Clin Inf Dis.* 2008;46:1664-1672
18. Stockman C, Ampofo K, Byington CL, et al. Pneumococcal meningitis in children: epidemiology, serotypes, and outcomes from 1997-2010 in Utah. *Pediatrics.* 2013;132:421-428
19. Licensure of a 13-valent pneumococcal conjugate vaccine (PCV13) and recommendations for use among children—Advisory Committee on Immunization Practices (ACIP), 2010. *MMWR.* 2010;59:258-261
20. Levy C, Varon E, Picard C, et al. Trends of pneumococcal meningitis in children after introduction of the 13-valent pneumococcal conjugate vaccine in France. *Pediatr Infect Dis J.* 2014;1216-1221
21. Advisory Committee on Immunization Practice (ACIP). Recommended immunization schedule for persons aged 0 through 18 years, United States, 2015. Available at: www.cdc.gov/vaccines/schedules/hcp/imz/child-adolescent.html. Accessed September 5, 2015
22. Harris, JG, Maletta, KI, Ren B, et al. Improving pneumococcal vaccination in pediatric rheumatology patients. *Pediatrics.* 2015;136:e680-e686
23. Thompson MD, Ninis N, Perera A, et al. Clinical recognition of meningococcal disease in children and adolescents. *Lancet.* 2006;367:397-403

24. World Health Organization. Meningococcal meningitis (fact sheet no. 141). February 2015 (updated). Available at: www.who.int/mediacentre/factsheets/fs141/en. Accessed October 15, 2015

25. Granoff DM, Pelton S, Harrison LH. Meningococcal vaccines. In: Plotkin SA, Orenstein WA, Offit PA, eds. *Vaccines*. 6th ed. Philadelphia: Saunders Elsevier; 2012:388-418

26. Meyer S. Epidemiology of meningococcal disease outbreaks in the United States. Presented at Advisory Committee on Immunization Practices Meeting, Atlanta, GA, June 26, 2014

27. Turner JC. College health and infectious diseases. Presented at IDC NY 2014, New York, November 22-23, 2014

28. Centers for Disease Control and Prevention. Active bacterial core surveillance (ABCs) cases from 1993-2012. Available at: www.cdc.gov/meningococcal/surveillance/index.html. Accessed September 8, 2015

29. Wang X, Shutt KA, Vuong JT, et al. Changes in the population structure of invasive *Neisseria meningitidis* in the United States after quadrivalent meningococcal conjugate vaccine licensure. *J Infect Dis*. 2015;211:1887-1894

30. MacNeil JR, Rubin L, McNamara L, et al. Use of Men ACWY-CRM vaccine in children aged 2 through 23 months at increased risk for meningococcal disease: recommendations of the Advisory Committee on Immunization Practices (ACIP), 2013. *MMWR*. 2014;63:527-530

31. American Academy of Pediatrics Committee on Infectious Disease. Updated recommendations on the use of meningococcal vaccines. *Pediatrics*. 2014;134:400-403

32. Centers for Disease Control and Prevention. Interim guidance for control of serogroup B meningococcal disease outbreaks in organizational settings. Available at: www.cdc.gov/meningococcal/downloads/interim-guidance.pdf. Accessed September 9, 2015

33. Folaranmi T, Rubin L, Martin SW. et al. Use of serogroup B meningococcal vaccine in persons aged ≥10 years at increased risk for serogroup B meningococcal disease: recommendations of the Advisory Committee on Immunization Practices, 2015. *MMWR*. 2015;64:608-612

34. Cohn AC, MacNeil JR, Clark TA, et al. Prevention and control of meningococcal disease: recommendations of the Advisory Committee on Immunization Practices (ACIP). *MMWR*. 2013; 62:1-28

35. McNamara LA, Shumate AM, Johnsen P, et al. First use of a serogroup B meningococcal vaccine in the US in response to a university outbreak. *Pediatrics*. 2015;135:798-803

36. Soeters HM, McNamara LA, Whaley M. Serogroup B meningococcal disease outbreaks and carriage evaluation at a college: Rhode Island, 2015. *MMWR*. 2015;64:606-607

37. Wallgren A. Etiology of meningoencephalitis in children, especially the syndrome of acute aseptic meningitis. *Acta Paediatr*. 1951;40:541-565

38. Khetsuriani N, Lamonte-Fowlkes A, Oberst S, et al. Centers for Disease Control and Prevention. Enterovirus surveillance—United States, 1970-2005. *MMWR*. 2006;55:1-20

39. Sawyer MH. Enterovirus infections: diagnosis and treatment. *Semin Pediatr Infect Dis*. 2002; 13:40-47

40. Nicolosi A, Hauser WA, Beghi E, et al. Epidemiology of central nervous system infections in Olmsted County, Minnesota, 1950-1981. *J Infect Dis*. 1986;154:399-408

41. Rantakallio P, Leskinen M, von Wendt L. Incidence and prognosis of central nervous system infections in a birth cohort of 12,000 children. *Scand J Infect Dis*. 1986;18:287-294

42. Sharp J, Harrison CJ, Puckett K, et al. Characteristics of young infants in whom human parechovirus, enterovirus or neither were detected in cerebrospinal fluid during sepsis evaluations. *Pediatr Infect Dis J*. 2013;32:213-216

43. Esposito S, Rahamat-Langendoen J, Ascolese B, et al. Pediatric parechovirus infections. *J Clin Virol*. 2014;60:84-89

44. Cabrerizo M, Trallero G, Pena MJ, et al. Comparison of epidemiology and clinical characteristics of infections by human parechovirus vs. those by enterovirus during the first month of life. *Eur J Pediatr*. 2015 [Epub ahead of print]

45. Julian KG, Mullins JA, Olin A, et al. Aseptic meningitis epidemic during a West Nile virus avian epizootic. *Emerging Infect Dis*. 2003;9:1082-1088

46. Wolthers KC, Benschop KSM, Schinkel J, et al. Human parechoviruses as an important viral cause of sepsis-like illness and meningitis in young children. *Clin Infect Dis.* 2008;47:358-363

47. Felsenstein S, Yang S, Eubanks N, et al. Human parechovirus central nervous system infections in southern California children. *Pediatr Infect Dis J.* 2014;33:e87-e91

48. Selvarangan R, Nzabi M, Selvaraju SB, et al. Human parechovirus 3 causing sepsis-like illness in children from midwestern United States. *Pediatr Infect Dis J.* 2011;30:238-242

49. Rorabaugh ML, Berlin LE, Heldrich F, et al. Aseptic meningitis in infants younger than 2 years of age: acute illness and neurologic complications. *Pediatrics.* 1993;92:206-211

50. Stellrecht KA, Harding I, Hussain FM, et al. A one-step RT-PCR assay using an enzyme-linked detection system for the diagnosis of enterovirus meningitis. *J Clin Virol.* 2000;17:143-149

51. Gartzonika C, Vrioni G, Levidiotou S. Evaluation of a commercially available reverse transcription-PCR enzyme immunoassay (Enterovirus Consensus kit) for the diagnosis of enterovirus central nervous system infections. *Clin Microbiol Infect.* 2005;11:131-137

52. Kost CB, Rogers B, Oberste MS, et al. Multicenter beta trial of the GeneXpert enterovirus assay. *J Clin Microbiol.* 2007;45:1081-1086

53. Abzug MJ. Presentation, diagnosis, and management of enterovirus infections in neonates. *Paediatr Drugs.* 2004;6:1-10

54. Desmond RA, Accortt NA, Talley L, et al. Enteroviral meningitis: natural history and outcome of pleconaril therapy. *Antimicrob Agents Chemother.* 2006;50:2409-2414

55. Abzug MJ, Cloud G, Bradley J, et al. Double blind placebo-controlled trial of pleconaril in infants with enterovirus meningitis. *Pediatr Infect Dis J.* 2003;22:335-341

56. Davis LE, Beckham JD, Tyler KL. North American encephalitic arboviruses. *Neurol Clin.* 2008;26:727-757

57. Romero JR, Simonsen KA. Powassan encephalitis and Colorado tick fever. *Infect Dis Clin North Am.* 2008;22:545-559

58. Sung S, Wurcel AG, Whittier S, et al. Powassan meningoencephalitis, New York, New York, USA. *Emerging Infect Dis.* 2013;19:1549-1551

59. Hinten SR, Beckett GA, Gensheimer KF, et al. Increased recognition of Powassan encephalitis in the United States, 1999-2005. *Vector Borne Zoonotic Dis.* 2008;8:733-740

60. Yendell SJ, Fischer M, Staples JE. Colorado tick Fever in the United States, 2002-2012. *Vector Borne Zoonotic Dis.* 2015;15:311-316

61. Lindsey NP, Lehman JA, Staples JE, et al. West Nile Virus and other arboviral diseases—United States, 2013. *MMWR Morb Mortal Wkly Rep.* 2014;63:521-526

62. Kramer LD, Li J, Shi P-Y. West Nile Virus. *Lancet Neurol.* 2007;6:171-181

63. Marfin AA, Gubler DJ. West Nile encephalitis: an emerging disease in the United States. *Clin Infect Dis.* 2001;33:1713-1719

64. Lindsey NP, Hayes EB, Staples JE, et al. West Nile Virus disease in children, United States, 1999-2007. *Pediatrics.* 2009;123:e1084-e1049

65. Murray K, Walker C, Herrington E, et al. Persistent infection with West Nile Virus years after initial infection. *J Infect Dis.* 2010;201:2-4

66. Gibney KB, Lanciotti RS, Sejvar JJ, et al. West Nile Virus RNA not detected in urine of 40 people tested 6 years after acute West Nile virus disease. *J Infect Dis.* 2011;203:344-347

67. Centers for Disease Control and Prevention (CDC). West Nile Virus and other arboviral diseases—United States, 2012. *MMWR.* 2013;62:513-517

68. Gaensbauer JT, Lindsey NP, Messacar K, et al. Neuroinvasive arboviral disease in the United States: 2003 to 2012. *Pediatrics.* 2014;134:e642-e650

69. Roehrig JT, Nash D, Maldin B, et al. Persistence of virus-reactive serum immunoglobulin m antibody in confirmed West Nile Virus encephalitis cases. *Emerging Infect Dis.* 2003;9:376-379

70. Johnson AJ, Karabatsos N, Lanciotti RS. Detection of Colorado tick fever virus by using reverse transcriptase PCR and application of the technique in laboratory diagnosis. *J Clin Microbiol.* 1997;35:1203-1208

71. Bloch KC, Glaser C. Diagnostic approaches for patients with suspected encephalitis. *Curr Infect Dis Rep.* 2007;9:315-322

72. Holden EM, Eagles AY, Stevens JE. Mumps involvement of the central nervous system. *JAMA.* 1946;131:382-385

73. Lepow ML, Coyne N, Thompson LB, et al. A clinical, epidemiologic and laboratory investigation of aseptic meningitis during the four-year period, 1955-1958. II. The clinical disease and its sequelae. *N Engl J Med.* 1962;266:1188-1193

74. Centers for Disease Control and Prevention (CDC). Mumps outbreak on a university campus—California, 2011. *MMWR.* 2012;61:986-989

75. Centers for Disease Control and Prevention (CDC). Update: mumps outbreak—New York and New Jersey, June 2009–January 2010. *MMWR.* 2010;59:125-129

76. Dayan GH, Quinlisk MP, Parker AA, et al. Recent resurgence of mumps in the United States. *N Engl J Med.* 2008;358:1580-1589

77. Arisoy ES, Demmler GJ, Thakar S, et al. Meningitis due to Parainfluenza virus type 3: report of two cases and review. *Clin Infect Dis.* 1993;17:995-997

78. Hänninen P, Arstila P, Lang H, et al. Involvement of the central nervous system in acute, uncomplicated measles virus infection. *J Clin Microbiol.* 1980;11:610-613

79. Uchida K, Shinohara M, Shimada S-I, et al. Rapid and sensitive detection of mumps virus RNA directly from clinical samples by real-time PCR. *J Med Virol.* 2005;75:470-474

80. Kreis S, Schoub BD. Partial amplification of the measles virus nucleocapsid gene from stored sera and cerebrospinal fluids for molecular epidemiological studies. *J Med Virol.* 1998;56:174-177

81. Poggio GP, Rodriguez C, Cisterna D, et al. Nested PCR for rapid detection of mumps virus in cerebrospinal fluid from patients with neurological diseases. *J Clin Microbiol.* 2000;38:274-278

82. Connelly KP, DeWitt LD. Neurologic complications of infectious mononucleosis. *Pediatr Neurol.* 1994;10:181-184

83. Fujimoto H, Asaoka K, Imaizumi T, et al. Epstein-Barr virus infections of the central nervous system. *Intern Med.* 2003;42:33-40

84. Rafailidis PI, Kapaskelis A, Falagas ME. Cytomegalovirus meningitis in an immunocompetent patient. *Med Sci Monit.* 2007;13:CS107-CS109

85. Deibel R, Flanagan TD. Central nervous system infections. Etiologic and epidemiologic observations in New York State, 1976-1977. *N Y State J Med.* 1979;79:689-695

86. Echevarría JM, Casas I, Tenorio A, et al. Detection of varicella-zoster virus-specific DNA sequences in cerebrospinal fluid from patients with acute aseptic meningitis and no cutaneous lesions. *J Med Virol.* 1994;43:331-335

87. Science M, MacGregor D, Richardson SE, et al. Central nervous system complications of varicella-zoster virus. *J Pediatr.* 2014;165:779-785

88. Pasedag T, Weissenborn K, Wurster U, et al. Varicella zoster virus meningitis in a young immunocompetent adult without rash: a misleading clinical presentation. *Case Rep Neurol Med.* 2014;2014:686218

89. Kangath RV, Lindeman TE, Brust K. Herpes zoster as a cause of viral meningitis in immunocompetent patients. *BMJ Case Rep.* January 9, 2013

90. Aberle SW, Aberle JH, Steininger C, et al. Quantitative real time PCR detection of varicella-zoster virus DNA in cerebrospinal fluid in patients with neurological disease. *Med Microbiol Immunol.* 2005;194:7-12

91. Wang AS, Ann Nguyen T, Krakowski AC. V1-distributed herpes zoster and meningitis in a two-year old. *J Clin Aesthet Dermatol.* 2015;8:53-54

92. Jhaveri R, Sankar R, Yazdani S, Cherry JD. Varicella-zoster virus: an overlooked cause of aseptic meningitis. *Pediatr Infect Dis J.* 2003;22:96-97

93. Schleede L, Bueter W, Baumgartner-Sigl S, et al. Pediatric herpes simplex virus encephalitis: a retrospective multicenter experience. *J Child Neurol.* 2013;28:321-331

94. Miller S, Mateen FJ, Aksamit AJ. Herpes simplex virus 2 meningitis: a retrospective cohort study. *J Neurovirol.* 2013;19:166-171

95. Terni M, Caccialanza P, Cassai E, et al. Aseptic meningitis in association with herpes progenitalis. *N Engl J Med.* 1971;285:503-504

96. Shalabi M, Whitley RJ. Recurrent benign lymphocytic meningitis. *Clin Infect Dis.* 2006; 43:1194-1197

97. Bergström T, Vahlne A, Alestig K, et al. Primary and recurrent herpes simplex virus type 2-induced meningitis. *J Infect Dis.* 1990;162:322-330

98. Mollaret P. Benign multi-recurrent endothelio-leukocytic meningitis. *Rev Neurol (Paris).* 1977;133:225-244

99. Mollaret P, Cateigne G. Unreported case of benign multi-recurrent endothelio-leukocytic meningitis; discussion on the viral origin. *Rev Neurol (Paris).* 1955;93:257-266

100. Teot LA, Sexton CW. Mollaret's meningitis: case report with immunocytochemical and polymerase chain reaction amplification studies. *Diagn Cytopathol.* 1996;15:345-348

101. Farazmand P, Woolley PD, Kinghorn GR. Mollaret's meningitis and herpes simplex virus type 2 infections. *Int J STD AIDS.* 2011;22:306-307

102. Picard FJ, Dekaban GA, Silva J, et al. Mollaret's meningitis associated with herpes simplex type 2 infection. *Neurology.* 1993;43:1722-1727

103. Fazili T, Hussain F, Fogle M. Mollaret's meningitis caused by herpes simplex virus type 2: case report and review of literature. *J Okla State Med Assoc.* 2008;101:237-238

104. Abu Khattab M, Soub AH, Maslamani AM, et al. Herpes simplex virus type 2 (Mollaret's) meningitis: a case report. *Int J Infect Dis.* 2009;13:e476-e479

105. Min Z, Baddley JW. Mollaret's meningitis. *Lancet Infect Dis.* 2014;14:1022

106. Abou-Foul AK, Buhary TM, Gayed SL. Herpes simplex virus type 2-associated recurrent aseptic (Mollaret's) meningitis in genitourinary medicine clinic: a case report. *Int Med Case Rep J.* 2014;7:31-33

107. Steel JG, Dix RD, Baringer JR. Isolation of herpes simplex virus type I in recurrent (Mollaret) meningitis. *Ann Neurol.* 1982;11:17-21

108. Prandota J. Mollaret meningitis may be caused by reactivation of latent cerebral toxoplasmosis. *Int J Neurosci.* 2009;119:1655-1692

109. Capouya JD, Berman DM, Dumois JA. Mollaret's meningitis due to human herpesvirus 6 in an adolescent. *Clin Pediatr.* 2006;45:861-863

110. Mikdashi J, Kennedy S, Krumholz A. Recurrent benign lymphocytic (Mollaret) meningitis in systemic lupus erythematosus. *Neurologist.* 2008;14:43-45

111. Shimizu M, Araki R, Niida Y, et al. Mollaret meningitis associated with occipital dermal sinus. *J Pediatr.* 2009;155:757.e1

112. Mpayo LL, Liu X-H, Xu M, et al. Extramedullary spinal teratoma presenting with recurrent aseptic meningitis. *Pediatr Neurol.* 2014;50:655-657

113. Childs JE, Glass GE, Korch GW, et al. Lymphocytic choriomeningitis virus infection and house mouse (Mus musculus) distribution in urban Baltimore. *Am J Trop Med Hyg.* 1992;47:27-34

114. Bonthius DJ. Lymphocytic choriomeningitis virus: an under-recognized cause of neurologic disease in the fetus, child, and adult. *Semin Pediatr Neurol.* 2012;19:89-95

115. Sosa LE, Gupta S, Juthani-Mehta M, et al. Meningitis in a college student in Connecticut, 2007. *J Am Coll Health.* 2009;58:12-14

116. Barton LL, Hyndman NJ. Lymphocytic choriomeningitis virus: reemerging central nervous system pathogen. *Pediatrics.* 2000;105:E35-E35

117. Lehmann-Grube F, Kallay M, Ibscher B, et al. Serologic diagnosis of human infections with lymphocytic choriomeningitis virus: comparative evaluation of seven methods. *J Med Virol.* 1979;4:125-136

118. Cordey S, Sahli R, Moraz M-L, et al. Analytical validation of a lymphocytic choriomeningitis virus real-time RT-PCR assay. *J Virol Methods.* 2011;177:118-122

119. McCormick JB, King IJ, Webb PA, et al. Lassa fever. Effective therapy with ribavirin. *N Engl J Med.* 1986;314:20-26

120. Mendenhall M, Russell A, Juelich T, et al. T-705 (favipiravir) inhibition of arenavirus replication in cell culture. *Antimicrob Agents Chemother.* 2011;55:782-787

Adolesc Med 026 (2015) 675–691

Adolescent Dating Violence in the Emergency Department: Presentation, Screening, and Interventions

Quyen M. Epstein-Ngo, PhD[a,b,c]*,
Emily Rothman, ScD[d,e]

[a]University of Michigan Institute for Research on Women and Gender, Ann Arbor, Michigan; [b]University of Michigan Institute for Clinical and Health Research, Ann Arbor, Michigan; [c]Injury Research Center, University of Michigan, Ann Arbor, Michigan; [d]School of Public Health, Boston University, Boston, Massachusetts; [e]School of Medicine, Boston University, Boston, Massachusetts

INTRODUCTION

Adolescent dating violence (ADV) is a significant public health concern. More than 1 in 3 youth experienced some form of dating violence in the past year.[1,2] Dating violence includes physical aggression (eg, punching, kicking), emotional or psychological aggression (eg, being verbally threatening, demeaning), sexual aggression (eg, forced sex, unwanted touching or groping), and stalking (eg, recurring harassing behavior resulting in fear) that is perpetrated against a current or former dating partner.[1,3] Studies using nationally representative data indicate that 1 in 10 adolescents experience physical dating violence victimization during high school, and slightly more than 1 in 11 adolescents report dating violence perpetration.[1,4] In some areas, the prevalence rate of ADV perpetration may be as high as 20%.[5] There is controversy in the field about gender disparities in ADV victimization. Some studies show that males report as much or more physical dating violence victimization as females, although females report higher rates of sexual dating violence victimization.[1,6] Moreover, males seem to perpetrate more extreme physical violence, and females are more likely to be injured as a result of dating violence.[7-9] Overall, the rates of dating violence have remained relatively stable over the last decade.[1,10,11]

*Corresponding author
E-mail address: qen@umich.edu

ADOLESCENT DATING VIOLENCE AS DISTINCT FROM ADULT INTIMATE PARTNER VIOLENCE

Although ADV and adult intimate partner violence (IPV) may be linked in that the former is associated with the latter,[12,13] there are important distinctions because of the inherent differences between adolescence and adulthood in terms of independence and socioemotional development. Consequently, the power dynamics involved in most ADV situations differ from those in many adult relationships characterized by IPV. First, adolescents are less likely to be living with their dating partners, which may result in less social isolation and increase the likelihood that another person will become aware of the potential for harm. This decreased likelihood of adolescent dating partners sharing a primary residence also decreases the amount of time they spend alone together. Second, adolescents are less likely to be financially tied to their dating partners. Typically adolescents do not have shared bank accounts or financial obligations that could make separating more difficult. Third, adolescents may be less likely to share children with their dating partners. The need to co-parent a child would require that adolescent dating partners be in contact with each other, at some level, unless 1 of the parents lost or gave up parental rights. Moreover, ADV is often reciprocal, with both partners perpetrating aggression.[14-16] Finally, adolescents' motivations for perpetrating dating violence seems to be related to them being in a bad mood, jealousy, or anger.[17-20] As a result, it could be difficult to determine what kind of services a youth needs and where to refer him or her. This is not to say that no adolescent relationships mirror the "intimate terrorism" of some violent adult relationships; only that there may need to be a broader perspective when it comes to the dynamics involved in violence in adolescent dating relationships.

ADOLESCENT DATING VIOLENCE AND ASSOCIATED RISK FACTORS

Adolescent dating violence is associated with numerous adverse sequelae, including poor school functioning (for youth still attending school), psychological distress, suicidal ideation, substance abuse, injury, later involvement in IPV, and mortality.[1,10-12,21]

Cross-Sectional Correlates

Ten-year trends using data from the Youth Risk Behavior Surveys found that physical teen dating violence for males was associated with sadness and hopelessness, repeated fighting, and risky sexual behaviors.[11] A parallel study using data from the Youth Risk Behavior Surveys examined 10-year trends for female victims of physical dating violence.[10] In this national sample of youth, physical dating violence victimization among female adolescents was associated with sadness and hopelessness, suicidal ideation, engagement in physical fights, and sexual risk behaviors.[10] In terms of sexual dating violence victimization among adult women, experiences with this type of violence are associated with adverse health symptoms, depression, severe injuries, chronic health problems, and death.[22,23] However, the research regarding adolescent sexual dating violence victimization is sparse, particularly studies with nationally representative samples. Two studies have measured sexual dating victimization in a national sample. Hamby et al[24] explored overlap in occurrences of adolescent physical dating violence with other forms of dating violence victimization. They found that youth who reported physical dating violence victimization were much more likely to report other types of victimization, including sexual dating violence victimization. In contrast, Wolitzky-Taylor et al[25] combined physical and sexual dating violence victimization and found that this combined measure of ADV was associated with older age, female sex, experiences of other traumatic events, and recent life stressors. More research is needed to understand adolescent sexual dating violence victimization, associated negative sequelae, and how it is related to other forms of dating violence victimization.

Longitudinal Correlates

Beyond cross-sectional correlates of ADV, several studies have also examined longitudinal associations between ADV and adverse health outcomes.[26-29] Two studies using the National Longitudinal Study of Adolescent Health (Add Health) found ADV to be associated with later health risk behaviors, IPV, and risk for human immunodeficiency virus infection.[27,28] A recent study by Exner-Cortens et al[12] used data from a national sample to conduct gender-stratified analyses examining longitudinal associations between ADV and adverse health outcomes 5 years after victimization. Using data from 2 waves of the National Longitudinal Study of Adolescent Health, the researchers found longitudinal associations between adolescent psychological dating violence victimization among males and increased antisocial behaviors, odds of suicidal ideation, marijuana use, and adult IPV victimization.[12] Among female adolescents, psychological dating violence victimization was associated with increased odds of heavy episodic drinking and adult IPV victimization. For male adolescent survivors of both psychological and physical dating violence, there were longitudinal associations with increased adult IPV victimization and a borderline association with depressive symptoms 5 years after incidence. Female adolescent survivors of both psychological and physical dating violence had greater depressive symptoms, as well as increased odds of suicidal ideation, smoking, and adult IPV victimization. The number of youth affected by ADV and the associated significant adverse outcomes make this a crucial factor affecting adolescent health.

PRESENTATION OF ADV IN THE EMERGENCY DEPARTMENT

Whereas national annual prevalence rates of adolescent physical dating violence have remained consistent at approximately 10% for the last decade, there is mounting evidence that rates among youth seeking care in hospital emergency departments (EDs) are significantly higher.[1,4,6,10,11,17,30,31] Rates of physical dating violence among adolescents presenting to urban EDs have been reported to range from 52% to 76% in the 6 months before ED treatment, with a higher prevalence among females than males.[17,30,31] One study of adolescents seeking treatment at an academic ED found lower rates of dating violence than those found in urban ED settings but still higher than the rates found in national samples (12% for males and 18% for females).[32] More studies are needed to determine whether there are differences in rates of ADV found in EDs in different locations (eg, urban, suburban, rural).

Given the higher likelihood of injury for female adolescents involved in dating violence, it seems more likely that females would seek treatment in the ED for injuries related to dating violence.[8,9,17,33] One study that provides such evidence examined 599 youth seeking treatment in an urban ED.[17] The study oversampled for youth seeking treatment for violent injuries as a result of interpersonal conflicts. Of the 143 female adolescents seeking treatment for a violent injury, 44% (n = 63) of the violent injuries were the result of dating violence. In contrast, of the 206 male adolescents seeking treatment for a violent injury, only 7% (n = 14) of the violent injuries were the result of dating violence. In another study of 327 youth seeking treatment in an urban pediatric ED, female youth were 5 times more likely to report fear of sustaining serious physical injuries as a result of dating violence.[30] However, rates for males reporting ADV involvement (victimization and perpetration) in the 6 months before ED treatment were also greater than 50%, indicating that males and females both should be assessed for this risk factor.[17,30,31] Moreover, youth seeking ED treatment who report dating violence are more likely to report depressive symptoms, screen positive for alcohol problems, smoke marijuana, use illicit drugs, and carry a weapon than youth who do not report ADV.[32,33] Research findings also indicate that youth seeking ED treatment are more likely to have used alcohol on days on which ADV occurs than on days with no ADV.[17,31] This may be particularly relevant to treatment in the ED given the increased likelihood for injury with alcohol use. The high rates of dating violence reported among adolescent ED patients as well as the associated negative health effects, coupled with the fact that youth involved in dating violence seek treatment in the ED for a wide variety of reasons, highlight the importance of universal screening for dating violence among male and female adolescents seeking treatment in EDs.

REVIEW OF ED SCREENING AND INTERVENTIONS FOR DATING VIOLENCE

Methods

This literature review used rapid review methods as described by Khangura et al.[34] Rapid review is an emerging method of synthesizing literature on a topic of interest. These reviews are designed to summarize what is known for a brief report and to inform a policy decision or a clinical decision. They can be compiled relatively quickly (ie, within 6 weeks vs 6-24 months typically required for a systematic review).[34] Rapid reviews cull information from previously published reviews and from literature searches, and provide a narrative description of findings rather than meta-analytic statistics.

The present rapid review was conducted by the 2 authors. Each searched PubMed, ISI World of Science, and PsychInfo databases for peer-reviewed published research on ED-based interventions that addressed IPV among adults or adolescents. To be considered eligible for inclusion, articles had to be published in English between 2000 and 2015 and relay outcome findings related to the delivery of an ED-based intervention that went beyond mere screening for IPV victimization. Using the search terms "violence" and "intervention" and "emergency," a total of 240 publications were identified. After reviewing abstracts to eliminate articles that did not present the results of intervention research in which the participants were patients, 23 articles were selected for abstract review. Of these, 10 publications were selected for inclusion in this review (Table 1).[35-43] In addition, to enrich understanding of the topic, the authors reviewed the literature on ED-based community violence and substance use interventions for youth.[44-49] One manuscript that relays the results of an ED-based ADV intervention that is not yet published, but is under review, was also included in the synthesis.[50]

Do ED-Based Interventions for Partner Violence Endanger Victims?

When considering whether to implement an ED-based intervention to address dating violence, the first question health care professionals are likely to face is: Will victims be at increased risk for harm as a result of an intervention? Of the 7 studies included in this review that screened ED patients for IPV victimization and the 2 that screened patients for IPV perpetration, 3 assessed whether the screening or intervention procedures caused adverse events or harm for patients.[37,43,50] None of these 3 studies reported any harm related to IPV screening, either for victimization or perpetration, in the ED setting. One of the 3 studies (Houry et al[37]) did report that 1 adverse event occurred among the enrolled 548 patients during the study period, but that event was not related to study participation. Moreover, 95% of patients who participated in Houry's intervention study reported that the intervention conferred some benefit. Thus, research results favor the potential benefit of ED-based interventions for ADV over the theoretical risks, although strong protections for patient safety are unquestionably important. Chief among the theoretical concerns about safety are that survivors of partner violence could be retaliated against for having spoken about their victimization to a health care professional, were it discovered by an abusive partner. In addition, there is concern that amateur counseling efforts could result in unintended consequences. For example, exhortation by a health care professional to leave an abusive partner in the absence of any "safety plan" or a sufficiently

Table 1
Summary information from studies about ED-based interventions for adult or ADV prevention

Study authors (year)	Sample	Year and site of data collection	Study design	Intervention description	Follow-up period	Retention rate	Results
Interventions designed to reduce victimization							
Houry et al (2008)	N = 548 61% female Age 18-55 year	2004-2006; US urban ED	One-group follow-up	Computer screening assessment Computer-generated resource information	1 week 12 weeks	51% (at 12 weeks)	70% of eligible patients agreed to participate 26% of patients in a relationship in the past year disclosed DV victimization 35% of participants used any resources at 3-month follow-up 44% of participants made a safety plan 95% of participants stated the intervention benefitted them Screening resulted in no harm to victims from partners
Kendall et al (2009)	N = 360 97% female Age ≥12 years	2002-2004; US urban ED	One-group follow-up	1-hour training for ED staff Linkage with local DV agency Consult with DV counselor Make 5-point safety plan	12 weeks	44%	10% of eligible patients agreed to participate in intervention 96% of participants reported improved safety Participants completed 49%-59% of items on safety plan Safety plan completion not related to age, race, income, or length of relationship

Koziol-McLain et al. (2010)	N = 399 100% female Age ≥16 years	2007; New Zealand urban ED	RCT	Patient screening Provide information Risk assessment Referral to resources Social worker spoke with high-risk women	12 weeks	86%	5% of eligible patients agreed to participate 10% of those who received the intervention could not recall having received it at follow-up No effect of intervention on victimization; 13.6% of control group and 12.0% of intervention group reported revictimization at follow-up New safety behaviors: OR 1.41 (95% CI 0.71-2.81) Resource use: aOR 4.57 (95% CI 1.36-15.37)
Krasnoff and Moscati (2002)	N = 528 100% female Age 18-65 years	1997-1999; US urban ED	One-group follow-up (authors refer to it as "observational case study")	Screening Intervention by local crisis worker Telephone counseling by community crisis worker	3-10 weeks	48%	2% of female ED patients reported past-year IPV victimization 84% of those who were eligible agreed to intervention with crisis worker 54% of those who met with crisis worker linked with the community agency for follow-up 49% of those who embarked on follow-up were determined to be not at risk for continued violence 64% of patients who participated in the intervention had ended their relationship with the abusive partner by follow-up
MacMillan et al (2009)	N = 6743 100% female Age 18-64 years	2005-2008; Canada 11 EDs, 15 other outpatient settings	RCT	Screening for IPV victimization Physician recommendations	18 months	47%	46% of screened women and 53% of women not screened for IPV reported IPV recurrence at 18-month follow-up Women reported no harm from screening Quality-of-life improvement scores not different for screened vs not-screened women

(continued)

Table 1
Summary information from studies about ED-based interventions for adult or ADV prevention (continued)

Study	Sample	Year; Setting	Design	Intervention	Follow-up	Retention	Results
Schrager et al (2013)	N = 154 100% female Age ≥18 years	2008-2009; US 3 urban EDs	One-group follow-up	Computer-based information kiosk in waiting room; Provide information about IPV; Referral to resources; Assessed victims' readiness to change per the transtheoretical model (TTM)	12 weeks	41%	44% of patients agreed to be screened at kiosk; 18% of those screened were positive for DV; 59% of DV victims agreed to participate in study; Younger age increased chance of loss to follow-up; At 12 weeks, 73% had taken at least 1 protective action; Of those who took protective action, 70% had ended their relationship, 33% had moved out, 50% had made a safety plan, 25% started carrying a weapon, 13% obtained a restraining order, and 33% sought counseling
Trautman et al (2007)	N = 411 100% female Age ≥18 years	2003; US urban ED	Three-group follow-up	Computer screening for DV victimization; Computer screening compared to "usual care," which is screening by physicians if they choose; Referrals to social work made by practitioners if computer screen was positive	Immediate	100%	73% of those eligible chose to participate in study; Participants who completed a computer-based survey about DV were more likely to be identified as having experienced DV than those who received usual care; 88% of participants reported that they liked answering computer questions; 19% of patients who were screened were positive for DV; 53% of those who screened positive were referred to social work; social work referrals were made more often if the DV screening was done by computer instead of by physician; Computers are a more effective way to screen for DV than nurses or physicians in the ED setting

Interventions designed to reduce perpetration (and victimization)

Study	Sample	Year; location	Design	Intervention	Follow-up	Retention	Results
Cunningham et al (2013)	N = 397 64% female Age 14-18 years	2006-2009; US urban ED	RCT	Role play designed to reduce ADV; available in either computer-only or computer-and-therapist formats, which were each compared with a no-intervention condition Brief intervention to reduce peer violence and alcohol use part of intervention	3 months 6 months 12 months	76%-86% (at 12 months)	88% of those eligible chose to participate in study Decreased ADV victimization at 3 and 6 months but not at 12 months for those with "moderate" vs "severe" ADV at baseline Modality of intervention (computer-only or computer-and-therapist) did not produce different results for most of the participants; however, among victims with more than 8 prior ADV incidents in the past year at baseline, the computer-and-therapist modality made larger improvements than computer-only at 3 and 6 months Neither type of intervention had an effect on severe ADV victimization, moderate ADV perpetration, or severe ADV perpetration at 3, 6, or 12 months
Rothman et al (Unpublished)	N = 36 78% female Age 16-21 years	2012; US urban ED	RCT	Brief motivational interview-style intervention Referral to resources Booster call follow-up	1 month	75%	At 1-month follow-up, 76% of those in the control group and 50% of those in the intervention group reported ADV perpetration in the past month 80% of participants reported that the intervention helped them 0% reported that participating was harmful Significantly more intervention group participants followed up with a doctor for additional help than did participants in the control group (5 participants vs 2 participants, Fisher exact $P <.05$)

(continued)

Table 1
Summary information from studies about ED-based interventions for adult or ADV prevention (*continued*)

Interventions designed to educate the public (ie, primary prevention)					
Ernst et al (2011)	N = 240 40% female Age ≥18 years	2007; US urban ED	Two-group follow-up	Compared a video depicting DV scenarios in which a person intervenes with a friend to a set of PowerPoint slides providing the same information Designed to improve DV-related knowledge; decrease victim-blaming attitudes and acceptability of DV; and increase intentions to intervene as a bystander	Immediate	100%	88% of eligible patients participated On average, 13% age point increase from pretest to posttest on the Knowledge, Attitudes, and Practices 46% of patients had a perfect score on pretest so they could not improve Men improved scores by 18%; women by 12% (NS) Men who watched the video improved more than did men who saw the PowerPoint slides (29% vs 6%, $P < .05$) No difference in video vs slides for women or for patients who were victims or perpetrators of DV

ADV, adolescent dating violence; aOR, adjusted odds ratio; CI, confidence interval; DV, domestic violence; ED, emergency department; IPV, intimate partner violence; NS, not statistically significant; OR, odds ratio; RCT, randomized controlled trial; US, United States.

resourced relocation plan could result in harm to the person or their children. Therefore, although the literature supports the use of IPV screening and intervention programs in the ED setting, research procedures should be carefully crafted to reflect best practices for violence-related data collection and patient safety.

Do ED-Based Interventions Interfere with Patient Care ("Flow")?

The issue of "flow," or streamlining health care services to be maximally efficient, is particularly important in the fast-paced ED setting. Physicians considering interventions for adolescents to reduce ADV in the ED setting may be concerned that such programs could disrupt usual care or patient care flow.[51,52] This is a reasonable consideration and one that cannot be addressed uniformly. Available evidence suggests that a variety of brief interventions can be implemented in the ED setting, ranging from a few minutes to over an hour, without interrupting patient care flow.[51,53] A few factors can improve flow when interventions are implemented in the ED setting. First, for interventions delivered by specialists who are not usual ED personnel (ie, advocates who are not ED social workers, nurses, or physicians), it can be helpful to identify a private space where the interventionist could deliver the intervention if the patient needs to vacate the treatment room. If it is impossible to identify a space where the interventionist can meet privately with the patient, it is possible that patient self-administered screening via computer tablet or semiprivate information kiosks may be feasible.[36,54] For example, Ernst et al conducted a randomized control trial of a simulation video for a bystander intervention that could be easily self-administered.[36] Rhodes et al conducted a randomized control trial of an intervention using a self-administered computer tablet-based health risk assessment to collect information on patients' health risk behaviors and to provide tailored, patient-requested health information. Information provided to patients receiving the tablet-based intervention was more likely to be retained than information provided to control patients receiving usual care.[54]

Do Eligible Patients Want to Participate in ED-Based IPV Interventions?

Most of the evidence suggests that a large proportion of patients who are eligible for IPV interventions will want to participate in them, although participation rates have varied widely. Among studies included in this rapid review, participation rates ranged from 5% to 84% (Table 1). Factors that may influence patients' propensity to participate in IPV interventions for which they are eligible include how they feel about the personnel conducting the intervention, how long they expect the intervention to take, and safety concerns (eg, whether their partner has accompanied them to the ED or whether they think their partner may find out about their participation). To enhance participation, providers are encouraged to hire, when appropriate, intervention staff who are from or represent the same community as patients (ie, the same geographic or racial/ethnic community as most patients),[44] who are close to the patients' age (eg, young adults to deliver ADV interventions), who are outgoing, and who have experience working with IPV victims or perpetrators. Providing adequate training and supervision for interventionists also enhances their capacity to recruit patients effectively.

Does Participating in ED-Based Violence Interventions Benefit Adolescent Patients?

The data about the success of ED-based brief interventions for youth are mixed. Data from hospital-based community violence programs are mounting, and the results of those studies suggest that advocacy programs for survivors of peer or community violence are effective.[45,47] However, these programs are not limited to adolescents, so it is not clear whether the interventions are any more or less successful for younger patients. Moreover, many of the community violence interventions may begin with a patient encounter in the ED but evolve to include multiple follow-up interactions, which may improve effect sizes. The results of trials of ED-based substance abuse brief interventions for youth are mixed or inconclusive,[46] and the data from assessments of ED-based IPV interventions for adults are inconsistent. For example, 1 study of an ED-based IPV brief intervention found no effect,[39] other studies found small effects,[43] and still others used non-experimental designs that make it impossible to attribute effects to the interventions.[37,38,40-42] Two studies conducted in the ED setting have addressed youth violence specifically. The larger, a Michigan-based trial, targeted peer violence but also found a positive effect on dating violence victimization but not perpetration.[35] The pilot study based in Boston found that a brief intervention for ADV perpetration reduced self-reported perpetration at 1-month follow-up by half and twice as effectively as those in a control condition, but the sample was small and the follow-up period was short.[50] Currently there is insufficient data to claim that ED-based interventions for ADV are effective or ineffective.

As additional research studies are conducted to assess the effect of ED-based interventions for ADV, researchers should plan to collect sufficient data to undertake subanalyses to determine whether the programs are more effective for certain subsets of patients, for example, by age, gender, sexual orientation, race, nativity, socioeconomic status, or severity of ADV victimization or perpetration. As Choo et al[55] recently discovered while analyzing ED-based brief intervention data on substance use, presenting the overall effect rates for the ED patient population can mask important differences that may be present for subsets. Also of interest is whether computer-delivered or interventionist-delivered interventions work equally well, and what kind of booster contact with patients seems to extend the effect of the intervention for as long as possible. If interventions are delivered by people (not computers), it will be important to determine whether patients experience more behavior change when the interventionist is of similar age or is more senior, is of the same gender or race, or whether these factors are immaterial. Assessing the cost-benefit or cost-effectiveness of ED-based ADV interventions will be of paramount importance. Hospitals and insurance companies are unlikely to invest in programs that are unable to demonstrate cost-effectiveness. One study of the cost-effectiveness of a community violence prevention program in an ED setting found that the cost of preventing a youth violence injury might range from $3 to $54, which is significantly less than the cost of placing a single intravenous line if an injury occurs.[56] Additional cost-effectiveness data that pertain to ADV interventions will benefit the field.

The Make-or-Break Factor: The Agencies To Which Patients Are Referred

The one feature that all of the ED-based interventions reviewed had in common was that they sought, ultimately, to refer patients to community-based resources that could continue to help them after the ED visit. This is a logical and expected component of the Screening, Brief Intervention, and Referral to Treatment (SBIRT) model, which has been established as an evidence-based intervention for the reduction of substance use.[57] However, for IPV, looking to community-based crisis and advocacy programs to provide "treatment" may not be as uniformly effective as it is in substance abuse treatment.[58] Although some evidence supports the positive effect of domestic violence shelter-based counseling and advocacy, the quality and availability of local domestic violence services vary widely.[59] Some agencies may not have the capacity to serve IPV victims who do not seem to be in immediate danger. Effective batterer intervention programs may be unavailable. Establishing working relationships with a variety of community-based resources, including mental health professionals who work on a sliding scale or accept state health insurance, is a critical element of implementing an ED-based ADV intervention. In short, the intervention will only be as effective as the community resources to which patients are referred. When community organizations are stressed beyond capacity, there is the potential for patients to have negative experiences when they follow through on the referrals, which could worsen, rather than improve, their condition. Building successful partnerships with community-based agencies may take significant investments of time and good will.

Alternatives to referring patients who screen positive for ADV to community-based organizations include enrolling them in a text messaging-based behavioral intervention,[60] referring them to therapy, or prescribing medication.[48] One recent study found that as many as 50% of adolescents treated in an urban ED expressed a preference for text messaging-based behavioral intervention as opposed to a human interactive intervention.[61] Some evidence suggests that each of these strategies may be effective with adolescent patients who have experienced community violence victimization, although there are no data on the effect of these types of interventions on ADV victimization or perpetration rates.

CONCLUSION

Adolescent dating violence is a significant public health concern with serious risks and consequences. A considerable proportion of youth seeking treatment in EDs report violence within dating relationships. As such, the ED represents a potentially important venue in which to engage adolescents in dating violence interventions. However, physical space, time, and resource limitations present challenges. Referral to community services may not be effective if there are not adequate and appropriate community resources for treatment. The research on effective adolescent dating violence interventions is emergent, and much more work is needed in order to provide effective, systemically sustainable treatment for youth who experience violence in dating relationships.

ACKNOWLEDGEMENTS

This research was supported by research grants from the Michigan Institute for Clinical Health Research, a National Center for Advancing Translational Sciences of the National Institutes of Health (2UL1TR000433) and the University of Michigan Injury Center, an Injury Control Research Center funded by the Centers for Disease Control and Prevention (CDC R49CE002099) (Epstein-Ngo). This research was also supported by the National Institute on Alcohol Abuse and Alcoholism (NIAAA) Grants K23AA022641 (Epstein-Ngo) and K01AA017630 (Rothman). The views expressed in this article are those of the authors and do not necessarily represent the views of NIAAA, the National Institutes of Health, the Centers for Disease Control and Prevention, the University of Michigan, or Boston University.

References

1. Brooks-Russell A, Foshee VA, Reyes HLM. *Dating Violence. Handbook of Adolescent Behavioral Problems.* New York: Springer; 2015:559-576
2. Haynie DL, Farhat T, Brooks-Russell A, et al. Dating violence perpetration and victimization among U.S. adolescents: prevalence, patterns, and associations with health complaints and substance use. *J Adolesc Health.* 2013;53:194-201
3. Centers for Disease Control and Prevention. Teen Dating Violence. 2014. Available at: www.cdc.gov/violenceprevention/intimatepartnerviolence/teen_dating_violence.html. Accessed January 6, 2015
4. Kann L, Kinchen S, Shanklin SL, et al. Youth risk behavior surveillance—United States, 2013. *MMWR Surveill Summ.* 2014;63(Suppl 4):1-168
5. Rothman EF, Johnson RM, Young R, et al. Neighborhood-level factors associated with physical dating violence perpetration: results of a representative survey conducted in Boston, MA. *J Urban Health.* 2011;88:201-213
6. Hamby S, Turner H. Measuring teen dating violence in males and females: insights from the national survey of children's exposure to violence. *Psychol Violence.* 2013;3:323
7. Archer J. Sex differences in aggression between heterosexual partners: A meta-analytic review. *Psychol Bull.* 2000;126:651-680
8. Chermack ST, Grogan-Kaylor A, Perron BE, et al. Violence among men and women in substance use disorder treatment: a multi-level event-based analysis. *Drug Alcohol Depend.* 2010;112:194-200

9. Walton MA, Cunningham RM, Chermack ST, et al. Correlates of violence history among injured patients in an urban emergency department: gender, substance use, and depression. *J Addict Dis.* 2007;26:61-75

10. Howard DE, Debnam KJ, Wang MQ. Ten-year trends in physical dating violence victimization among US adolescent females. *J School Health.* 2013;83:389-399

11. Howard DE, Debnam KJ, Wang MQ, Gilchrist B. 10-Year trends in physical dating violence victimization among US adolescent males. *Int Q Commun Health Educ.* 2011;32:283-305

12. Exner-Cortens D, Eckenrode J, Rothman E. Longitudinal associations between teen dating violence victimization and adverse health outcomes. *Pediatrics.* 2013;131:71-78

13. Gómez AM. Testing the cycle of violence hypothesis: child abuse and adolescent dating violence as predictors of intimate partner violence in young adulthood. *Youth Soc.* 2011;43:171-192

14. Swahn MH, Alemdar M, Whitaker DJ. Nonreciprocal and reciprocal dating violence and injury occurrence among urban youth. *West J Emerg Med.* 2010;11:264-268

15. Walton MA, Cunningham R, Chermack ST, et al. Predictors of violence following emergency department visit for cocaine-related chest pain. *Drug Alcohol Depend.* 2009;99:79-88

16. Zweig JM, Dank M, Yahner J, Lachman P. The rate of cyber dating abuse among teens and how it relates to other forms of teen dating violence. *J Youth Adolesc.* 2013;42:1063-1077

17. Epstein-Ngo QM, Cunningham RM, Whiteside LK, et al. A daily calendar analysis of substance use and dating violence among high risk urban youth. *Drug Alcohol Depend.* 2013;130:194-200

18. Epstein-Ngo QM, Walton MA, Chermack ST, et al. Event-level analysis of antecedents for youth violence: Comparison of dating violence with non-dating violence. *Addict Behav.* 2014;39:350-353

19. Hettrich EL, O'Leary KD. Females' reasons for their physical aggression in dating relationships. *J Interpers Violence.* 2007;22:1131-1143

20. Foshee VA, Bauman KE, Linder F, Rice J, Wilcher R. Typologies of adolescent dating violence: identifying typologies of adolescent dating violence perpetration. *J Interpers Violence.* 2007;22:498-519

21. Banyard VL, Cross C. Consequences of teen dating violence: understanding intervening variables in ecological context. *Violence Against Women.* 2008;14:998-1013

22. Bonomi AE, Anderson ML, Rivara FP, Thompson RS. Health outcomes in women with physical and sexual intimate partner violence exposure. *J Womens Health.* 2007;16:987-997

23. Campbell JC, Soeken KL. Forced sex and intimate partner violence effects on women's risk and women's health. *Violence Against Women.* 1999;5:1017-1035

24. Hamby S, Finkelhor D, Turner H. Teen dating violence: co-occurrence with other victimizations in the National Survey of Children's Exposure to Violence (NatSCEV). *Psychol Violence.* 2012;2:111-124

25. Wolitzky-Taylor KB, Ruggiero KJ, Danielson CK, et al. Prevalence and correlates of dating violence in a national sample of adolescents. *J Am Acad Child Adolesc Psychiatry.* 2008;47:755-762

26. Ackard DM, Eisenberg ME, Neumark-Sztainer D. Long-term impact of adolescent dating violence on the behavioral and psychological health of male and female youth. *J Pediatr.* 2007;151:476-481

27. Roberts TA, Klein JD, Fisher S. Longitudinal effect of intimate partner abuse on high-risk behavior among adolescents. *Arch Pediatr Adolesc Med.* 2003;157:875-881

28. Teitelman AM, Ratcliffe SJ, Dichter ME, Sullivan CM. Recent and past intimate partner abuse and HIV risk among young women. *J Obstet Gynecol Neonat Nurs.* 2008;37:219-227

29. Van Dulmen MH, Klipfel KM, Mata AD, et al. Cross-lagged effects between intimate partner violence victimization and suicidality from adolescence into adulthood. *J Adolesc Health.* 2012;51:510-516

30. Carroll BC, Raj A, Noel SE, Bauchner H. Dating violence among adolescents presenting to a pediatric emergency department. *Arch Pediatr Adolesc Med.* 2011;165:1101-1106

31. Rothman EF, Stuart GL, Winter M, et al. Youth alcohol use and dating abuse victimization and perpetration: a test of the relationships at the daily level in a sample of pediatric emergency department patients who use alcohol. *J Interpers Violence.* 2012;27:2959-2979

32. Singh V, Walton MA, Whiteside LK, et al. Dating violence among male and female youth seeking emergency department care. *Ann Emerg Med.* 2014;64:405-412

33. Walton MA, Cunningham RM, Goldstein AL, et al. Rates and correlates of violent behaviors among adolescents treated in an urban emergency department. *J Adolesc Health*. 2009;45:77-83

34. Khangura S, Konnyu K, Cushman R, Grimshaw J, Moher D. Evidence summaries: the evolution of a rapid review approach. *Syst Review*. 2012;1:1-9

35. Cunningham RM, Whiteside LK, Chermack ST, et al. Dating violence: outcomes following a brief motivational interviewing intervention among at-risk adolescents in an urban emergency department. *Acad Emerg Med*. 2013;20:562-569

36. Ernst AA, Weiss SJ, Hobley K, et al. Brief intervention for perpetration of intimate partner violence (IPV): simulation versus instruction alone. *South Med J*. 2011;104(6):446-455

37. Houry D, Kaslow NJ, Kemball RS, et al. Does screening in the emergency department hurt or help victims of intimate partner violence? *Ann Emerg Med*. 2008;51:433-442

38. Kendall J, Pelucio MT, Casaletto J, et al. Impact of emergency department intimate partner violence intervention. *J Interpers Violence*. 2009;24:280-306

39. Koziol-McLain J, Garrett N, Fanslow J, et al. A randomized controlled trial of a brief emergency department intimate partner violence screening intervention. *Ann Emerg Med*. 2010;56:413-423

40. Krasnoff M, Moscati R. Domestic violence screening and referral can be effective. *Ann Emerg Med*. 2002;40:485-492

41. Schrager JD, Smith LS, Heron SL, Houry D. Does stage of change predict improved intimate partner violence outcomes following an emergency department intervention? *Acad Emerg Med*. 2013;20:169-177

42. Trautman DE, McCarthy ML, Miller N, Campbell JC, Kelen GD. Intimate partner violence and emergency department screening: computerized screening versus usual care. *Ann Emerg Med*. 2007;49:526-534

43. MacMillan HL, Wathen CN, Jamieson E, et al. Screening for intimate partner violence in health care settings: a randomized trial. *JAMA*. 2009;302:493-501

44. James TL, Bibi S, Langlois BK, Dugan E, Mitchell PM. Boston violence intervention advocacy program: a qualitative study of client experiences and perceived effect. *Acad Emerg Med*. 2014;21:742-751

45. Neville FG, Goodall CA, Williams DJ, Donnelly PD. Violence brief interventions: a rapid review. *Aggress Violent Behav*. 2014;19:692-698

46. Newton AS, Dong K, Mabood N, et al. Brief emergency department interventions for youth who use alcohol and other drugs a systematic review. *Pediatr Emerg Care*. 2013;29:673-684

47. Snider C, Lee J. Youth violence secondary prevention initiatives in emergency departments: a systematic review. *Can J Emerg Med*. 2009;11:161-168

48. Zatzick D, Russo J, Lord SP, et al. Collaborative care intervention targeting violence risk behaviors, substance use, and posttraumatic stress and depressive symptoms in injured adolescents a randomized clinical trial. *JAMA Pediatr*. 2014;168:532-539

49. Becker MG, Hall JS, Ursic CM, Jain S, Calhoun D. Caught in the crossfire: the effects of a peer-based intervention program for violently injured youth. *J Adolesc Health*. 2004;34:177-183

50. Rothman E, Evans E. An emergency department-based intervention to prevent adolescent dating violence perpetration: results of a pilot RCT (Unpublished Manuscript)

51. Akin J, Johnson JA, Seale JP, Kuperminc GP. Using process indicators to optimize service completion of an ED drug and alcohol brief intervention program. *Am J Emerg Med*. 2015;33:37-42

52. Bray JW, Mallonee E, Dowd W, et al. Program- and service-level costs of seven screening, brief intervention, and referral to treatment programs. *Subst Abuse Rehabil*. 2014;5:63-73

53. Sise MJ, Sise CB, Kelley DM, Simmons CW, Kelso DJ. Implementing screening, brief intervention, and referral for alcohol and drug use: The trauma service perspective. *J Trauma Injury Infect Crit Care*. 2005;59:S112-S118

54. Rhodes KV, Lauderdale DS, Stocking CB, et al. Better health while you wait: a controlled trial of a computer-based intervention for screening and health promotion in the emergency department. *Ann Emerg Med*. 2001;37:284-291

55. Choo EK, McGregor AJ, Mello MJ, Baird J. Gender, violence and brief interventions for alcohol in the emergency department. *Drug Alcohol Depend*. 2013;127:115-121

56. Sharp AL, Prosser LA, Walton M, et al. Cost analysis of youth violence prevention. *Pediatrics.* 2014;133:448-453
57. Substance Abuse and Mental Health Services Administration. White Paper on Screening, Brief Intervention and Referral to Treatment (SBIRT) in Behavioral Healthcare. April 2011. Available at: www.samhsa.gov/sites/default/files/sbirtwhitepaper_0.pdf. Accessed October 19, 2015
58. Klevens J, Kee R, Trick W, et al. Effect of screening for partner violence on women's quality of life a randomized controlled trial. *JAMA.* 2012;308:681-689
59. Bybee DI, Sullivan CM. The process through which an advocacy intervention resulted in positive change for battered women over time. *Am J Commun Psychol.* 2002;30:103-132
60. Ranney ML, Choo EK, Cunningham RM, et al. Acceptability, language, and structure of text message-based behavioral interventions for high-risk adolescent females: a qualitative study. *J Adolesc Health.* 2014;55:33-40
61. Ranney ML, Choo EK, Spirito A, Mello MJ. Adolescents' preference for technology-based emergency department behavioral interventions: does it depend on risky behaviors? *Pediatr Emerg Care.* 2013;29:475-481

Adolesc Med 026 (2015) 692–711

Syncope in Children and Adolescents

Khalil Kanjwal, MD, FHRS, FACC, CCDS[a]*,
Sundus Masudi, BS[b],
Blair P. Grubb, MD, FACC[c]

[a]*Assistant Professor of Medicine, Central Michigan University, Staff Cardiac Electrophysiologist, Michigan Cardiovascular Institute, Saginaw, Michigan;* [b]*St Mary's of Michigan, Saginaw, Michigan;* [c]*Professor of Medicine, University of Toledo Medical Center, Toledo, Ohio*

INTRODUCTION

Syncope is not a disease but a symptom of various disease processes. The word is derived from the Greek word *synkoptein*, meaning "to cut short." Syncope is defined as a transient, self-limited loss of consciousness and postural tone. Recovery is spontaneous, rapid, prompt, and complete without any neurologic sequelae. Most often syncope leads to a fall. The mechanism invariably is insufficient blood and oxygen supply to the brain.[1-4]

In a population-based study, syncope accounted for 126 of 100,000 children coming to medical attention.[1-4] One of every 2000 emergency department visits is because of syncope. Syncope has been reported to occur more commonly in girls and has a peak incidence between the ages of 15 and 19 years. It has been reported that almost 15% of children will experience at least 1 episode of syncope before the age of 18.[4-8]

Vasovagal syncope (VVS), also called neurocardiogenic syncope (NCS), has been reported to be the most common cause of syncope (75%), followed by cardiac disease in 10% and psychogenic or unexplained syncope of unknown cause in 8% to 17% of cases. [2,4,7]

Seizure disorder can mimic syncope in children and accounts for almost 5% of episodes that were presumed to be caused by syncope.[8] In this article we will discuss some of the most common causes of syncope in children.

---

*Corresponding author
E-mail address:* khalilkanjwal@yahoo.com

Various terms are related to syncope, and one must be familiar with them in order to understand what these terms imply. *Presyncope* refers to the aura of syncope without actually having syncope. Symptoms may include dizziness, nausea, warm or cold sensation, and rarely, visual changes.[1,7-9] Patients often report feeling that they will "pass out." Syncope can occur without aura or with minimal or no warning signs, and the episodes often lead to severe injuries and morbidity.[9-12] *Reflex syncope* is often triggered by a stimulus such as pain or the sight of blood. Syncope that occurs only on standing is usually the result of one of the many forms of orthostatic intolerance, especially vasodepressor syncope. Rarely syncope leads to convulsive movements and is often termed *convulsive syncope*.[12] In children it can be challenging to differentiate episodes of convulsive syncope from seizure disorder. In this article we will follow a simple classification of syncope into 3 categories; autonomic, cardiac, and non-cardiac.

AUTONOMIC SYNCOPE

The last 2 decades have witnessed a substantial growth in our understanding of this category of syncope, which is the most common cause of syncope in children. Once thought of as a single entity, we now know that this group comprises a series of abnormalities in autonomic control.[12,13]

Neurocardiogenic Syncope

Neurocardiogenic syncope is also referred to as vasovagal syncope or a "common faint." Triggers associated with the development of neurally mediated syncope include orthostatic stress such as prolonged standing, a hot shower, or an emotional stress such as the sight of blood. It has been proposed that NCS results from a paradoxical reflex (Bezold-Jarisch reflex) that is initiated when ventricular preload is reduced by venous pooling.[12-18] This reduction leads to decreased cardiac output and blood pressure, which is sensed by arterial baroreceptors. The resultant increased catecholamine levels, combined with reduced venous filling, lead to a vigorously contracting volume-depleted ventricle. The heart itself is involved in this reflex through mechanoreceptors, or C-fibers, which consist of nonmyelinated fibers found in the atria, ventricles, and pulmonary artery. It has been proposed that vigorous contraction of a volume-depleted ventricle leads to activation of these receptors in susceptible individuals. These afferent C-fibers project centrally to the dorsal vagal nucleus of the medulla, leading to a "paradoxical" withdrawal of peripheral sympathetic tone and an increase in vagal tone, which, in turn, cause vasodilation and bradycardia.[18] The ultimate clinical consequence is syncope or presyncope. Not all neurally mediated syncope results from activation of mechanoreceptors. In humans, the sight of blood or extreme emotion can trigger syncope, suggesting that higher neural centers also participate in the pathophysiology of VVS. In addition, central mechanisms can contribute to the production of neurally mediated syncope. It is interesting that anemia lowers the threshold for NCS, so on a physiologic basis it is oxygen delivery rather than mere cerebral perfusion that leads to eventual syncope. Patients suffering from NCS usually have an aura or warning signs (grayout spells), which allow them to take evasive measures to prevent injuries from falls that can result from syncope with minimal or no warning signs (blackout spells).

Dysautonomic Syncope

Standing displaces up to 500 mL of blood to the abdomen and lower extremities as a result of gravity, leading to an abrupt drop in venous return to the heart.[19-21] This drop leads to decreased cardiac output and stimulation of aortic, carotid, and cardiopulmonary baroreceptors that trigger a reflex increase in sympathetic outflow. As a result, heart rate, cardiac contractility, and vascular resistance increase to maintain a stable systemic blood pressure on standing. Although these disorders are often seen in adults, they have also been recognized in adolescents with increasing frequency.[12-17] Usually the symptoms appear during periods of rapid growth. Some investigators believe that the predominance of parasympathetic over sympathetic tone that may coincide with periods of rapid growth may result in predisposition to bradycardia and hypotension in affected individuals. Orthostatic intolerance is a term used to refer to the signs and symptoms of abnormality in any portion of this blood pressure control system. Symptoms of orthostatic intolerance include syncope, light-headedness, presyncope, tremulousness, weakness, fatigue, palpitations, diaphoresis, and blurred or tunnel vision. Many adolescents may also have acral cyanosis resulting from excess venous pooling. Orthostatic hypotension is defined as a 20 mm Hg drop in systolic blood pressure or a 10 mm Hg drop in diastolic blood pressure within 3 minutes of standing.[12-14] Orthostatic hypotension can be asymptomatic, or it can be associated with the symptoms of orthostatic intolerance. These symptoms are often worse immediately on arising in the morning or after meals or exercise. Initial orthostatic hypotension is defined as a more than 40 mm Hg decrease in blood pressure immediately on standing, with rapid return to normal in less than 30 seconds. In contrast, delayed progressive orthostatic hypotension is characterized by a slow progressive decrease in systolic blood pressure on standing.[12-17]

Dysautonomic syncope has also been reported to occur in patients with joint hypermobility syndrome.[13, 22-24] Symptoms include syncope, presyncope, palpitations, chest discomfort, fatigue, heat intolerance, orthostatic hypotension, postural orthostatic tachycardia syndrome (POTS), and uncategorized orthostatic intolerance. Joint hypermobility syndrome is one of the most common heritable collagen disorders. It is currently believed that the connective tissue laxity seen in patients with hypermobility syndrome allows for a greater than normal degree of vascular dispensability, leading to exaggerated blood pooling in the lower extremities during upright posture.[22-24]

Orthostatic hypotension can also result from neurogenic causes, which can be subclassified into primary and secondary autonomic failure. Primary causes are generally idiopathic, whereas secondary causes are associated with a known biochemical or structural anomaly or are part of a particular disease or syndrome.[25]

Another form of inherited dysautonomia which usually affects children of Ashkenazi Jewish ancestry is familial dysautonomia (FD), also called Riley-Day syndrome.[26] The FD gene has been identified as *IKBKAP*. Mutations result in tissue-specific expression of mutant IκB kinase-associated protein (IKAP).[25] Familial dysautonomia belongs to the group of hereditary sensory motor neuropathy type III.[26] Clinical features reflect widespread involvement of sensory and autonomic neurons. Patients with FD present in infancy with failure to thrive, poor sucking and swallow difficulties, thermoregulatory disturbances, breath-holding spells, sleep disturbances, and seizures. Dysautonomic syncope as a result of postural hypotension is usually seen in adolescents. Almost 60% of FD patients suffer from breath-holding spells during their first 5 years of life.[25] Some patients suffer autonomic crises such as hypertension, tachycardia, excessive sweating, and erythematous blotching of the skin.[27]

Postural Orthostatic Tachycardia Syndrome

Postural orthostatic tachycardia syndrome is currently defined as symptoms of orthostatic intolerance associated with heart rate increases of 30 bpm or more (or rate >120 bpm) that occur within the first 10 minutes of standing or upright tilt in the absence of other chronic debilitating conditions such as protracted periods of bed rest or use of medications known to affect vascular or autonomic function.[28-32] The estimated number of patients with POTS in the United States is at least 500,000.[31] Some patients have no change, a small decline, or even a modest increase in blood pressure on standing. Abnormalities of heart rate are only one manifestation of autonomic dysfunction in such patients, who may also suffer from disturbances in sweating, temperature regulation, and bowel and bladder function. Early descriptions of the disorder focused on a group of patients who had been previously healthy until a sudden febrile illness (presumably viral) brought on an abrupt onset of symptoms.[28-32] Recent research has shown that POTS can have variants resulting from multiple etiologies, including partial dysautonomic, centrally mediated hyperadrenergic stimulation, norepinephrine transporter dysfunction,[33] autoimmune antibody against cholinesterase receptors,[34] POTS associated with deconditioning,[35] and hypervolemia.[36] A recently published study reported that POTS may be a manifestation of autonomic cardiac neuropathy.[37] Postural orthostatic tachycardia syndrome has been reported to be associated with trauma,[38] Lyme disease,[39] electrocution,[40] multiple sclerosis,[41] and mitochondrial cytopathy,[42] and to occur after slow pathway ablation for treatment of atrioventricular nodal reentrant tachycardia.[43]

Breath-holding Spells

This group of disorders is usually seen in children and can be broadly subdivided into 2 groups. (1) The cyanotic form usually occurs around 6 months of age, peaks around 2 years, and completely disappears by 5 years.[44] The episode begins with the child making a loud cry, followed by apnea. The child turns pale or cyanotic. There may be associated jerky or myoclonic movements or opisthotonus, followed by limpness. The whole episode may last less than 1 minute and ends with gasping breaths and sudden deep inspirations with return of normal color and consciousness.[45] However, in some severe episodes, recovery is delayed because the child remains drowsy for a few moments. (2) The other form of the disorder is called pallid breath-holding spells or reflex anoxic seizures. It is usually seen in children between the ages of 12 and 24 months. It is similar to the cyanotic form, which is usually brought on by injury, pain such as a head bump, or sudden startle. The child suddenly stops breathing but, in contrast to the cyanotic form, the child does not cry and loses consciousness quickly. The child becomes deadly pale and hypotonic, and develops rhythmic muscular contractions. The episodes are associated with severe bradycardia or asystole on monitoring. The frequency of episodes is highly variable, ranging from 2 to 4 episodes per day to once per year. Almost 30% of the children have a history of similar episodes in a family member.[44-46] No specific treatment is needed for these breath-holding spells; only a correct diagnosis and reassurance for the patient and parents are required. Almost 50% of the children have complete resolution of symptoms by age 4, and 100% of patients will never experience additional episodes after age 8. However, it has been reported that up to 25% of people who suffered breath-holding spells as children may develop NCS and concentration problems later in life. This association has led some to believe that breath-holding spells are infantile forms of NCS.[46]

Blood Injury Phobia

Most phobias lead to a hyperadrenergic state, and patients usually have tachycardia. However, a specific group of children who suffer from blood injury phobia (BIP) have a paradoxical bradycardia or a severe asystole in response to an initial transient tachycardia.[47,48] This often leads to presyncope or syncope. Over time, these children, like other children who suffer from phobic disorders, learn to avoid situations in which they are exposed to their triggers because they perceive these injuries or blood sightings as quite unpleasant. However, unlike those with other phobic disorders, children with BIP do not have an increased association with other psychiatric disorders such as depression. Some children develop NCS later on, and there is some evidence of clinical overlap between BIP and breath-holding spells.[46] Deconditioning by exposure is often helpful, and the tendency toward syncope can be prevented by tensing the muscles and by inducing anger.[49]

Fainting Lark

Fainting lark is a game or trick played by older children in schools or colleges. The game starts with the person squatting with the knees fully bent while breathing rapidly and taking 20 deep breaths. This is followed by standing up suddenly and performing forced expiration against closed glottis (Valsalva). In a similar version, another person pushes on the chest of the subject and pushes him against the wall. Some children with autism and learning disabilities suffer from compulsive Valsalva and may develop syncope, especially convulsive syncope, which often mimics seizure disorder.[50,51]

CARDIAC SYNCOPE

Cardiac syncope is responsible for almost 10% of syncope seen in children and young adults. Cardiovascular causes include obstruction of blood flow, myocardial dysfunction, and arrhythmia.[52]

Obstructive Causes

Hypertrophic Cardiomyopathy

Hypertrophic cardiomyopathy affects approximately 0.2% of the general population.[53] Although a significant number of patients suffer spontaneous mutations, both autosomal dominant and recessive variants also exist. Hypertrophic cardiomyopathy is usually characterized by asymmetric septal hypertrophy, which produces dynamic left ventricular outflow tract obstruction.[53] Symptoms include dyspnea, fatigue, palpitations, near syncope, and syncope (either from abnormal blood pressure responses during exercise or from serious ventricular tachyarrhythmia). Although syncope occurs in up to 20% of patients, it is less common in the pediatric population.[54] Syncope in children carries a more ominous prognosis. Early onset of the disease in infancy carries the worst prognosis, with most infants (85%) dying by age 1 year.[53-55] The aim of therapy is to provide symptomatic relief and decrease the risk of sudden cardiac death from ventricular tachycardia. Negative inotropes such as beta blockers, calcium channel blockers, and disopyramide may provide symptomatic relief. Surgical myotomy and myomectomy may help relieve symptoms but carry an operative mortality of almost 2%. An implantable cardioverter-defibrillator (ICD) is now commonly used in patients with recurrent syncope, ventricular arrhythmia, or a family history of sudden cardiac death.[55]

Aortic Stenosis

Aortic valve stenosis causes a fixed obstruction to blood flow. Congenital aortic stenosis accounts for almost 5% of congenital cardiac anomalies in children.[56] Bicuspid aortic valve is more common and is seen in up to 2% of the general population.[56] More severe cases of aortic stenosis are seen in pediatric patients suffering from unicommissural aortic valve. Almost 25% of these patients have another cardiac anomaly, such as aortic coarctation.[56] As the disease progresses and the stenosis becomes severe, patients may develop syncope from reduced cardiac output and cerebral perfusion. They are also at increased risk for sudden cardiac death from ischemia, which results from both increased demand as well as decreased supply from hypotension. Therapy consists of either balloon valvuloplasty or surgical correction.[57,58]

Primary Pulmonary Hypertension

Primary pulmonary hypertension is a diagnosis of exclusion. It is defined as mean pulmonary artery pressure greater than 25 mm Hg at rest and greater than 30 mm Hg during exercise.[59] It affects 1 to 2 in 1,000,000 persons in western countries and has a greater female predominance, which may be seen even in early childhood. Up to 50% of children with pulmonary hypertension suffer syncope.[60] Syncope may result from both arrhythmia and obstruction to blood flow. Vasodilators including calcium channel blockers and prostaglandins are used to alleviate symptoms. Most patients are also treated with anticoagulation.[61]

Primary Myocardial Dysfunction

Cardiomyopathies are rarely seen in children, and syncope in these patients may be the result of ischemia, arrhythmia, or an inflammatory process.[8] Neuromuscular dystrophies such as Duchenne, Becker, and Emery-Dreifuss may present as myocardial dysfunction as well as bradyarrhythmia from atrioventricular block.[52] Myocarditis resulting in ventricular tachycardia may present as syncope in children, and unrecognized myocarditis may be an important cause of sudden unexplained death in children. Myocardial ischemia is rarely seen in children. It usually results from anomalous left main coronary artery arising from a pulmonary trunk or an interarterial course of the left coronary artery between the aorta and pulmonary artery, making it vulnerable to compression. Patients usually have exercise-related syncope because blood flow to both the aorta and pulmonary artery increases during exercise, making the left coronary artery more vulnerable to compression. Another rare condition seen in children younger than 5 years is Kawasaki disease.[62] Syncope may occur, especially during acute myocarditis from ventricular arrhythmias. Arrhythmogenic right ventricular dysplasia can result in ventricular tachycardia and syncope. It should be suspected in children with exercise-induced syncope and left bundle branch block pattern of ventricular tachycardia. This disorder usually manifests in the third to fourth decade of life but rarely earlier. Cardiac magnetic resonance imaging shows classic involvement of the right ventricle. Many patients may require an ICD. Other causes of syncope include Eisenmenger syndrome, tetralogy of Fallot, pulmonary stenosis, and right ventricular outflow tract obstruction.[63,64]

Arrhythmias as a Cause of Syncope

Cardiac rhythm disturbances in the absence of structural heart disease rarely cause syncope in children.[63-65] However, patients with long QT syndrome (Figures 1 and 2), Brugada syndrome (Figure 3), or short QT syndrome (Figure 4) essentially have a structurally normal heart but may be at risk for syncope and sudden cardiac death. *Long QT syndrome* usually manifests as syncope associated with emotion or exercise in individuals with a structurally normal heart.

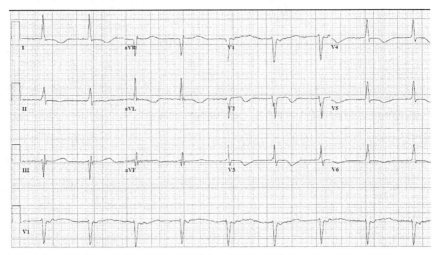

Fig 1. Electrocardiogram from a patient with long QT interval.

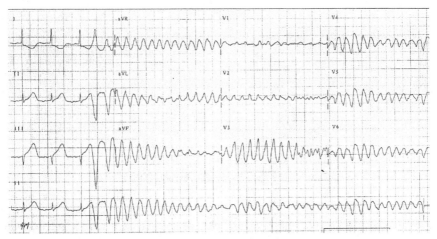

Fig 2. Torsades de pointes, a polymorphic ventricular tachycardia, in a patient with long QT interval.

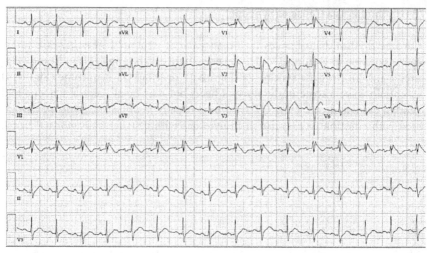

Fig 3. Electrocardiogram from a patient with Brugada syndrome.

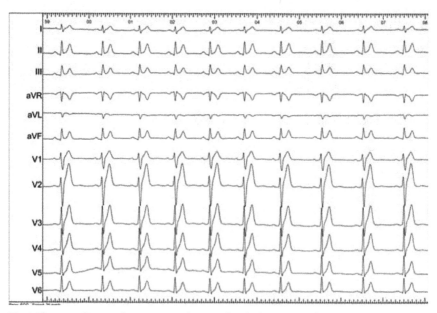

Fig 4. Electrocardiogram from a patient diagnosed with short QT syndrome.

Patients are prone to develop polymorphic ventricular tachycardia (torsades de pointes), which can lead to hemodynamic compromise and subsequent syncope. They may also suffer abrupt onset of syncope in response to a fright or awakening because of a loud noise (eg, an alarm clock). Usually patients exhibit symptoms during the second decade of life.[66-69] Beta-blocker therapy may reduce mortality, from 70% in untreated patients to 7%.[70] Some patients may be candidates for ICD implantation. Sympathetic ganglionectomy has been reserved for treatment of severe refractory cases. *Brugada syndrome* is a hereditary disorder that results from a mutation in an alpha-subunit of the sodium channel protein of the *SC5NA* gene. It manifests as incomplete right bundle branch block and ST elevation in leads V_1 to V_3. Patients are at risk for syncope and sudden cardiac death from polymorphic ventricular tachycardia. Many patients with Brugada syndrome have a normal electrocardiogram (ECG) and manifest the typical Brugada pattern only after a drug challenge with either ajmaline or procainamide.[71] In an earlier published study on a population of children with Brugada syndrome, fever was the most important precipitating factor for any arrhythmic event, and the risk of fatal arrhythmias was significantly higher in previously symptomatic patients and in those demonstrating a spontaneous type I ECG (60% vs 7%).[71,72] These patients should receive an ICD if they have a cardiac arrest, documented ventricular tachycardia even without cardiac arrest, or a spontaneous type I ECG with syncope.[71,72] *Catecholaminergic polymorphic ventricular tachycardia* is a rare inherited arrhythmic disorder that affects up to 1 in 10,000 people. It is an autosomal dominant disorder resulting from mutation in the ryanodine receptor 2 (*RYR2*) gene. Less commonly, the autosomal recessive variant has resulted from the *CASQ2* gene. Patients suffer from disruption of calcium handling within cardiac myocytes, which leads to ventricular tachycardia especially after exercise and emotional stress.[73] They may present with bidirectional ventricular tachycardia as well. Beta blockers are the only proved therapy for these patients, and ICDs have been used especially in patients with recurrent cardiac arrest on beta blockers.[73]

Arrhythmias may also result from repaired or palliated structural heart disease. Sinus node dysfunction has been reported to occur after atrial repair surgery.[74-76] In severe cases, patients may suffer symptomatic bradycardia and syncope. Atrioventricular block in pediatric patients can be either congenital (seen in maternal lupus), which may not require pacing, or acquired, from an infection such as diphtheria, endocarditis, Lyme disease, or Rocky Mountain spotted fever. Ventricular tachycardia is rare but has been reported to occur in patients with corrected tetralogy of Fallot. Usually the tachycardia originates close to the ventricular path, especially in the septum and outflow tract. Supraventricular tachycardia, as in adults, rarely presents as syncope in children. The most common causes of supraventricular tachycardia, including atrioventricular reciprocating tachycardia and atrioventricular reentrant tachycardia, have clinical presentations similar to those seen in adults.

NON-CARDIAC CAUSES OF SYNCOPE

In some individuals, global cerebral hypoxia results not only in loss of consciousness but in convulsive activity as well. These episodes of convulsive syncope may be difficult to distinguish from seizures resulting from epilepsy.[77,78]

Autonomically mediated forms of reflex syncope (eg, NCS, VVS) may produce sudden episodes of profound hypotension and bradycardia resulting in loss of consciousness and occasionally convulsive activity. It has been reported that as many as one-third of patients initially diagnosed with epilepsy actually had a cardiovascular cause of convulsive episodes.[77,78] However, in contrast to convulsive syncope, convulsions in epileptic disorders are prolonged (>1 minute), rhythmic, and usually not provoked by the stimuli that commonly provoke syncope. Seizures (especially neonatal seizures and complex partial seizures with minimal convulsive activity) may be confused with true syncope. It may be difficult to differentiate these 2 entities, especially when minimal or no convulsive activity (akinetic seizures) is observed. Ictal electroencephalography (EEG) may be the only method to differentiate these seizures from syncope. In cases of syncope, the EEG may be normal, or it may demonstrate diffuse slowing of background activity. However, in cases of seizure, an abnormal increase in background activity will be seen.

Another group of disorders that may closely mimic both syncope and seizures is loss of consciousness in the setting of complex migraine headaches or basilar migraines, which are sometimes referred to as "brainstem attacks."[79] Loss of consciousness can also occur in patients suffering from hydrocephalus who experience a sudden increase in intracranial pressure. If hydrocephalus is suspected, neuroimaging may reveal structural abnormalities such as a tumor or brainstem herniation with dilated ventricles.[79]

Advances in our understanding of the causes of syncope combined with advances in diagnostic technology have greatly reduced the number of patients with recurrent syncope of unknown origin. However, in at least 10% of patients with syncope the cause remains unidentified after traditional cardiac and neurologic workups. Physicians should exercise great caution before labeling any syncope as "psychogenic" in origin because a potential treatable cardiac cause can be uncovered only by prolonged and diligent cardiac monitoring in these patients.[80]

EVALUATION OF SYNCOPE

The cause of syncope can be successfully identified by detailed history and comprehensive physical examination in almost half of patients. Unlike the case with adults, obtaining a history from children may be difficult, and often the history is obtained from the parents or eyewitnesses. When obtaining information from these sources, a detailed account of the circumstances and activity occurring immediately before the event, identified triggers or precipitating factors, situations surrounding the period of syncope, whether the syncope occurred during standing or lying down, and any symptoms or warning signs that occurred before the event should be diligently recorded. Information about convulsive movements, loss of bladder and bowel control, tongue bite, and whether the recovery was quick or delayed provides important clues to the diagnosis. While obtaining the history, it is also important to recognize patients who may be at risk for sudden cardiac death. The group of patients who may be considered high risk and thus require additional cardiac workup include those with syncope during peak exercise, a family history of sudden cardiac death, convulsive or traumatic syncope, chest pain preceding syncope, a family history of deafness, syncope with structural heart disease in children, syncope with abnormal cardiovascular examination, or syncope with focal neurologic defects.[81]

A comprehensive cardiovascular examination including supine, sitting, and standing blood pressures and heart rate should be recorded and repeated at 2-, 5-, and 10-minute intervals in the standing position. Close attention should be paid to a complete cardiac examination, including the presence of murmurs, clicks, gallops, and any rhythm disturbances. A comprehensive neurologic examination should be performed, with attention paid to focal neurologic abnormalities.

Laboratory Blood Tests

Routine blood tests, such as serum electrolytes, cardiac enzymes, glucose, and hematocrit levels, are of low diagnostic value in patients with syncope. Complete blood count and a pregnancy test are routinely performed in girls.

Electrocardiography

A 12-lead ECG should be obtained for all patients with loss of consciousness, especially that occurring after exercise. Particular attention should be paid to QT interval, preexcitation, bundle branch block, ventricular hypertrophy, and any evidence of atrioventricular block.

Evaluation of the ECG is particularly important if long QT syndrome is a possibility. If events appear to be related to exercise or stress and the results of standard ECG are normal, an exercise ECG should be performed. An echocardiogram is usually obtained in children in whom the physical examination warrants the imaging or in whom structural heart disease is suspected.

Video-Assisted Recording

Video recording has allowed physicians to see the actual episode and, when combined with physical monitoring that includes continuous ECG and EEG, may improve the diagnostic yield.[82]

Ambulatory ECG Monitoring

Ambulatory ECG monitoring has allowed greater symptom rhythm correlation in patients suffering from frequent syncope. External digital monitoring may help reveal the potential rhythm disturbance at the time of syncope. However, in patients with infrequent episodes, implantable loop monitors can allow for prolonged monitoring up to 3 years.[83]

Head-Up Tilt-Table Testing

Head-up tilt-table testing (HUTT) is generally performed for 30 to 45 minutes after a 20-minute horizontal pretilt stabilization phase, at an angle between 60 and 80 degrees (with 70 degrees the most common). The sensitivity of the test can be increased (but with an associated decrease in specificity) with longer tilt durations, steeper tilt angles, and use of provocative agents such as isoproterenol and nitroglycerin.[84-86] Head-up tilt-table testing has been safely performed in children older than 6 years. It can also be performed in younger children if they are cooperative. In contrast to studies in adult patients, only a few studies on the use of HUTT in pediatric patients have been reported. Given the lack of extensive data on the use of HUTT in pediatric patients, most of the consensus recommendations for pediatric patients derive from adult HUTT data. However, the issue of HUTT duration has not been assessed in the pediatric population. In addition, gravity-induced orthostatic stress during HUTT is less pronounced in children than in adults given their lower size and body surface area. A more prolonged HUTT or use of a provocative agent (isoproterenol) during HUTT may be necessary in pediatric patients. Head-up tilt-table testing may not be necessary for further evaluation of syncope in pediatric patients who present with a normal physical examination, absence of abnormal laboratory findings, and a medical history characteristic of VVS.

Echocardiography

Echocardiograms are commonly used to evaluate patients with syncope who have an abnormal ECG or abnormal cardiovascular examination. It should be performed in all patients suspected of having structural heart disease.

Imaging

Neuroimaging is not performed routinely when evaluating children and young adults with syncope unless abnormalities on neurologic examination indicate signs of increased intracranial pressure or focal neurologic defects. Cardiac imaging including cardiac magnetic resonance may rarely be needed to evaluate a patient suspected of having an anomalous coronary artery.

TREATMENT

The approach to treatment of a patient with syncope depends largely on the cause and mechanism of syncope. We will discuss the management of NCS, the most common cause of syncope in children.

Education and Reassurance

Treatment of syncope resulting from VVS begins with a careful history, paying particular attention to identifying precipitating factors, quantifying the degree of salt intake and current medication use, and determining whether the patient has any prior conditions that may alter the approach to treatment. For most patients with neurally mediated syncope, particularly those with infrequent episodes associated with an identifiable precipitant, education and reassurance are sufficient.[87]

1. Physical countermaneuvers. If used early at the onset of NCS symptoms, physical maneuvers may help abort the episode. The easiest of these maneuvers is assumption of a supine posture. Subsequent leg elevation may lead to increased venous return to the heart. Sitting and squatting may augment peripheral vascular resistance and improve venous return to the heart. Increase in venous return to the heart subsequently increases cardiac output, blood pressure, and cerebral perfusion and aborts the syncope. The combination of leg crossing and tensing of the thigh and abdominal musculature has been shown to be highly effective in preventing reflex syncope in young patients.[88] In cooperative patients, progressively prolonged periods of enforced upright posture or tilt training may reduce the recurrence of NCS by lowering vascular compliance in the compartments most responsible for venous pooling. Raising the head of the bed during sleep (>10 degrees) also contributes to symptom improvement. Compression stockings may be helpful but must be waist high and provide at least 30 mmHg of ankle counterpressure in order to be effective. The European Guidelines on Management of Syncope identify the following physical measures as class 2 treatments of neurally mediated syncope: (1) tilt training, (2) head-up tilt sleeping (>10 degrees), (3) isometric leg and arm counterpressure maneuvers, and (4) moderate aerobic and isometric exercise.[88,89] It has been reported that 2 minutes of an isometric hand grip maneuver initiated at the onset of symptoms during tilt testing rendered two-thirds of patients asymptomatic.[88] Other studies have demonstrated that tilt (standing) training is effective for treatment of neurally mediated syncope.[87,89] Standing training involves leaning against a wall with the heel 10 inches from the wall for progressively longer periods over 2 to 3 months. Standing time initially should be 5 minutes twice per day with a progressive increase to 40 minutes twice daily. Although the results of nonrandomized studies of standing training have been positive, the results of randomized trials suggest that standing training may have only limited effectiveness.[89]

2. Paced breathing. In some cooperative patients, respiratory training with paced breathing has been shown to prevent tilt-induced NCS.[90] Paced breathing is a deeper, slower method of breathing. It involves filling the lungs to full capacity when inhaling and then pushing out as much air as possible when exhaling. Paced breathing was shown to inhibit HUTT-induced syncope in 1 study.[90]

3. Fluid therapy. Increasing oral fluid and salt intake can be a highly effective measure to prevent an episode of VVS. Patients are advised to drink about 2 L of fluid per day and ingest 2 to 4 g of salt or to increase fluid intake until the urine is clear and colorless. In 1 study, acute oral therapy with 200 to 250 mL of water was found to prevent HUTT-induced syncope in 78% of patients who demonstrated a positive HUTT before fluid therapy.[87]

4. Pharmacologic treatment. Currently, no therapy is approved by the US Food and Drug Administration (FDA) for patients with NCS, and there is a paucity of evidence supporting any pharmacologic therapy. In contrast to physical maneuvers, the value of pharmacologic agents is less certain. Medications that are generally used to treat VVS include beta-blockers, fludrocortisone, serotonin reuptake inhibitors, and midodrine.[87] Despite the widespread use of these pharmacologic agents, none has been demonstrated to be effective in multiple large prospective randomized clinical trials. Although many previously considered beta blockers to be effective therapy, recent studies have reported that the beta blockers metoprolol, propranolol, and nadolol are no more effective than placebo.[91-93]

5. Pacemaker therapy. In some patients with HUTT-induced episodes of profound bradycardia and sometimes asystole, it seems logical that permanent pacemaker placement might be of benefit in preventing syncope. However, an important concern is whether these tilt-induced asystolic events accurately reflect what occurred during the spontaneous episodes. Although there were questions regarding the use of pacemakers for treatment of patients with severe NCS and documented asystole, the recent ISSUE-3 trial has appeared to confirm their effectiveness.[94] When considering device implantation for patients with NCS, pacemakers that provide specialized pacing algorithms, such as rate drop hysteresis or closed loop stimulation, are often selected. Closed loop stimulation is a form of rate adaptive pacing that responds to myocardial contraction dynamics by measuring variations in right ventricular intracardiac impedance. When an incipient NCS episode is detected, pacing rate is increased. Although no prospective randomized clinical trials have determined which pacing feature is superior, several recent nonrandomized or retrospective trials suggest that close-look stimulation may be preferable.[95,96] Further research in this evolving approach to management of NCS is needed.

6. Cardioneuroablation. Recently, there have been reports on the use of radiofrequency energy[97] (similar to ablation of atrial fibrillation) in patients with refractory NCS, targeting the ganglionic plexi in right and left atria and thus abolishing the Bezold-Jarisch reflex. Initial reports from a few centers on the use of this procedure, referred to as cardioneuroablation, are encouraging, with markedly reduced recurrences in patients with refractory syncope reported.[97-100] However, these results need to be confirmed in large randomized controlled trials.

FUTURE PERSPECTIVES

Given the paucity of literature on syncope in children and adolescents, most of the management strategies in children reflect the data from studies involving the adult population. Children are not merely young adults, so studies specifically of children and adolescents suffering from recurrent syncope are needed. To date there is no FDA-approved therapy for NCS, which is the most common cause of syncope in both adults and children. We have found that none of the clinical trials of pharmacotherapy for NCS have shown benefit over placebo. One potential reason is that most of the trials were flawed or the endpoints were not reasonable. Most of these clinical trials looked at the "time to first syncope," which may not be a reasonable endpoint to assess the success of any therapy. Neurocardiogenic syncope should be considered a chronic condition because, as with other chronic diseases, the aim of therapy should be to decrease the recurrence of syncope rather than complete elimination of syncope. More reasonable endpoints such as "syncope burden" are needed when devising new clinical trials. We look forward to more data on the pharmacotherapy of NCS and it variants, including POTS and other dysautonomic syncopes, from future studies.

References

1. Brignole M, Alboni P, Benditt DG, et al. Guidelines on management (diagnosis and treatment) of syncope—update 2004. *Europace*. 2004;6:467-537
2. Kapoor WN. Syncope. *N Engl J Med*. 2000;343:1856-1862
3. Lewis DA, Dhala A. Syncope in the pediatric patient. The cardiologist's perspective. *Pediatr Clin North Am*. 1999;46:205-219
4. Pratt JL, Fleisher GR. Syncope in children and adolescents. *Pediatr Emerg Care*. 1989;5:80-82
5. Massin MM, Bourguignont A, Coremans C, et al. Syncope in pediatric patients presenting to an emergency department. *J Pediatr*. 2004;145:223-228
6. Gillette PC, Garson A Jr. Sudden cardiac death in the pediatric population. *Circulation*. 1992;85:I64-I69
7. Strickberger SA, Benson DW, Biaggioni I, et al. AHA/ACCF Scientific Statement on the evaluation of syncope: from the American Heart Association Councils on Clinical Cardiology, Cardiovascular Nursing, Cardiovascular Disease in the Young, and Stroke, and the Quality of Care and Outcomes Research Interdisciplinary Working Group; and the American College of Cardiology Foundation: in collaboration with the Heart Rhythm Society: endorsed by the American Autonomic Society. *Circulation*. 2006;113:316
8. Driscoll DJ, Jacobsen SJ, Porter CJ, et al. Syncope in children and adolescents. *J Am Coll Cardiol*. 1997;29:1039-1045
9. Stephenson JBP. *Fits and Faints*. London: Mac Keith Press; 1990
10. Horrocks IA, Nechay A, Stephenson JB, et al. Anoxic-epileptic seizures: observational study of epileptic seizures induced by syncopes. *Arch Dis Child*. 2005;90:1283-1287
11. Gastaut H. Syncopes: generalised anoxic cerebral seizures. In: Vinken PJ, Bruyn GW, eds. *Handbook of Clinical neurology, Volume 15: The Epilepsies*. Amsterdam: North-Holland Publishing; 1974;15:815-835
12. Grubb BP, Friedman R. Syncope in child and adolescent. In: Grubb BP, Olshansky B, eds. *Syncope: Mechanisms and Management*. 2nd ed. Malden, MA: Blackwell Press; 2005:273-286
13. Grubb BP. Dysautonomic (orthostatic) syncope. In: Grubb BP, Olshansky B, eds. *Syncope: Mechanisms and Management*. 2nd ed. Malden, MA: Blackwell Press; 2005:72-91

14. Stewart JM. Orthostatic intolerance in pediatrics. *J Pediatr.* 2002;140:404-411
15. Stewart JM, Gewitz MH, Weldon A, et al. Patterns of orthostatic intolerance: the orthostatic tachycardia syndrome and adolescent chronic fatigue. *J Pediatr.* 1999;135:218-225
16. Stewart JM. Chronic orthostatic intolerance and the postural tachycardia syndrome (POTS). *J Pediatr.* 2004;145:725-730
17. Wieling W. Standing, orthostatic stress and autonomic function. In: Bannister R, Mathias C, eds. *Autonomic Failure: A Textbook of Clinical Disorders of the Autonomic Nervous System.* Oxford, UK: Oxford University Press; 1992:308-320
18. Grubb BP. Clinical practice. Neurocardiogenic syncope. *N Engl J Med.* 2005;352:1004-1010
19. Wieling W, VanLieshout JJ. Maintenance of postural normotension in humans. In: Low P, ed. *Clinical Autonomic Disorders.* Philadelphia: Lippincott Williams & Wilkins; 2008:57-67
20. Thompson WO, Thompson PK, Dailey ME. The effect of upright posture on the composition and volume of the blood in man. *J Clin Invest.* 1988;5:573-609
21. Consensus Committee of the American Autonomic Society and the American Academy of Neurology. Consensus statement on the definition of orthostatic hypotension, pure autonomic failure and multiple system atrophy. *Neurology.* 1996;46:1470-1471
22. Rowe PC, Barron DF, Calkins H, et al. Orthostatic intolerance and chronic fatigue syndrome associated with Ehlers-Danlos syndrome. *J Pediatr.* 1999;135:494-499
23. Rowe PC, Barron DF, Calkins H, et al. Ehlers-Danlos syndrome. *J Pediatr.* 1999;135:513
24. Gazit Y, Nahir M, Grahame R, Jacob G. Dysautonomia in the joint hypermobility syndrome. *Am J Med.* 2003;115:33-40
25. Shohat M, Halpern GJ. Familial dysautonomia. In: Pagon RA, Bird TD, Dolan CR, Stephens K, Adam MP, eds. GeneReviews [Internet]. Seattle, WA: University of Washington, Seattle; 1993-2003 [Updated October 22, 2007]
26. Dong J, Edelmann L, Bajwa AM, Kornreich R, Desnick RJ. Familial dysautonomia: detection of the IKBKAP IVS20(+6T→C) and R696P mutations and frequencies among Ashkenazi Jews. *Am J Med Genet.* 2002;110:253-257
27. Mathias C, Bannister R. Clinical features and evaluation of the primary autonomic failure syndromes. In: Mathias C. Bannister R. (eds.) *Autonomic Failure: A Textbook of Clinical Disorders of the Autonomic Nervous System* 4th ed. Oxford, England: Oxford University Press; 1999: 307–520
28. Low PA, Opfer-Gehrking TL, Textor SC, et al. Postural tachycardia syndrome (POTS). *Neurology.* 1995;45:S19-S25
29. Schondorf R, Low PA. Idiopathic postural orthostatic tachycardia syndrome: an attenuated form of acute pandysautonomia? *Neurology.* 1993;43:132-137
30. Jacob G, Biaggioni I. Idiopathic orthostatic intolerance and postural orthostatic tachycardia syndrome. *Am J Med Sci.* 1999;317:88-101
31. Robertson D. The epidemic of orthostatic tachycardia and orthostatic intolerance. *Am J Med Sci.* 1999;317:75-77
32. Thieben M, Sandroni P, Sletten D et al. Postural orthostatic tachycardia syndrome—Mayo Clinic experience. *Mayo Clin Proc.* 2007;82:308-313
33. Jordan J, Shannon JR, Diedrich A, Black BK, Robertson D. Increased sympathetic activation in idiopathic orthostatic intolerance: role of systemic adrenoreceptor sensitivity. *Hypertension.* 2002;39:173-178
34. Vernino S, Low PA, Fealey RD, et al. Autoantibodies to ganglionic acetylcholine receptors in autoimmune autonomic neuropathies. *N Engl J Med.* 2000;343:847-855
35. Levine BD, Zuckerman JH, Pawelczyk JA. Cardiac atrophy after bed-rest deconditioning: a nonneural mechanism for orthostatic intolerance. *Circulation.* 1997;96:517-525
36. Raj SR, Robertson D. Blood volume perturbations in the postural tachycardia syndrome. *Am J Med Sci.* 2007;334:57-60
37. Haensch CA, Lerch H, Schlemmer H, et al. Cardiac neurotransmission imaging with 123I-meta-iodobenzylguanidine in postural tachycardia syndrome. *J Neurol Neurosurg Psychiatry.* 2010; 81:339-343
38. Kanjwal K, Karabin B, Kanjwal Y, Grubb BP. Autonomic dysfunction presenting as postural tachycardia syndrome following traumatic brain injury. *Cardiol J.* 2010;17:482-487

39. Kanjwal K, Karabin B, Kanjwal Y, Grubb BP. Postural orthostatic tachycardia syndrome following Lyme disease. *Cardiol J.* 2011;18:63-66

40. Kanjwal K, Karabin B, Kanjwal Y, Grubb BP. Postural orthostatic tachycardia syndrome: a rare complication following electrical injury. *Pacing Clin Electrophysiol.* 2010;33:e59-e61

41. Kanjwal K, Karabin B, Kanjwal Y, Grubb BP. Autonomic dysfunction presenting as postural orthostatic tachycardia syndrome in patients with multiple sclerosis. *Int J Med Sci.* 2010;7:62-67

42. Kanjwal K, Karabin B, Kanjwal Y, Saeed B, Grubb BP. Autonomic dysfunction presenting as orthostatic intolerance in patients suffering from mitochondrial cytopathy. *Clin Cardiol.* 2010;33:626-629

43. Kanjwal K, Karabin B, Sheikh M, Kanjwal Y, Grubb BP. New onset postural orthostatic tachycardia syndrome following ablation of AV node reentrant tachycardia. *J Interv Card Electrophysiol.* 2010;29:535-536

44. Lombroso CT, Lerman P. Breathholding spells (cyanotic and pallid infantile syncope). *Pediatrics.* 1967;39:563-581

45. Stephenson JB. Reflex anoxic seizures ('white breath-holding'): nonepileptic vagal attacks. *Arch Dis Child.* 1978;53:193-200

46. DiMario FJ Jr. Prospective study of children with cyanotic and pallid breath-holding spells. *Pediatrics.* 2001;107:265-269

47. Marks I. Blood-injury phobia: a review. *Am J Psychiatry.* 1988;145:1207-1213

48. Connolly J, Hallam RS, Marks IM. Selective association of fainting with blood-injury-illness fear. *Behav Ther.* 1976;7:8-13

49. Ost LG, Lindahl IL, Sterner U, et al. Exposure in vivo vs applied relaxation in the treatment of blood phobia. *Behav Res Ther.* 1984;22:205-216

50. Howard P, Leathart GL, Dornhorst AC, Sharpey-Schafer EP. The mess trick and the fainting lark. *Br Med J.* 1951;2:382-384

51. Wieling W, van Lieshout JJ. The fainting lark. *Clin Auton Res.* 2002;12:207

52. Massin MM, Malekzadeh-Milani S, Benatar A. Cardiac syncope in pediatric patients. *Clin Cardiol.* 2007;30:81-85

53. Nishimura RA, Holmes DR, Hypertrophic obstructive cardiomyopathy. *N Engl J Med.* 2004; 350:1320-1327

54. Colan SD. Hypertrophic cardiomyopathy in childhood. *Heart Fail Clin.* 2010;6:433-444

55. Ostman-Smith I. Hypertrophic cardiomyopathy in childhood and adolescence strategies to prevent sudden death. *Fundam Clin Pharmacol.* 2010;24:637-652

56. Hoffman JI, Kaplan S. The incidence of congenital heart disease. *J Am Coll Cardiol.* 2002;39: 1890-1900

57. Maskatia SA, Ing FF, Justino H, et al. Twenty-five year experience with balloon aortic valvuloplasty for congenital aortic stenosis. *Am J Cardiol.* 2011;108:1024-1028

58. Karamlou T, Jang K, Williams WG, et al. Outcomes and associated risk factors for aortic valve replacement in 160 children: a competing-risks analysis. *Circulation.* 2005;112:3462-3469

59. Pfammatter JP. [Needle in the haystack: potentially dangerous syncope in childhood]. *Praxis (Bern 1994).* 2011;100:1487-1491

60. Douwes JM, van Loon RL, Roothooft MT, Berger RM. [Pulmonary arterial hypertension in childhood]. *Ned Tijdschr Geneeskd.* 2011;155:A3901

61. Barst RJ, McGoon MD, Elliott CG, et al. Survival in childhood pulmonary arterial hypertension: insights from the registry to evaluate early and long-term pulmonary arterial hypertension disease management. *Circulation.* 2012;125:113-122

62. Burns JC, Shike H, Gordon JB, et al. Sequelae of Kawasaki disease in adolescents and young adults. *J Am Coll Cardiol.* 1996;28:253-257

63. Garson A Jr. Arrhythmias in pediatric patients. *Med Clin North Am.* 1984;68:1171-1210

64. Rocchini AP, Chun PO, Dick M. Ventricular tachycardia in children. *Am J Cardiol.* 1981;47: 1091-1097

65. Garson A Jr, Smith RT, Moak JP, et al. Ventricular arrhythmias and sudden death in children. *J Am Coll Cardiol.* 1985;5:130B-133B

66. Schwartz PJ, Moss AJ, Prolonged QT interval: what does it mean? *J Cardiovasc Med.* 1982;7:1317

67. Priori SG, Schwartz PJ, Napolitano C, et al. Risk stratification in the long QT syndrome. *N Engl J Med.* 2003;348:19:1866-1874
68. Schwartz PJ, Stramba-Badiale M, Segantini A, et al. Prolongation of the QT interval and the sudden infant death syndrome. *N Engl J Med.* 1998;338:1709-1714
69. Vincent GM. The long-QT syndrome: bedside to bench to bedside. *N Engl J Med.* 2003;348: 1837-1838
70. Moss AJ, Zareba W, Hall WJ, et al. Effectiveness and limitations of beta-blocker therapy in congenital long-QT syndrome. *Circulation.* 2000;101:616-623
71. Probst V, Denjoy I, Meregalli PG, et al. Clinical aspects and prognosis of Brugada syndrome in children. *Circulation.* 2007;115:2042-2048
72. Sarkozy A, Boussy T, Kourgiannides G, et al. Long-term follow-up of primary prophylactic implantable cardioverter-defibrillator therapy in Brugada syndrome. *Eur Heart J.* 2007;28:334-344
73. Sy RW, Gollob MH, Klein GJ, et al. Arrhythmia characterization and long-term outcomes in catecholaminergic polymorphic ventricular tachycardia. *Heart Rhythm.* 2011;8:8648-71
74. Hamilton RM, Fidler L. Right ventricular cardiomyopathy in the young: an emerging challenge. *Heart Rhythm.* 2009;6:571-575
75. Celik M, Santas B, Tatar T, et al. Risk factors for postoperative arrhythmia in patients with physiologic univentricular hearts undergoing Fontan procedure. *Anadolu Kardiyol Derg.* 2012;12: 347-351
76. Stephenson EA, Lu M, et al; Pediatric Heart Network Investigators. Arrhythmias in a contemporary Fontan cohort: prevalence and clinical associations in a multicenter cross-sectional study. *J Am Coll Cardiol.* 2010;56:890-896
77. Joensen P. Prevalence, incidence, and classification of epilepsy in the Faroes. *Acta Neurol Scand.* 1986;74:150-155
78. Zaidi A, Clough P, Cooper P, et al. Misdiagnosis of epilepsy: many seizure-like attacks have a cardiovascular cause. *J Am Coll Cardiol.* 2000;36:181-184
79. Rossi LN. Headache in childhood. *Childs Nerv Syst.* 1989;5:129-134. Erratum in: *Childs Nerv Syst.* 1990;6:58
80. Kanjwal K, Kanjwal Y, Karabin B, Grubb BP. Psychogenic syncope? A cautionary note. *Pacing Clin Electrophysiol.* 2009;32:862-865
81. Strieper MJ. Distinguishing benign syncope from life-threatening cardiac causes of syncope. *Semin Pediatr Neurol.* 2005;12:32-38
82. Sheth RD, Bodensteiner JB. Effective utilization of home-video recordings for the evaluation of paroxysmal events in pediatrics. *Clin Pediatr (Phila).* 1994;33:578-582
83. Al Dhahri KN, Potts JE, Chiu CC, Hamilton RM, Sanatani S. Are implantable loop recorders useful in detecting arrhythmias in children with unexplained syncope? *Pacing Clin Electrophysiol.* 2009;32:1422-1427
84. Lin P, Wang C, Cao MJ, et al. [Application of the head-up tilt table test in children under 6 years old]. *Zhongguo Dang Dai Er Ke Za Zhi.* 2012;14:276-278
85. Yilmaz S, Gokben S, Levent E, Serdarofülu G. Syncope or seizure? The diagnostic value of synchronous tilt testing and video-EEG monitoring in children with transient loss of consciousness. *Epilepsy Behav.* 2012;24:93-99
86. Dietz S, Murfitt J, Florence L, Thakker P, Whitehouse WP. Head-up tilt testing in children and young people: a retrospective observational study. *J Paediatr Child Health.* 2011;47:292-298
87. Brignole M, Alboni P, Benditt DG, et al; Task Force on Syncope, European Society of Cardiology. Guidelines on management (diagnosis and treatment) of syncope—update 2004. *Europace.* 2004;6:467-537
88. Krediet CT, van Dijk N, Linzer M, et al. Management of vasovagal syncope: controlling or aborting faints by leg crossing and muscle tensing. *Circulation.* 2002;106:1684-1689
89. Di Girolamo E, Di Iorio C, Leonzio L, Sabatini P, Barsotti A. Usefulness of Tilt training program for prevention of refractory neurocardiogenic syncope in adolescents: A controlled study. *Circulation.* 1999;100(17):1798-1780

90. Jauregui-Renaud K, Marquez MF, Hermosillo AG, et al. Paced breathing can prevent vasovagal syncope during head-up tilt testing. *Can J Cardiol.* 2003;19:698-700

91. Scott WA, Pongiglione G, Bromberg BI, et al. Randomized comparison of atenolol and fludrocortisone acetate in the treatment of pediatric neurally mediated syncope. *Am J Cardiol.* 1995;76: 400-402

92. Qingyou Z, Junbao D, Chaoshu T. The efficacy of midodrine hydrochloride in the treatment of children with vasovagal syncope. *J Pediatr.* 2006;149:777-880

93. Madrid AH, Ortega J, Rebollo JG, et al. Lack of efficacy of atenolol for the prevention of neurally mediated syncope in a highly symptomatic population: a prospective, double-blind, randomized and placebo-controlled study. *J Am Coll Cardiol.* 2001;37:554-559

94. Brignole M, Menozzi C, Moya A et al. Pacemaker therapy in patients with neurally-medicated syncope and documented asystole. Third International Study on Syncope of Uncertain Etiology (ISSUE-3): a randomized trial. *Circulation.* 2012;125:2566-2571

95. Kanjwal K, Karabin B, Kanjwal Y, Grubb BP. Preliminary observations on the use of closed-loop cardiac pacing in patients with refractory neurocardiogenic syncope. *J Interv Card Electrophysiol.* 2010:1:69-73

96. Palmisano P, Zaccaria M Luzzi G, et al. Closed-loop cardiac pacing vs. conventional dual-chamber pacing with specialized sensing and pacing algorithms for syncope prevention. *Europace.* 2012;14:1038-1043

97. Rebecchi M, de Ruvo E, Strano S, et al. Ganglionated plexi ablation in right atrium to treat cardio-inhibitory neurocardiogenic syncope. *J Interv Card Electrophysiol.* 2012;34:231-235

98. Liang Z, Jiayou Z, Zonggui W, Dening L. Selective atrial vagal denervation guided by evoked vagal reflex to treat refractory vasovagal syncope. *Pacing Clin Electrophysiol.* 2012;35:e214-e218

99. Yao Y, Shi R, Wong T, et al. Endocardial autonomic denervation of the left atrium to treat vasovagal syncope: an early experience in humans. *Circ Arrhythm Electrophysiol.* 2012;5:279-286

100. Pachon JC, Pachon EI, Cunha Pachon MZ, et al. Catheter ablation of severe neurally meditated reflex (neurocardiogenic or vasovagal) syncope: cardioneuroablation long-term results. *Europace.* 2011;13:1231-1242

Note: Page numbers of articles are in **boldface** type. Page references followed by "*f*" and "*t*" denote figures and tables, respectively.

1,1-difluoroethane, 574, 576
2C compounds, 577
2,5-Hexanedione, 576
13-valent pneumococcal vaccine (PCV13), 660
25C-NBOMe, 577

A

Abacavir, 636*t*
Abnormal uterine bleeding (AUB), 479–481
Acculturation and social integration, 591
Acculturative gaps, 591
Acculturative stress, 591
Acquired immune deficiency syndrome
        (AIDS). *See* Human immunodeficiency
        virus (HIV)
Acquired LCMV infection, 669
Acral cyanosis, 694
Acute concussion evaluation tool, 499
Acute epididymitis, 486
Acute HIV infection (AHI), 622, 626–627
Acute pericarditis, 541
Acutely painful scrotum, 484–485. *See*
        also Adolescent male genitourinary
        emergencies
Adenosine, 536
Adenosine triphosphate (ATP), 494
Adolescent chest pain, **528–551**
    admission to hospital, 548
    agitated patients, 543–544
    approach to child with chest pain, 547*t*
    cardiac disease, 532–544
    cocaine, 542–543
    differential diagnosis, 529*t*
    follow-up, 548
    gastrointestinal disorders, 530
    history, 544–545
    hypertrophic cardiomyopathy (HCM),
        536–537
    illicit drug use, 542–543
    indications for diagnostic testing, 547*t*
    laboratory studies, 546–547
    management, 548
    methamphetamine, 543
    musculoskeletal disorders, 530
    myocarditis, 537–539
    non-cardiac causes of chest pain, 530–532
    pericarditis, 539–541
    physical examination, 545–546, 545*t*
    psychogenic disturbances, 530

    pulmonary disorders, 530–531
    referral, 548, 548*t*
    supraventricular tachycardia (SVT),
        533–536
Adolescent dating violence (ADV), **675–691**
        See also Adolescent sexual assault patient
    cross-sectional correlates, 676–677
    do ED-based interventions endanger
        victims?, 679, 685
    do ED-based interventions interfere with
        patient care?, 685
    effectiveness of ED-based interventions,
        686–687
    intimate partner violence, distinguished,
        676
    longitudinal correlates, 677
    patient participation in ED-based
        interventions, 685–686
    presentation of ADV in emergency
        department, 677–678
    referral to community services, 687
    research studies and findings, 680–684*t*
    text messaging-based behavioral
        intervention, 687
Adolescent gynecologic emergencies, **473–483**
    abnormal uterine bleeding (AUB), 479–481
    confidential interview, 473–474
    differential diagnosis (vaginal bleeding),
        480*t*
    ectopic pregnancy, 474–476
    emergency contraception (EC), 481
    ovarian torsion, 476–477
    PID, 477–479
    prevention of unplanned pregnancy, 481
    tubo-ovarian abscess (TOA), 478–479
Adolescent male genitourinary emergencies,
        484–490
    acutely painful scrotum, 484–485
    anatomy, 484
    appendix epididymis, 487
    bell-clapper deformity, 485
    blue dot sign, 488
    cremasteric reflex, 485
    epididymitis, 486–487
    incarcerated inguinal hernia, 488
    mumps orchitis, 488–489
    orchitis, 488–489
    testicular torsion, 485–486
    torsion of the appendix testis, 487–488
    trauma, 488

Adolescent sexual assault patient, **647–657**. *See also* Adolescent dating violence (ADV)
  date rape drugs, 652
  discharge and follow-up, 656
  drug testing, 653
  ED evaluation, 649
  educational programs, 657
  emergency severity index (ESI), 649
  forensic evidence collection, 650, 652–653
  history, 649–650
  HIV prophylaxis, 654–655
  injuries indicative of penetrating trauma, 651
  physical examination, 650–652
  pregnancy prophylaxis, 655
  pregnancy testing, 653
  preservation of evidence, 652
  quality improvement programs, 657
  rape shield laws, 653
  reporting, 655
  research study findings, 647–649
  sexual assault response team, 648, 656
  statutory rape, 655
  STI testing, 653
  therapeutic interventions, 654
  triage and presentation, 649
Adrenergic drugs, 556*t*
ADV. *See* Adolescent dating violence (ADV)
AED. *See* Automatic external defibrillator (AED)
Afterload reducers, 539
Agitated patients, 543–544, 561–563, 564*t*
AHI. *See* Acute HIV infection (AHI)
AIDS. *See* Human immunodeficiency virus (HIV)
Alcohol septal ablation, 510
Aldosterone inhibitors, 539
Alpha-PVP, 577
Ambulatory ECG monitoring, 703–704
Amphetamine, 556*t*
Amphetamine salts, 577
Ampicillin/sulbactam, 479*t*
Angina, 533
Angioedema, 576
Anomalous anterior left coronary artery (LCA), 512*f*
Anomalous circumflex, 512*f*
Anomalous interarterial left coronary artery (LCA), 512*f*
Anomalous posterior left coronary artery (LCA), 512*f*
Antacids, 548
Anti-N-methyl-D-aspartate receptor encephalitis, 558
Anticholinergic drugs, 556*t*
Antihistamine, 556*t*, 562
Antiretroviral medications, 635, 636*t*, 640
Aortic coarctation, 698
Aortic stenosis, 697–698
Apolipoprotein E, 497

Appendix epididymis, 487
Appendix testis, 484, 487
Arbovirus, 665–667
Arenavirus, 669
Arrhythmia, 699–701
Arrhythmic right ventricular dysplasia, 698
Arrhythmogenic right ventricular cardiomyopathy/dysplasia (ARVC/D), 513–514, 519*t*
Arrhythmogenic ventricular cardiomyopathy (AVC), 513–514, 519*t*
ARVC/D. *See* Arrhythmogenic right ventricular cardiomyopathy/dysplasia (ARVC/D)
Aseptic meningitis, 664. *See also* Meningitis
Ashkenazi Jews, 695
Aspirin, 543
Asthma, 530
Atazanavir, 636*t*
ATP. *See* Adenosine triphosphate (ATP)
Atrial repair surgery, 701
Atrioventricular block, 701
Atrioventricular reentrant tachycardia (AVRT), 533, 534
Atypical neuroleptics, 563
AUB. *See* Abnormal uterine bleeding (AUB)
Automatic external defibrillator (AED), 508–509
AVC. *See* Arrhythmogenic ventricular cardiomyopathy (AVC)
Azithromycin, 663

B

Bacterial enteric infection, 632*t*
Bacterial epididymitis, 486
Bacterial meningitis, 658–659. *See also* Meningitis
Bacterial pericarditis, 541
Bacterial respiratory disease, 633*t*
Bagging, 574. *See also* Hydrocarbons
Barbiturate, 556*t*
Bartonella species, 635
Baseball (line drives to third base), 508
"Bath salts," 543, 577
Beck triad, 540
Becker muscular dystrophy, 698
Behavioral disorders. *See* Mental health and behavioral disorders
Bell-clapper deformity, 485
Benzodiazepines
  agitated patients, 543–544, 562
  chemical restraint, 562
  cocaine-induced chest pain, 543
  inhalation abuse, 576
  phenylethylamine derivatives, 579
  synthetic cannabinoids, 573
Beta blockers
  arrhythmia, 700–701
  cocaine-induced chest pain, 543

CPVT, 518, 701
HCM, 510
inhalation abuse, 576
LQTS, 521
neurocardiogenic syncope (NCS), 706
Bexsero, 662, 663
Bezold-Jarisch reflex, 693, 706
Bicuspid aortic valve, 697
Bilateral pneumothorax, 532f
BIP. *See* Blood injury phobia (BIP)
Blood injury phobia (BIP), 696
Blue dot sign, 488
Brainstem attack, 702
Breath-holding, 535
Breath-holding spells, 696
Brucella spp., 486
Brugada syndrome, 522, 523f, 700f, 701
Burkitt lymphoma, 638

C

C trachomatis, 477, 486
Calcium channel blockers, 510, 698
Calsequestrin gene *CASQ2,* 515
Campylobacter, 632t
Candida albicans, 637
Candidiasis, 631t
Cannabinoid hyperemesis syndrome, 573
Cannabinoid receptor agonists, 570. *See also*
    Synthetic cannabinoids (SCs)
Cardiac diseases, 507. *See also* Sports-related
    sudden cardiac death
Cardiac ischemia, 513f
Cardiac magnetic resonance imaging, 537
Cardiac rhythm disturbances, 699
Cardiac syncope, 697-701
Cardiomyopathies, 698
Cardioneuroablation, 706
Carotid sinus massage, 535
CASQ2 gene, 515, 701
Catecholamine-sensitive polymorphic
    ventricular tachycardia (CPVT), 516-518,
    519t, 524, 701
Cathinones, 577, 578
CB_1 receptors, 572
CB_2 receptors, 572
CCR5 antagonist, 636t
CD4 count, 629, 632t, 633t, 635, 638, 639
Cefotaxime, 663
Cefotetan, 479t
Cefoxitin, 479t
Ceftriaxone
    epididymitis, 487
    meningitis, 663
    PID, 479t
Cerebral blood flow, 494-495
Cerebral glucose metabolism, 495
Chemical pneumonitis, 576
Chemical restraint, 562

Chest pain. *See* Adolescent chest pain; Sports-
    related sudden cardiac death
Chlamydia, 637
Chlamydia trachomatis, 477, 486
Cholinergic/anticholinesterase, 556t
Chronic epididymitis, 486, 487
Chronic post-concussion syndrome, 501
Chronic traumatic encephalopathy (CTE), 501
Ciprofloxacin, 663
Clindamycin, 479t
Clopidogrel, 543
Clostridium difficile, 637
Club drugs, 577
CNS lymphoma, 640
Cocaine, 542-543, 556t
Coccidiodes immitis, 631t
CogSport, 499
Collagen vascular disorders, 532, 540
Colorado tick fever virus, 666t
Combivir, 642t
Common faint, 693
Commotio cordis, 508-509
Compendium of State HIV Testing Laws, 625
Compression stockings, 705
Concussion, 491, 492. *See also* Sports-related
    head injuries
Concussion Care for Kids: Minds Matter, 502
Concussion modifiers, 498, 498t
Concussion symptoms, 496, 496t
Condyloma lata, 637
Confidentiality
    HIV, 628
    vulnerable and marginalized youth, 590
Congenital aortic stenosis, 697
Congenital LCMV infection, 669
Conjugated HIB vaccine, 659
Consent
    HIV, 624-625
    vulnerable and marginalized youth, 590
Convulsive syncope, 693, 701-702
Copper IUD, 481
Coronary abnormalities, 511-513
Coronary artery anomalies, 511-512, 512f,
    519t
Coronary magnetic resonance angiography,
    512
Corticosteroids, 541
Corynebacterium spp., 486
Costochondritis, 530
Coxsackie virus infection, 532, 540
CPVT. *See* Catecholamine-sensitive
    polymorphic ventricular tachycardia
    (CPVT)
Crack cocaine, 542
Cremasteric reflex, 485
Crixivan, 636t
Cryptococcal meningitis, 637
Cryptococcosis, 638
Cryptococcus, 486

Cryptococcus neoformans, 631*t*
Cryptosporidium, 631*t*
Cryptosporidium parvum, 637
"Crystal Dex," 580
Crystal methamphetamine (Ice), 543
CTE. *See* Chronic traumatic encephalopathy
    (CTE)
Cystic fibrosis, 530
Cytomegalovirus, 486

D

Darunavir, 636*t*, 642*t*
Date rape drugs, 652
Dating violence. *See* Adolescent dating
    violence (ADV); Adolescent sexual
    assault patient
Decongestant, 556*t*
Defective desmosome hypothesis, 513
Delayed progressive orthostatic hypotension,
    694
Delta-9-THC, 571
Depression, 555–557
Detorsion, 486
Dextroamphetamine, 577, 579
Dextromethorphan (DXM), 580–582
Dextrorphan (DOR), 580
Diazepam, 573, 576
Didanosine, 636*t*
Diffuse axonal injury, 495
Diffuse tensor imaging, 503
1,1-difluoroethane, 574, 576
Diphenhydramine, 564*t*
Diphenidine, 580, 581
Disseminated *Mycobacterium avium* complex
    (MAC) disease, 630*t*
Diuretics, 510, 539
Dolutegravir, 636*t*
Dopamine, 575
Doppler ultrasound
    acutely painful scrotum, 485
    epididymitis, 487
    ovarian torsion, 477
    scrotal trauma, 488
DOR. *See* Dextrorphan (DOR)
Downregulation of CB receptors, 573
Doxycycline
    epididymitis, 487
    PID, 479*t*
Droperidol, 564*t*
Drug abuse. *See* Substance abuse
Duchenne muscular dystrophy, 698
DXM. *See* Dextromethorphan (DXM)
Dysautonomic syncope, 694–695

E

E coli, 486
Eastern equine encephalitis, 666*t*
EC. *See* Emergency contraception (EC)

ECG. *See* Electrocardiography (ECG)
Echocardiography, 512, 515, 537, 541, 704
Echovirus, 540
Ecobiodevelopmental framework, 589
Ecstasy (MDMA), 543, 577–579
Ectopic pregnancy, 474–476
Edurant, 636*t*
EEG. *See* Electroencephalography (EEG)
Efavirenz, 636*t*
Eisenmenger syndrome, 698
Electrocardiography (ECG), 703
Electroencephalography (EEG), 702
Elvitegravir, 636*t*
Emergency contraception (EC), 481, 655
Emergency severity index (ESI), 649
Emery-Dreifuss muscular dystrophy, 698
Emtricitabine, 636*t*
Emtriva, 636*t*
Endometritis, 477
Energizing Aromatherapy, 543
Enfuvirtide, 636*t*
Enterovirus, 664–665
Epidemiologic paradox, 594
Epididymis, 484
Epididymitis, 486–487
Epivir, 636*t*
EPS. *See* Extrapyramidal symptoms (EPS)
Escherichia coli, 486
ESI. *See* Emergency severity index (ESI)
Esophagitis, 548, 637
Ethanol, 556*t*
Ethnic identity development, 591
Etravirine, 636*t*
Exercise-induced syncope, 698
Exotic dancing, 607. *See also* Sexually
    exploited youth
External digital monitoring, 703–704
Extracorporeal membrane oxygenation, 539
Extrapyramidal symptoms (EPS), 563

F

Fainting. *See* Syncope
Fainting lark, 697
Familial dysautonomia (FD), 695
Favipiravir, 669
FD. *See* Familial dysautonomia (FD)
Fibro-fatty infiltrates, 513
Fitz-Hugh and Curtis perihepatitis, 478
Flecainide, 518
Fluoroquinolone, 487
Foreign-born youth. *See* Immigrant and
    refugee youth
Forensic evidence collection, 650,
    652–653
Fosamprenavir, 636*t*
Foscarnet, 638
Foster care youth, 598–599, 600*t*
Fuseon, 636*t*
Fusion inhibitors, 636*t*

G

Gag reflex, 535
Ganciclovir, 638
Gas chromatography, 571
Gastrointestinal disorders, 530
Genitourinary emergencies. *See* Adolescent
    male genitourinary emergencies
Giardia lamblia, 637
Glial fibrillary acidic protein, 497
Global cerebral hypoxia, 701
Gonorrhea, 637
Guidelines for the Prevention and Treatment
    of Opportunistic Infections in HIV-
    infected Adults and Adolescents, 640
Guidelines for the Use of Antiretroviral Agents
    in Adolescents and Adults, 640
Guttmacher Institute, 624
Gynecologic emergencies. *See* Adolescent
    gynecologic emergencies

H

H influenzae, 540
Haemophilus influenza B (HIB), 659
Haloperidol, 564*t*
hCG test. *See* Serum human chorionic
    gonadotropin (hCG) test
HCM. *See* Hypertrophic cardiomyopathy
    (HCM)
Head Impact Telemetry system, 493
Head-up tilt-table testing (HUTT), 704
Heads Up (CDC), 502
HEADSS/HEADSSSS, 554
Healthy immigrant effect, 594
Heart transplantation, 510
Hemophilus influenzae, 540
Heptavalent protein-polysaccharide
    pneumococcal conjugate vaccine (PCV7),
    659–660
HERG mutation, 519
Herpes simplex virus, 637
Herpes simplex virus type 2 (HSV-2), 668
Herpes zoster, 638
Herpesvirus, 668
2,5-Hexanedione, 576
HIB. *See Haemophilus influenza B* (HIB)
High-potency neuroleptics, 562–563
Histoplasma capsulatum infection, 631*t*
HIV-1 RNA, 622, 624, 625*t*
HIV infection. *See* Human immunodeficiency
    virus (HIV)
Hodgkin lymphoma, 638
Holiday heart, 515
Holter monitoring
    CPVT, 517
    SVT, 535
    ventricular tachycardia, 518*f*
    WPW syndrome, 515

Homeless and street-involved youth, 566,
    602–608
    acute physical health presentations, 604–605
    barriers and challenges to care, 606–607
    classification, 602–604
    key health considerations, 602–606
    mental health disorders, 605
    pregnancy, 605
    protective factors and strategies, 607
    recommendations for emergency care, 608*t*
    STIs, 605
    substance abuse, 605–606
    unstable housing status screening tool, 606*f*
hRyR2 gene, 515, 701
HSV-2. *See* Herpes simplex virus type 2
    (HSV-2)
Huffing, 574. *See also* Hydrocarbons
Human chorionic gonadotropin. *See* Serum
    human chorionic gonadotropin (hCG)
    test
Human immunodeficiency virus (HIV),
    619–646
    acute HIV infection (AHI), 622, 626–627
    antiretroviral medications, 635, 636*t*
    ART, complications of, 635, 636*t*
    CD4 count, 629, 632*t*, 633*t*, 635, 638, 639
    chest radiography, 639
    complete blood count (CBC), 639
    confidentiality, 628
    consent laws, 624–625
    counseling, 625–626
    delivery of HIV test results, 626, 628*t*
    dermatologic disease, 638
    DHHS guidelines, 640
    diagnostic evaluation, 639–640
    fever/lymphadenopathy, 635
    genitourinary disease, 637–638
    hematologic and oncologic disease, 638
    history, 628–629
    HIV-1 RNA, 622, 624, 625*t*
    immune reconstitution inflammatory
        syndrome (IRIS), 635
    laboratory testing, 622–626
    linkage to care (referral, etc.), 626, 627, 643
    medication side effects, 635, 636*t*
    neurologic disease, 637
    newly proposed CDC/APHL testing
        algorithm, 623, 623*f*
    ophthalmologic disease, 638
    opportunistic infections (OIs), 630–634*t*,
        640
    oral and gastrointestinal disease, 637
    physical examination, 629
    postexposure prophylaxis (PEP), 640–643
    pulmonary disease, 635
    rapid antibody tests, 624
    screening, 620–622
    statistics/factoids, 620
    up-to-date treatment recommendations, 640
HUTT. *See* Head-up tilt-table testing (HUTT)

Hydrocarbons, 574–577
  abuse via inhalation of vapors, 574
  clinical presentation, 575–576
  pharmacology, 574–575
  at risk for later abuse of hallucinogens,
    cocaine, etc., 574
  summary comments, 576–577
  treatment, 576
Hydroxyzine, 564*t*
Hypertrophic cardiomyopathy (HCM),
    509–511, 519*t*, 524, 536–537, 697

I

I_{Kr}, 519
I_{Na}, 519, 522
IκB kinase-associated protein (IKAP), 695
ICD. *See* Implantable cardioverter-defibrillator
    (ICD)
Ice (crystal meth), 543
ICP. *See* Intracranial pressure (ICP)
Ictal electroencephalography (EEG), 702
IKAP. See IκB kinase-associated protein
    (IKAP)
Illicit drugs. *See* Substance abuse
Immigrant and refugee youth, 591–595,
    596–597*t*
  acculturation problems, 591, 594
  barriers and challenges to care, 595
  family-related factors, 594, 595
  healthy immigrant effect, 594
  key health considerations, 591–595
  protective factors and strategies, 595
  recommendations for emergency care,
    596–597*t*
  suicidality, 594
Immigrant paradox, 594
Immune reconstitution inflammatory
    syndrome (IRIS), 635
ImPACT, 499
Implantable cardioverter-defibrillator (ICD),
    509, 697, 698, 701
Incarcerated inguinal hernia, 488
Indinavir, 636*t*
Influenza, 634*t*
Inguinal hernia, 488
Inhalant abuse. *See* Hydrocarbons
Inherited dysautonomia, 695
Initial orthostatic hypotension, 694
"Insect repellent," 543
Insecticide, 556*t*
INSTIs. *See* Integrase strand transfer inhibitors
    (INSTIs)
Integrase strand transfer inhibitors (INSTIs),
    636*t*
Intelence, 636*t*
Intergenerational cultural conflicts, 594
Intimate partner violence (IPV), 676. *See also*
    Adolescent dating violence (ADV)

Intracranial pressure (ICP), 495
Intrauterine device (IUD)
  ectopic pregnancy, 474
  emergency contraception (EC), 481
  PID, 478
Invirase, 636*t*
Involuntary psychiatric hospitalization,
    565–566
Ion channelopathies, 507, 522
IRIS. *See* Immune reconstitution inflammatory
    syndrome (IRIS)
Isentress, 636*t*
Isoproterenol, 704
Isospora belli, 637
ISSUE-3 trial, 706
IUD. *See* Intrauterine device (IUD)
Ivory Wave, 543

J

JC virus, 632*t*, 637
Jervell and Lange-Nielsen syndrome, 518
Jewish people, 695
Joint hypermobility syndrome, 694
Juvenile justice-involved youth, 598–599,
    600*t*

K

K2, 559, 570
Kaletra, 636*t*
Kaposi sarcoma, 638
Kawasaki disease, 533, 545, 698
KCNQ1 gene, 518
Ketamine, 580, 581
King-Devick test, 499

L

La Crosse virus (LCV), 666*t*, 667
Lamivudine, 636*t*
Lamivudine/zidovudine, 642*t*
Laparoscopy, 477
LCA. *See* Left coronary artery (LCA)
LCMV. *See* Lymphocytic choriomeningitis
    virus (LCMV)
LCV. *See* La Crosse virus (LCV)
LCx. *See* Left circumflex artery (LCx)
Left circumflex artery (LCx), 511, 512*f*
Left coronary artery (LCA), 511, 512*f*
Lesbian, gay, bisexual, transgender, and
    questioning (LGBTQ) youth, 566–567,
    600–602, 603*t*
Levonorgestrel, 481, 655
Lexiva, 636*t*
LGBTQ youth, 566–567, 600–602, 603*t*
Long QT syndrome (LQTS), 518–521, 519*t*,
    524, 699–701, 699*f*
Long QT syndrome (LQTS), type 1, 518, 521*f*

Long QT syndrome (LQTS), type 2, 518–519, 521*f*
Long QT syndrome (LQTS), type 3, 520–521, 522*f*
Lopinavir/ritonavir, 636*t*
Lorazepam, 564*t*
Loss of consciousness (brainstem attack), 702
LQTS. *See* Long QT syndrome (LQTS)
Lymphocytic choriomeningitis virus (LCMV), 669

M

MAB-CHMINACA, 571
MAC. *See Mycobacterium avium* complex (MAC)
Magnetic resonance spectroscopy, 503
Male genitourinary emergencies. *See* Adolescent male genitourinary emergencies
Marfan syndrome, 530, 531
Marginalized youth. *See* Vulnerable and marginalized youth
Marijuana, 570
Marviroc, 636*t*
Mass spectrometry, 571
Mature minor legislation, 590
MDMA (Ecstasy), 543, 577–579
MDPV, 577
Measles, mumps, and rubella (MMR) vaccine, 489
Medroxyprogesterone acetate, 481
MenB, 662, 663
MenHibrix, 662
Meningitis, **658–674**
   arbovirus, 665–667
   arenavirus, 669
   aseptic/viral, defined, 664
   at-risk persons, 660*t*, 662*t*
   enterovirus, 664–665
   Haemophilus influenza B (HIB), 659
   herpesvirus, 668
   La Crosse virus (LCV), 666*t*, 667
   lymphocytic choriomeningitis virus (LCMV), 669
   Mollaret, 668–669
   mumps, 667
   Neisseria meningitidis, 660–663
   Neisseria meningitidis serogroups, 661*t*
   parainfluenza virus, 668
   paramyxovirus, 667–668
   parechovirus, 665
   picornaviridae, 664–665
   postexposure chemoprophylaxis, 663, 663*t*
   recommended vaccine and booster, 662
   Streptococcus pneumoniae, 659–660
   vaccines, 659–663
   viral causes of aseptic meningitis, 664*t*
   West Nile virus (WNV), 666–667, 666*t*

Meningococcal vaccination, 662–663
Mental health and behavioral disorders, **552–569**
   agitated patients, 561–563, 564*t*
   depression, 555–557
   goals of emergency treatment, 553, 553*t*
   HEADSS/HEADSSSS, 554
   homeless youth, 566, 567, 605
   LGBTQ youth, 566–567
   medical clearance, 559
   mental status examination, 556, 557*t*
   patient assessment, 554–555
   physical examination, 555
   psychosis, 557–558
   psychosomatic disorders, 559–560
   schizophrenia, 557, 558
   screening test for medical illness, 560*t*
   self-injurious behaviors, 566
   sexual minority youth, 566–567
   substance abuse, 558–559
   suicidal behaviors, 563–566
   toxidromes, 556*t*
   urine toxicology screening tests, 558–559
   VITAMINS, 555
Mental status examination, 556, 557*t*
Methamphetamine, 543, 577
Methoxetamine (MXE), 580–582
Methoxphenidine (MXP), 580, 581
Methylene chloride, 576
Methylenedioxymethamphetamine (MDMA), 543, 577–579
Methylphenidate, 577–579
Metoprolol, 706
MI. *See* Myocardial infarction (MI)
Midazolam, 573, 576
Mild traumatic brain injury (mTBI), 491, 492*t. See also* Sports-related head injuries
Minds Matter: Concussion Care for Kids, 502
MMR vaccine. *See* Measles, mumps, and rubella (MMR) vaccine
Mollaret cells, 668
Mollaret meningitis, 668–669
mTBI. *See* Mild traumatic brain injury (mTBI)
Mumps meningitis, 667
Mumps orchitis, 488–489
Musculoskeletal disorders, 530
Mutant IκB kinase-associated protein (IKAP), 695
MXE. *See* Methoxetamine (MXE)
MXP. *See* Methoxphenidine (MXP)
Mycobacterium avium complex (MAC), 630*t*, 635
Mycobacterium spp., 486
Mycobacterium tuberculosis infection (TB), 630*t*, 635
Myocardial infarction (MI), 533
Myocardial ischemia, 698
Myocarditis, 537–539, 698

N

N gonorrheae, 486
N-methyl-D-aspartate (NMDA) receptor
	antagonists, 579–582
	clinical presentation, 581
	pharmacology, 580–581
	summary comments, 582
	treatment, 581–582
NAAT. *See* Nucleic acid amplification test
	(NAAT)
Nadolol, 706
National Institute of Drug Abuse, 559
National Physicians' Consultation Center
	PEPline, 641
NCS. *See* Neurocardiogenic syncope (NCS)
Neck strength, 502
Neisseria gonorrheae, 486
Neisseria meningitidis, 660–663
Neisseria meningitidis serogroups, 661*t*
Nelfinavir, 636*t*
Neoplastic pericarditis, 540
Neurocardiogenic syncope (NCS), 692,
	693–694, 707
Neuroleptics, 562–563
Neuromuscular dystrophies, 698
Neuron-specific enolase, 497
Nevirapine, 636*t*
Nitroglycerine, 543
NMDA receptor antagonists. *See* N-methyl-D-
	aspartate (NMDA) receptor antagonists
NNRTIs. *See* Non-nucleoside reverse
	transcriptase inhibitors (NNRTIs)
"No-suicide" contract, 566
Non-nucleoside reverse transcriptase
	inhibitors (NNRTIs), 636*t*
Non-steroidal anti-inflammatory drugs
	(NSAIDs)
	epididymitis, 487
	head injury, 499
	pericarditis, 541
	torsion of the appendix testis, 488
NRTIs. *See* Nucleoside reverse transcriptase
	inhibitors (NRTIs)
NSAIDs. *See* Non-steroidal anti-inflammatory
	drugs (NSAIDs)
Nucleic acid amplification test (NAAT)
	arbovirus, 667
	HIV, 622–624, 625*f*
	paramyxovirus, 668
	West Nile virus (WNV), 667
Nucleoside reverse transcriptase inhibitors
	(NRTIs), 636*t*

O

Oculomotor training, 499
OIs. *See* Opportunistic infections (OIs)
Olanzapine, 564*t*

Oophoritis, 477
Opioid toxidrome, 556*t*
Opportunistic infections (OIs), 630–634*t,* 640
Orchiectomy, 486
Orchitis, 488–489
Orthostatic hypotension, 694, 695
Orthostatic intolerance, 694
Ovarian torsion, 476–477

P

Paced breathing, 705
Pacemaker, 706
Pallid breath-holding spells, 696
Paradoxical IRIS, 635
Parainfluenza virus, 668
Paramyxovirus, 667–668
Parechovirus, 665
Pause-dependent ventricular arrhythmias,
	519–520
PCP. *See* Phencyclidine (PCP); *Pneumocystis
	jirovecii* pneumonia (PCP)
PCV7. *See* Heptavalent protein-polysaccharide
	pneumococcal conjugate vaccine (PCV7)
PCV13. *See* 13-valent pneumococcal vaccine
	(PCV13)
PE. *See* Pulmonary embolism (PE)
Pelvic inflammatory disease (PID), 474, 477–479
Pelvic peritonitis, 477
Penicillin, 663
PEP. *See* Postexposure prophylaxis (PEP)
Pericardial effusion, 541
Pericardiocentesis, 541
Pericarditis, 539–541
Pericardium, 540
Permanent post-concussion syndrome, 501
Phencyclidine (PCP), 580–582
Phenothiazine, 556*t*
Phenylethylamine derivatives, 577–579
Physical restraints, 544, 561, 562, 562*t*
Picornaviridae, 664–665
PID. *See* Pelvic inflammatory disease (PID)
Pill-induced esophagitis, 548
PIs. *See* Protease inhibitors (PIs)
"Plant food," 543
Pneumocystis jirovecii pneumonia (PCP), 630*t*
Pneumomediastinum, 531, 531*f,* 542
Pneumonia, 633*t*
Pneumothorax, 530, 531, 532*f,* 542
Poisoning (toxidromes), 556*t*
Polymorphic ventricular tachycardia, 522*f,* 700*f*
Postexposure prophylaxis (PEP), 640–643
Postural orthostatic tachycardia syndrome
	(POTS), 702
Potassium current $I_{K,}$ 519
POTS. *See* Postural orthostatic tachycardia
	syndrome (POTS)
Powassan virus, 666*t*
Precordial catch, 532

Pregnancy prophylaxis, 655
Prehn sign, 487
Presyncope, 693
Prevention of unplanned pregnancy, 481
Prezista, 636*t*
Primary myocardial dysfunction, 698
Primary pulmonary hypertension, 698
Probenecid, 479*t*
Progestin-only emergency contraceptive pills, 655
Progressive multifocal leukoencephalopathy infection, 632*t*
Prolonged QT syndrome, 518–523
Propranolol, 706
Prostaglandins, 698
Prostitution, 607. *See also* Sexually exploited youth
Protease inhibitors (PIs), 636*t*
Pseudomonas spp., 486
Psychiatric emergencies. *See* Mental health and behavioral disorders
Psychogenic disturbances, 530
Psychosis, 557–558
Psychosomatic disorders, 559–560
Pulmonary disorders, 530–531
Pulmonary embolism (PE), 531
Pulmonary stenosis, 698
Purulent pericarditis, 541

Q

QT interval (QTc), 520, 521*f*, 522*f*
Quetiapine, 564*t*

R

R-on-T phenomenon, 508
Raltegravir, 636*t*, 642*t*
Rape shield laws, 653
Rapid antibody tests, 624
Rapid review (of literature), 678–679
RCA. *See* Right coronary artery (RCA)
Red Dove, 543
Reflex anoxic seizure, 696
Reflex syncope, 693, 702
Reflux esophagitis, 530
Refugees. *See* Immigrant and refugee youth
Relatively homeless youth, 604. *See also* Homeless and street-involved youth
Restraint devices. *See* Chemical restraint; Physical restraints
Retrovir, 636*t*
Reyataz, 636*t*
Ribavirin, 669
Rifampin, 663
Right coronary artery (RCA), 511, 512*f*
Right ventricular outflow tract obstruction, 698
Riley-Day syndrome, 695

Rilpivirine, 636*t*
Risperidone, 564*t*
Ritonavir, 642*t*
Runaways, 604. *See also* Homeless and street-involved youth
Ruptured ectopic pregnancy, 474, 475
Ryanodine receptor gene *hRyR2*, 515, 701
RyR2 gene, 515, 701

S

s100B, 497
S aureus, 540
S pneumonia, 540
Safety baseball, 508
Salmonella, 632*t*, 637, 639
Salpingitis, 477
Saquinavir, 636*t*
SCD. *See* Sports-related sudden cardiac death
Schizophrenia, 557, 558
SCN5A gene, 519, 701
Scrotal anatomy, 484. *See also* Adolescent male genitourinary emergencies
Scrotal trauma, 488
SCs. *See* Synthetic cannabinoids (SCs)
Second impact syndrome, 495, 501
Sedative-hypnotic drugs, 556*t*
Seizure, 692, 702
Self-cutting, 566
Self-injurious behaviors, 566
Selzentry, 636*t*
Serotonin transporter (SERT), 578
Serum cardiac enzymes (troponins), 543
Serum human chorionic gonadotropin (hCG) test
    abnormal uterine bleeding (AUB), 481
    ectopic pregnancy, 475
Sexual assault. *See* Adolescent sexual assault patient
Sexual assault response team, 648, 656
Sexual minority youth, 566–567. *See also* LGBTQ youth
Sexually exploited youth, 607–610, 611*t*
Shigella, 632*t*, 637
Short QT syndrome, 700*f*
SIDECAPS mnemonic (depression), 557*t*
Sinus node dysfunction, 701
Sniffing, 574. *See also* Hydrocarbons
Social and environmental vulnerabilities. *See* Vulnerable and marginalized youth
Social determinants, 589
Sodium current I_{Na}, 519, 522
Solvent abuse. *See* Hydrocarbons
Spermatic cord, 484
Spice (drug of abuse), 559, 570
Sport concussion assessment tool 3, 499
Sports-related head injuries, **491–506**
    biomarkers, 497, 503
    chronic post-concussion syndrome, 501

Sports-related head injuries, *continued*
    chronic traumatic encephalopathy (CTE),
        501
    classification of traumatic brain injury
        severity, 492*t*
    concussion, defined, 492
    concussion modifiers, 498, 498*t*
    concussion symptoms, 496, 496*t*
    diagnosis, 495–497, 503
    epidemiology, 493
    future directions, 502–503
    imaging, 496–497
    long-term sequelae/complications, 500–501
    loss of consciousness (LOC), 496
    management, 497–500
    mechanism, 493
    moderate and severe TBI, 492*t*, 496, 500,
        502
    neck strength, 502
    neurocognitive testing, 499
    on-field evaluation, 495
    pathophysiology, 494–495
    pharmacologic therapy, 499–500
    prevention, 502
    prolonged recovery, 499
    return to learn, 497
    return to play, 497
    second impact syndrome, 495, 501
Sports-related sudden cardiac death, **507–527**
    AEDs, 508–509
    arrhythmogenic ventricular cardiomyopathy
        (AVC), 513–514, 519*t*
    Brugada syndrome, 522, 523*f*
    cardiac ischemia (ECG), 513*f*
    catecholamine polymorphic ventricular
        tachycardia (CPVT), 516–518, 519*t*
    common symptoms/signs, 519*t*, 524
    commotio cordis, 508–509
    coronary abnormalities, 511–513
    coronary artery anomalies, 511–512, 512*f*,
        519*t*
    defective desmosome hypothesis, 513
    defining feature of SCD, 507
    family history, 524
    holiday heart, 515
    hypertrophic cardiomyopathy (HCM),
        509–511, 519*t*
    ICD, 509
    LQTS, 518–521, 519*t*
    overview, 519*t*
    possible ECG findings, 519*t*
    preparticipation examination, 523–524
    prolonged QT syndrome, 518–523
    screening, 523–524
    Torsades de pointes, 520, 520*f*
    WPW syndrome, 514–515, 515*f*, 519*t*
Spotting the Signs, 610
St. Louis encephalitis, 666*t*
Staphylococcus aureus, 540

Statutory rape, 655
Stavudine, 636*t*
Stitch in the side, 532
Street-involved youth (SIY), 604. *See also*
        Homeless and street-involved youth
Street youth, 604
Streptococcus pneumoniae, 539, 635, 659–660
Stribild, 636*t*
Substance abuse, 558–559
    cocaine, 542–543
    homeless and street-involved youth,
        605–606
    methamphetamine, 543
    xenobiotic abuse. *See* Xenobiotic abuse
Sucralfate, 548
Sudden cardiac death (SCD), 507. *See also*
        Sports-related sudden cardiac death
Sudden sniffing death syndrome, 575–576
Suicidal gesture, 565
Suicide
    immigrant and refugee youth, 594
    juvenile justice-involved youth, 598
    suicidal behaviors, generally, 563–566
Supraventricular tachycardia (SVT),
        533–536
    case study (vignette), 533
    classifications, 533–534
    clinical features, 535
    defined, 533
    diagnosis, 535
    ECG, 534*f*
    pathophysiology, 534
    syncope, 701
    treatment and outcome, 535–536
    WPW syndrome, 514
Surgical septal myectomy, 510
Sustiva, 636*t*
SVT. *See* Supraventricular tachycardia (SVT)
Sympathetic ganglionectomy, 701
Syncope, **692–711**
    ambulatory ECG monitoring, 703–704
    aortic stenosis, 697–698
    arrhythmias, 699–701
    blood injury phobia (BIP), 696
    breath-holding spells, 696
    cardiac, 697–701
    cardioneuroablation, 706
    chest pain, 533
    convulsive, 693, 701–702
    defined, 692
    dysautonomic, 694–695
    ECG, 703
    echocardiography, 704
    exercise-induced, 698
    fainting lark, 697
    familial dysautonomia (FD), 695
    fluid therapy, 706
    future perspectives, 707
    HCM, 697

head-up tilt-table testing (HUTT), 704
high-risk patients, 703
history, 702–703
imaging, 704
laboratory blood tests, 703
loss of consciousness (brainstem attack), 702
neurocardiogenic syncope (NCS), 692, 693–694, 707
orthostatic hypotension, 694, 695
paced breathing, 705
pacemaker therapy, 706
pharmacologic treatment, 706, 707
physical countermaneuvers, 705
physical examination, 703
POTS, 695
presyncope, 693
primary myocardial dysfunction, 698
primary pulmonary hypertension, 698
seizure, contrasted, 702
sports-related sudden cardiac death, 524
video-assisted recording, 703
Syncope burden, 707
Synthetic cannabinoids (SCs), 559, 570–584
clinical presentation, 572–573
pharmacology, 572
summary comments, 573–574
treatment, 573
Syphilis, 637

T

Tau deposits (brain), 501
TB. *See Mycobacterium tuberculosis* infection (TB)
TBI. *See* Traumatic brain injury (TBI)
Tenofovir, 636*t*
Tenofovir/emtricitabine, 642*t*
Testicular torsion, 485–486
Testis (testes), 484
Tetralogy of Fallot, 511, 698
Texidor twinge, 532
Text messaging-based behavioral intervention, 687
Throwaways, 604. *See also* Homeless and street-involved youth
Thrush, 637
Tivicay, 636*t*
TOA. *See* Tubo-ovarian abscess (TOA)
Toluene, 575, 576
Torsades de pointes, 520, 520*f*, 699*f*, 700
Torsion of the appendix testis, 487–488
"Toxic stress," 589–590
Toxidromes, 556*t*
Toxoplasma, 640
Toxoplasma gondii encephalitis, 630*t*
Toxoplasmosis, 637
Tranquilizer, 556*t*
Transgender youth, 602

Transposition of the Great Arteries, 511
Transthoracic echocardiogram, 512
Traumatic brain injury (TBI), 491, 492*t. See also* Sports-related head injuries
Traumatic pericarditis, 540
Treponema pallidum, 637
Trichloroethylene, 576
Trichomoniasis, 637
Trigeminal neuralgia, 576
Troponins, 543
Trumenba, 662, 663
Truvada, 642*t*
Tubal surgery, 474
Tubo-ovarian abscess (TOA), 477, 478–479
Tunical vaginalis, 484

U

Ulipristal acetate, 481
Ultrasound. *See* Doppler ultrasound
Unplanned pregnancy, prevention of, 481
Unstable housing status screening tool, 606*f*
Urine nucleic acid amplification test, 487
Urine toxicology screening tests, 558–559

V

Vagal maneuvers, 535
Vaginal bleeding, differential diagnosis, 480*t*
Valsalva maneuver, 535
Varicella zoster virus (VZV), 638, 668
Vas deferens, 484
Vasodilators, 698
Vasovagal syncope (VVS), 692, 693. *See also* Neurocardiogenic syncope (NCS)
Ventricular arrhythmia, 511. *See also* Sports-related sudden cardiac death
Ventricular assist devices, 539
Ventricular ectopy, 515
Ventricular tachycardia, 518*f*, 698, 701
Verapamil, 518
Vestibular/ocular motor screening, 499
Videx, 636*t*
Violence. *See* Adolescent dating violence (ADV); Adolescent sexual assault patient
Viracept, 636*t*
Viral meningitis, 664. *See also* Meningitis
Viramune, 636*t*
Viread, 636*t*
VITAMINS, 555
Vulnerable and marginalized youth, **589–618**
confidentiality, 590
consent for health services, 590
foster care youth, 598–599, 600*t*
general recommendations for care, 592–593*t*
homeless and street-involved youth, 602–607, 608*t*
immigrant and refugee youth, 591–595, 596–597*t*

Vulnerable and marginalized youth, *continued*
   juvenile justice-involved youth, 598–599,
     600*t*
   LGBTQ youth, 600–602, 603*t*
   recommended clinician approach, 590, 612
   recommended health professional advocacy,
     612
   sexually exploited youth, 607–610, 611*t*
   youth in care, 598–599, 600*t*
VVS. *See* Vasovagal syncope (VVS)
VZV. *See* Varicella zoster virus (VZV)

W

West Nile virus (WNV), 666–667, 666*t*
WNV. *See* West Nile virus (WNV)
Wolff-Parkinson-White (WPW) syndrome,
   514–515, 515*f,* 519*t,* 534
WPW syndrome. *See* Wolff-Parkinson-White
   (WPW) syndrome

X

Xenobiotic abuse, **570–588**
   hydrocarbons, 574–577
   NMDA receptor antagonists, 579–582
   phenylethylamine derivatives, 577–579
   synthetic cannabinoids, 570–574

Y

Youth in care, 598–599, 600*t*
Yuzpe method, 481

Z

Zerit, 636*t*
Ziagen, 636*t*
Zidovudine, 636*t,* 638
Ziprasidone, 564*t*